Critical Thinking About Critical Periods

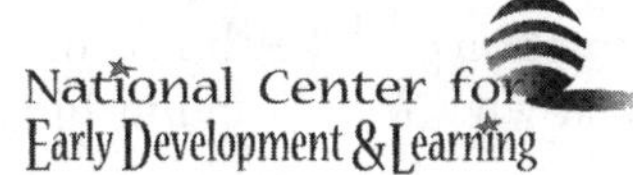

A Series from the National Center for Early Development & Learning

Series Editor: Donald B. Bailey, Jr., Ph.D.

This book is part of a series edited by Donald B. Bailey, Jr., Ph.D., and developed in conjunction with the National Center for Early Development & Learning (NCEDL). Books in this series are designed to serve as resources for sharing new knowledge to enhance the cognitive, social, and emotional development of children from birth through 8 years of age. For information on other books in this series, please refer to the Brookes web site at www.brookespublishing.com.

Other Books in this Series

The Transition to Kindergarten
Robert C. Pianta and Martha J. Cox

Infants and Toddlers in Out-of-Home Care
Debby Cryer and Thelma Harms

Critical Thinking About Critical Periods

edited by

Donald B. Bailey, Jr., Ph.D.
Frank Porter Graham Child Development Center
University of North Carolina at Chapel Hill

John T. Bruer, Ph.D.
James S. McDonnell Foundation
St. Louis, Missouri

Frank J. Symons, Ph.D.
University of Minnesota
Minneapolis, Minnesota

and

Jeff W. Lichtman, M.D., Ph.D.
Washington University School of Medicine
St. Louis, Missouri

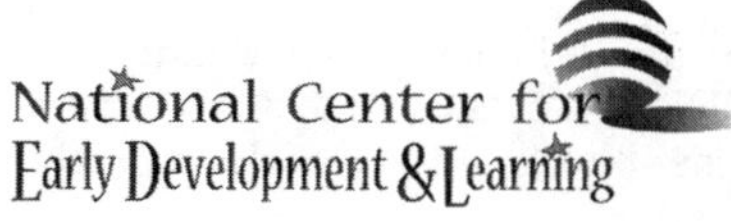

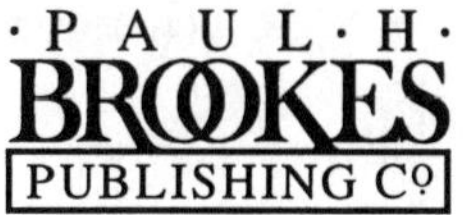

Baltimore • London • Toronto • Sydney

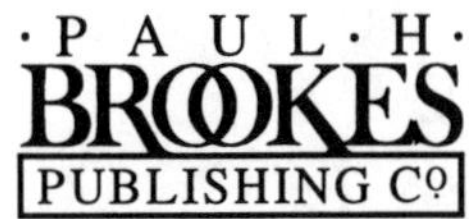

Paul H. Brookes Publishing Co.
Post Office Box 10624
Baltimore, Maryland 21285-0624

www.brookespublishing.com

Typeset by A.W. Bennett, Inc., Hartland, Vermont.
Manufactured in the United States of America by
Versa Press, East Peoria, Illinois.

The National Center for Early Development & Learning is supported under the Educational Research and Development Centers Program, PR/Award Number R307A60004, as administered by the Office of Educational Research and Improvement, U.S. Department of Education. However, no official endorsement by the federal government should be inferred.

Library of Congress Cataloging-in-Publication Data

Critical thinking about critical periods / edited by Donald B. Bailey . . . [et al.].
p. cm.
Includes bibliographical references and index.
ISBN 1-55766-495-1
1. Critical periods (Biology). 2. Developmental neurobiology.
I. Bailey, Donald B.
QP363.5 .C75 2001
612.8—dc21 00-049807

British Library Cataloguing in Publication data are available from the British Library.

Contents

About the Editors

Donald B. Bailey, Jr., Ph.D., Director, Frank Porter Graham Child Development Center, and Professor of Education, University of North Carolina at Chapel Hill, CB #8180, 105 Smith Level Road, Chapel Hill, North Carolina 27599

Dr. Bailey's research and publications have addressed a variety of issues related to early intervention of children with disabilities and their families, with a particular focus on family support, inclusion, early identification, and fragile X syndrome.

John T. Bruer, Ph.D., President, James S. McDonnell Foundation, 1034 South Brentwood Boulevard, Suite 1850, St. Louis, Missouri 63117

Dr. Bruer has been a foundation executive for more than 20 years, administering programs in education, psychology, and neuroscience. He is the author of *Schools for Thought* (MIT Press, 1993) and *The Myth of the First Three Years* (Free Press, 1999).

Frank J. Symons, Ph.D., Assistant Professor of Education, University of Minnesota, 238 Burton Hall, 178 Pillsbury Drive, S.E., Minneapolis, Minnesota 55455

Dr. Symons' primary research activities are supported by the National Institute of Child Health and Human Development (NICHD) and focus on improving the assessment and treatment of severe self-injurious behavior among individuals with developmental disabilities and pervasive developmental disorders. Dr. Symons was a research scientist at the Frank Porter Graham Child Development Center at the University of North Carolina at Chapel Hill and a postdoctoral fellow at the John F. Kennedy Center at the Peabody College of Vanderbilt University in Nashville, Tennessee. He is the co-author of *Behavioral Observation: Technology and Applications in Developmental Disabilities* (Paul H. Brookes Publishing Co., 2000).

Jeff W. Lichtman, M.D., Ph.D., Professor of Neurobiology, Washington University School of Medicine, 660 South Euclid Avenue, St. Louis, Missouri 63110

Dr. Lichtman uses new optical imaging techniques in living animals to study changes that occur as synaptic circuits remodel in response to experience. His work is focused on the naturally occurring elimination of synapses that takes place in early postnatal life. He is the co-author of *Principles of Neural Development* (Sinauer Press, 1985).

About the Contributors

Elinor W. Ames, Ph.D., Professor Emerita, Simon Fraser University, 8888 University Drive, Burnaby, British Columbia, Canada V5A 1S6

Dr. Ames taught developmental psychology at Canadian and American universities before her retirement in 1997. Her research specialties included infant perceptual development, infant crying, and the development of children adopted from Romanian orphanages.

Maria L. Boccia, Ph.D., Scientist, Frank Porter Graham Child Development Center, University of North Carolina at Chapel Hill, CB #8180, 105 Smith Level Road, Chapel Hill, North Carolina 27599

Dr. Boccia is a research associate, a professor of psychology, and a member of the graduate faculty in the neuroscience curriculum. She is well-known for her nonhuman primate research, which utilizes an animal model system to study the effects of early experience on social and emotional development and stress responsivity. She also engages in research that examines the role of central oxytocin systems in an animal model of autism.

Heather Bortfeld, Ph.D., Assistant Professor of Research, Brown University, 190 Thayer Street, Providence, Rhode Island 02912

Dr. Bortfeld completed her doctorate in experimental biology at State University of New York at Stony Brook in 1997. Her research addresses questions about the nature of lexical representation in both first and second language development. She is working on a model of phonological differentiation in collaboration with Dr. James Morgan of Brown University.

Kim Chisholm, Ph.D., Assistant Professor, St. Francis Xavier University, Post Office Box 5000, Antigonish, Nova Scotia, Canada B2G 2W5

Dr. Chisholm teaches courses in developmental psychology and psychology of gender. Her research interests include attachment in the preschool years, development of empathy, and development in children adopted from Romanian orphanages.

Dale C. Farran, Ph.D., Professor of Education, Vanderbilt University, Box 330, Nashville, Tennessee 37203

Dr. Farran is the director of the Susan Gray School for Children, an on-campus research and demonstration school and the largest early intervention program in Tennessee. She has been involved in research and intervention for children and youth at high risk for all of her professional career. She has conducted research at the Frank Porter Graham Child Development Center in Chapel Hill, North Carolina, and the Kamehameha Schools Early Education Project in Hawaii.

William T. Greenough, Ph.D., Professor of Psychology, University of Illinois–Beckman Institute, 405 N. Mathews Avenue, Urbana, Illinois 61801

Dr. Greenough is Professor of Psychology, Psychiatry, and Cell and Structural Biology at the University of Illinois. He also is a member of the National Academy of Sciences.

Kenji Hakuta, Ph.D., Professor of Education, Stanford University, CERAS Building, Stanford, California 94305

Dr. Hakuta teaches courses on language development, bilingual education, and research methods. He received his doctorate in experimental psychology from Harvard University in 1979. Dr. Hakuta's research is in the areas of psycholinguistics, bilingualism, language shift, and the acquisition of English in immigrant students.

Jonathan C. Horton, M.D., Ph.D., Associate Professor of Ophthalmology, Neurology, and Physiology, University of California at San Francisco (UCSF), 10 Kirkham Street, San Francisco, California 94143

Dr. Horton is a clinical neuro-ophthalmologist at the UCSF medical school where he also directs the Laboratory for Visual Neuroscience. He studies the neural basis of amblyopia and strabismus.

Robert B. McCall, Ph.D., Professor of Psychology, University of Pittsburgh, 121 University Place, Pittsburgh, Pennsylvania 15260

Dr. McCall has been a student of early experience and its contribution to child development for 35 years. He co-directs the University of Pittsburgh Office of Child Development, which promotes and operates university and community partnership projects in interdisciplinary education and applied research, human service demonstration projects, and program evaluation.

Helen J. Neville, Ph.D., Professor of Psychology and Neuroscience, University of Oregon, 1227 University of Oregon, Eugene, Oregon 97403

Dr. Neville studied at the University of British Columbia, Cornell University, and the University of California at San Diego. She directed the Human Neuropsychology Lab at the Salk Institute from 1977 to 1994 and now teaches and directs the Brain Development Lab at the University of Oregon.

Cort Pedersen, M.D., Professor of Psychiatry, University of North Carolina School of Medicine, Medical School Wing B, Chapel Hill, North Carolina 27599

Dr. Pedersen is an internationally recognized expert on the psychobiology of parental and sexual behavior. He has had federal grant support for animal studies in these areas for 2 decades and has published extensively. More recently, Dr. Pedersen's research interests have expanded to include investigation of brain mechanisms underlying early experience effects on the development of social behaviors and social attachments.

Bradford W. Plemons, M.S., Doctoral Candidate, University of Pittsburgh, 253 Langley Hall, Pittsburgh, Pennsylvania 15260

Mr. Plemons received his master's degree in psychology from Western Washington University. The title of his master's thesis was *A Cross-Validation of the Stanford Binet Intelligence Scales: Fourth Edition Across Age Groups.* His thesis has been presented at multiple conferences, including the Western Psychological Association Annual Conference and the Psychometric Society. Currently, he works as a research associate at the University of Maryland, conducting research on a substance abuse treatment outcome study involving more than 1,600 clients from 13 clinics. He also is in the process of completing his doctoral degree in psychology at the University of Pittsburgh, where he has pursued his interests of exploring the effects of poverty and welfare transitions on child health and development.

Ross A. Thompson, Ph.D., Carl A. Happold Distinguished Professor, University of Nebraska, 238 Burnett Hall, Lincoln, Nebraska 68588

Dr. Thompson is a developmental psychologist who studies early parent–child relationships, emotional growth, and the development of conscience in young children. As a psycholegal scholar, he also studies child and family policy problems concerning young children's relationships, including divorce and custody, child maltreatment, grandparent visitation rights, and child care policy. He currently is Associate Editor of the research journal *Child Development* and edits a series of specialized textbooks in developmental psychology for McGraw-Hill.

Lawrence Tychsen, M.D., Associate Professor of Ophthalmology and Visual Sciences, Pediatrics, Anatomy, and Neurobiology, Washington University, #1 Children's Place, St. Louis, Missouri 63110

Dr. Tychsen is a pediatric eye surgeon and visual neuroscientist, and his clinical and laboratory research focuses on development of brain circuits for binocular vision in infant humans and monkeys.

Grover J. Whitehurst, Ph.D., Leading Professor of Psychology, Professor of Pediatrics, State University of New York at Stony Brook, Stony Brook, New York 11794

Dr. Whitehurst's research focuses on the prevention of reading problems in children from low socioeconomic backgrounds and the nature and consequences of early language delay. He currently directs nationwide projects to enhance emergent literacy and prevent reading difficulties for the National Center for Learning Disabilities and the Public Library Association. He is a recipient of the Microsoft Innovators in Higher Education Award. The National Institutes of Health, the Pew Charitable Trusts, the Smith Richardson Foundation, and the Administration on Children, Youth and Families have supported his research.

Preface

One could distill popular understanding of the importance of brain science for child development in a single sentence: Following birth, there is a period of rapid brain reorganization that is *a/the* critical period in brain development during which children are most sensitive to environmental stimuli. Parents, educators, policy makers, and early childhood advocates share, with greater or lesser understanding, this concept of critical "windows of opportunity" early in development. Although the current interest in the implications of neuroscience for child and human development should be applauded, popular understanding of this developmental and neuroscientific phenomenon is not entirely consistent with what is now known about critical periods. The presentation and use of complex neuroscience findings within policy and education contexts can be easily misinterpreted or overgeneralized. To the extent that misinterpretations, misunderstandings, and overgeneralizations of this research occur and are accepted by the public and policy makers, there is the danger that we establish unrealistic expectations for programs and services. However, to the extent that our emerging understanding of the brain can contribute to our understanding of the mind, cognitive-emotional development, and learning, we may acquire new and powerful strategies for improving child rearing and education.

In 1999, the National Center for Early Development & Learning (NCEDL) under the auspices of the National Institute on Early Childhood Development and Learning and the U.S. Department of Education convened a working conference on *Critical Thinking About Critical Periods* that brought together recognized experts from the fields of basic neuroscience and early child development to begin the process of integrating the various domains of science and educational policy related to the study of early brain and child development. The conference participants were selected on the basis of their national and international recognition as leaders in their various fields of research; yet, it is safe to say many were unfamiliar with each other's work. Basic neuroscientists studying the process of molecular development of synapse formation listened to educational researchers talk about impoverished home environments and their deleterious effects on early attachment. Behavioral scientists and educational policy makers heard about the latest findings on cortical plasticity during early brain development and its implications for learning and memory. As each of the respective groups listened to one another, they began commenting on each other's work from different points of view and gradually developed insights into the potential relationships between their disparate views of early brain and child development. Recognizing the potential for continuing the conversations begun at the meeting, each of the experts agreed to contribute to this book.

The range of interests and perspectives in this book are enormous and exciting. The book presents a critical discussion of the neural and behavioral sciences that undergird the notion of "windows of opportunity" in early brain development. Although the notion of critical or sensitive periods originated in the field of embryology in the 1920s, it is most widely known from its use in psychology and animal behavior. Neuroscientific research on critical periods began in the mid-1950s and continues to this day, representing a stunning example of our progress in understanding brain development and function. It also provides a model of a successful research program that has answered many questions but has raised as many, if not more, new ones. Thus, research on critical periods provides an excellent example around which we can organize a discussion of what we know and do not know about brain development and the implications of brain science on early childhood policy and practice.

First, in this book, the early history of critical periods and evidence for the existence of critical periods in various domains of human cognition and learning are reviewed. After this introduction, subsequent chapters present concise summaries of research in various domains, describe the evidence, and discuss implications for research, training, policy, and practice. Although the importance of technical precision required for effective communication about theory and research cannot be overstated, we asked each contributor to avoid overly technical jargon. In general, our strategy was to begin each section with a chapter that lays the basic foundation for the area, followed by chapters providing clinical, applied, or educational examples of the implications of critical periods for practice. In all cases, the emphasis is on what we know, how we know it, and what we would like to know. We hope that this book will help all of us to realize the power of critical thinking and multiple perspectives in interaction.

I

Critical Periods

An Overview of Behavior and Biology

1

A Critical and Sensitive Period Primer

John T. Bruer

Since the mid-1990s, policy advocates, educators, and parents have come to believe that new breakthroughs in brain science have the imminent potential to revolutionize parenting, child care, and education. One major theme in this brain-based early childhood literature is the existence and significance of critical or sensitive periods in development (Bruer, 1997, 1998, 1999). This book examines the critical or sensitive period theme and assesses what the implications of critical period research might actually be for child development and early education.

In almost every popular article on brain development, we read about David Hubel and Torsten Wiesel's (1970) blind kittens. Kittens deprived of visual input to one eye for 6 weeks following birth remain permanently blind in that eye when visual input is restored to the eye. No amount of subsequent visual experience, these articles tell us, will restore normal function to the deprived eye.

Using Hubel and Wiesel's kittens as a model of a critical period, the brain and early childhood articles make claims about other critical or sensitive periods in development. Some of these articles tell us that there is a critical period from birth to age 3 years, during which the foundations for learning, emotional control, and social development must be established (Carnegie Corporation, 1994). Other articles extend this period from birth through age 6 or 12 years (Carnegie Corporation, 1996; Shore, 1997). Educators believe that there is a critical period for learning that lasts from age 3 to 10 years (Carnegie Corporation, 1996; Sousa, 1998; Wolfe & Brandt, 1998). All of us commonly accept the assertion that there is a critical period for acquiring a second language that ends at puberty.

Subsequent chapters discuss these and other critical periods. This introductory chapter attempts to present a brief primer on critical, or sensitive, period research to help nonspecialists understand what sensitive periods are (and are not) and to aid the nonspecialist in making his or her own reasoned judgments about the existence of specific sensitive periods and what the implications might be for development.

This chapter begins with a brief history of the critical period concept. This history is interesting in its own right, but from it we will see that the terms *critical period*, *sensitive period*, or *windows of opportunity* are used in a number of different scientific fields, with slightly different meanings. Unfortunately, we also will see that even within single scientific fields the terms are not used consistently.

Despite these varied, and sometimes conflicting, usages, a core scientific idea unites them. The core idea is that having a certain kind of experience at one point in development has a profoundly different impact on future behavior than having that same experience at any other point in development. This core idea places constraints on the kinds of experiments and evidence that are required to show that critical or sensitive periods exist. With this core idea in mind, we then look at four examples of popular critical or sensitive period claims and the experimental evidence that can be offered to support them. Forewarned about the semantic confusions and forearmed with an understanding of methodological issues associated with critical period research, readers will be prepared to evaluate other critical period claims and their possible implications for child development.

SOURCE OF THE CRITICAL AND SENSITIVE PERIOD CONCEPT: EMBRYOLOGY

Although Hubel and Wiesel's 1970 studies of the visual system may be the best known example of a critical period, the idea of a critical period in development has been used in various areas of science since the 1920s. There are numerous review articles on critical and sensitive period research that outline this interesting history (Bateson, 1979, 1981; Bornstein, 1989; Colombo, 1982; Connolly, 1972; Immelmann & Suomi, 1981; Nash, 1978; Sackett, Sameroff, Cairns, & Suomi, 1981). Researchers, educators, and early childhood advocates who take time to read these reviews will quickly appreciate that critical and sensitive periods are not nearly as simple as "windows of opportunity that open briefly and then slam shut."

The idea of a critical period first appeared neither in neuroscience nor in psychology. Its origin is in the field of embryology. Around 1920, Charles Stockard, an embryologist at Cornell Medical College, was studying the effects of exposing fish embryos to extreme temperatures and to toxic chemicals. In these experiments, Stockard tried to show that birth defects might arise as the result of disrupting normal embryonic development. Based on his experiments, he claimed that specific birth defects occurred when normal development was disturbed just at the time when a specific embryonic organ, for example the embryonic retina, was developing. He argued that the period of rapid cellular growth in an embryonic organ was a period, or moment, in the organ's development when disruptions could cause the greatest damage. Developmental disturbances before or after that period would cause no, or only slight, damage to the organ. Stockard wrote, "such particular sensitive periods during development I have termed 'critical moments'" (1921, p. 139).

Stockard used the terms *sensitive period* and *critical moment* synonymously to define the period during which an embryonic organ was most susceptible to damage by exposure to abnormal or toxic conditions. Critical periods, in Stockard's sense, were danger periods or periods of susceptibility during development.

In the 1930s, the idea of a critical period again appeared in embryology but with a slightly different meaning. A question of central interest to embryologists is, How can cells that are all identical early in development eventually differentiate into very specific and different kinds of cells (e.g., nerve cells, heart cells, skin cells)? In the 1930s, Hans Spemann and his colleagues transplanted cells from one site in the embryo to a different site (Spemann, 1938). They found that sometimes the transplanted cells matured like cells at the new site, but that at other times the cells would develop as they would have at their original site in the embryo. Further experiments revealed that the key variable that determined how the transplanted cells would develop was the time or stage in embryonic development when the transplantation occurred. That is, they found that before a certain stage in development, embryonic cells are highly plastic and their developmental future is open. They can become nerve cells, heart cells, or skin cells. However, at some later stage in development, the cells' developmental courses are determined. Their fates are sealed, and the cells are constrained to develop, for example, as a neuron or a heart cell. Spemann called this developmental phenomenon *cellular induction*.

Spemann's experiments also showed that this change from being highly plastic to being developmentally constrained was determined not by the cell itself but by the local environment in which the cell was embedded. Neighboring cells in the embryo send chemical messages that, in Spemann's usage, *induce* the cells to take one particular developmental path, rather than another. If a cell was transplanted before it received such an inducing signal, it could be induced to mature like the cells found at its new site. If it was transplanted after it received its inducing signal, it would develop as it would have at its original site. Once this determining signal has been sent to the cell, the cell becomes impervious to other signals. Spemann called the time during which embryonic cells were induced to take one developmental pathway rather than another the *critical period* in the cells' developmental histories. In Spemann's usage, critical periods were necessary and normal aspects of development, a time when changes had to occur for normal development to proceed.

A similar notion of *critical period* appears in current developmental neurobiology. A question that intrigues developmental neurobiologists is, How do neurons in the developing nervous system make appropriate connections among themselves? Are neural connections determined by information carried within the neurons themselves, or are connections determined, at least in part, by stimuli external to the cells? Roger Sperry (1963) investigated this question by studying how nerve cells in the eye make the correct connections with nerve cells in the visual area of the brain. He hypothesized that cells in both the retina and the brain's visual area acquire specific chemical markers by virtue of their relative positions in the retina and in the brain. When retinal cells send out axons to seek their target cells in the brain, axons and target cells find each other by means of these chemical markers. Sperry assumed that the neurons in the retina and the brain acquired the specific markers at certain times during development, that is, during the *critical period* in their development. If this were the case, then one could test this critical period hypothesis by transplanting cells into new sites in the retina. If the transplantation occurred before the critical period, the cell would make connections to the brain appropriate to its new retinal location. If it were transplanted after the critical period, it would make connections to the brain as if it were still at its original retinal location.

One of the easiest systems in which to test this hypothesis is the frog visual system. Marcus Jacobsen rotated the eye cups (all the retinal cells) in tadpoles 180° long before the neural connections between the eye and the brain developed (Jacobsen, 1968). He found that if he rotated the eye cups before Stage 29 (an early developmental stage) the eye formed a normal pattern of connections to the frog's brain. If, however, the rotation occurred at Stage 31 in development, a highly abnormal pattern of connections formed between the retina and the visual area of the frog's brain. Developmental Stage 31 occurs less than 24 hours after Developmental Stage 29 in the tadpole. Thus, developmental neurobiologists reason that the intercellular signaling, which determines the eventual pattern of retina–brain connections, occurs within a 24-hour period during frog development. As a leading neurobiological textbook described this experiment, "Stages 29 and 30, therefore, constitute a critical period in development after which retinal specification becomes irreversible. *Critical periods are a common feature of the development of the nervous system*" (Kandel & Schwartz, 1985, p. 747). The idea of a critical period as a decision point during development that sets nerve cells irreversibly on one path of differentiation or connectivity as opposed to another, is a fundamental one in developmental neurobiology (Kandel, Schwartz, & Jessell, 1991).

Spemann's use of the term *critical period* with respect to cellular induction and its closely related use in developmental neurobiology introduced three ideas that remain part of our modern popular (although not necessarily scientific) concept of critical periods. First, because embryological development occurs quite rapidly (e.g., the retinal connections in the frog are specified within a 24-hour developmental period), it would appear that critical periods are short in duration and that they begin and end quickly. Second, this concept of critical period brings with it the idea that outside stimulation or environmental influences exert particularly strong effects during a critical period. Third, it introduces the idea that the effects of critical periods are irreversible and permanent.

KONRAD LORENZ'S CRITICAL PERIODS IN THE DEVELOPMENT OF BEHAVIOR

Critical periods in embryonic development occur before birth and, as such, rely not at all on experience from the physical world. However, the term *critical period* also is used to describe how experience at a specific point in development is necessary for the normal emergence of *behaviors*, such as sexual identity, social competence, and sensory systems. Konrad Lorenz introduced the notion of critical period into studies of animal and, eventually, human behavior. He did so by drawing an analogy between his and Spemann's work.

Spemann published his ideas about critical periods in the 1930s, about the same time that Lorenz was publishing his work on the phenomenon of imprinting in birds. Lorenz, as well as some early students of animal behavior, had observed that hatchlings of certain bird species would fixate, or imprint, on the first large moving object that they saw. The hatchlings would follow this object around, as they would normally follow their mother. (Of course, in the wild, typically the first large moving object the hatchlings would see would be the mother.) However, within a few days of hatching, this tendency to imprint would disappear. Among the features of imprinting that were of most interest to Lorenz were that "the process is confined to a very definite period of individual life, a period that in many cases is of extremely short duration" and "the process, once accomplished, is totally irreversible, so that from then on, the reaction behaves exactly like an 'unconditioned' or purely instinctive response" (Lorenz, 1937, p. 264).

These features of imprinting, Lorenz pointed out, were analogous to the features of cellular induction that Spemann had identified during embryological development (Lorenz, 1937, pp. 265–266). According to Lorenz's analogy, imprinting and cellular induction are both critical period phenomena because environmental influences (cellular environment for induction and social environment for the hatchling) have effects that are confined to limited periods of development, and in both cases the results of this environmental influence are irreversible.

Lorenz's observations about critical periods in imprinting gave rise to decades of research on imprinting in the behavioral sciences. In this research, imprinting was understood as the process whereby an animal's social preferences could be influenced by experience during a critical period (Bateson, 1979). In addition to imprinting in birds, behavioral scientists studied a variety of animal behaviors, ranging from sociability in dogs to emotional development in monkeys, as made famous by the work of Harry Harlow and his colleagues (1958, 1959) at the University of Wisconsin. Scientists also studied critical periods in song-bird learning (Konishi, 1995). Others extended these ideas to human development: For example, critical periods in human socioemotional development and the establishment of secure attachments between infant and caregiver (see Chapter 5). In 1967, Eric Lenneberg argued that there was a critical period for acquiring one's first, or native, language.

Although the research program inspired by Lorenz tested many critical period hypotheses, we should note that, for the most part, this was behavioral research, not brain science. Also, for the most part, this research merely described critical periods and did not investigate the underlying mechanisms responsible for critical period effects. In this respect, Hubel and Wiesel's work on the visual system was an exception. They found a critical period during which visual experience affected how neural connections were made in the visual area of cat brains.

A LEGACY OF CRITICAL PERIOD RESEARCH: TERMINOLOGICAL CONFUSION

Some appreciation of what these decades of research on critical periods discovered is fundamental to understanding the implications of critical period phenomena for child development. For Lorenz, critical periods had two key features. First, animals' susceptibility to certain kinds of experience were restricted to short, well-defined periods in development. Second, critical period effects were permanent and irreversible. Decades of research on imprinting and other critical period effects, however, have provided behavioral scientists with sufficient evidence to seriously weaken, if not totally reject, Lorenz's original claims. Scientists now know that critical periods are rarely brief and seldom sharply defined; rather, during a critical period the impact of the experience peaks and then gradually declines (see Chapters 2 and 3).

Similarly, decades of research also have shown that critical period effects are not necessarily permanent and irreversible. Critical period phenomena from imprinting, to the development of the visual system, to the effects of maternal deprivation have been shown to be, if not totally, at least substantially reversible (Bateson, 1983; Colombo, 1982). As early as the mid-1970s, experiments had shown that Hubel and Wiesel's kittens did not have to remain functionally blind in their deprived eye. Visually deprived kittens forced to use the deprived eye in visual training tasks, even after the critical period was presumed to have ended, could learn to make discriminations between visual patterns and behaved as if they had sight in the deprived eye (Chow & Stewart, 1972; Harweth, Smith, Crawford, & van Noorden, 1989). Monkeys that have had one eye closed during the critical period can recover normal to near normal function if forced to use the deprived eye by having the normal eye sutured shut. Just as there are periods when abnormal visual experience can damage visual functions, there also are later periods when reverse deprivation can result in recovery of visual functions. As one review of critical period research noted,

> Fixity of outcome is widely thought to be one of the sensitive period's most salient characteristics. To many minds, the sensitive period's lasting effect is what stamps the phenomenon with its special character. Some outcomes do indeed seem to endure permanently. Research has shown, however, that many sensitive period outcomes are modifiable or even reversible. (Bornstein, 1989, p. 188)

In an attempt to avoid the connotations of Lorenz's narrow, rigid definition of *critical periods*, many scientists now favor using the terms *sensitive phase* or *sensitive period* when discussing phenomena such as imprinting, the development of perceptual and motor skills, and social-emotional development (Connolly, 1972; Immelmann & Suomi, 1981). The preferred *sensitive period* carries the implication of longer, ill-defined periods, when specific kinds of experiences have particularly pronounced effects on development, still allowing that these effects might be modifiable or reversible by subsequent experience.

Unfortunately, not all scientists in all fields adhere to this terminological preference. This can make reading articles and comparing conclusions about critical or sensitive periods a semantic nightmare. (Readers can find a listing of various other definitions of sensitive and critical periods in Freedman, 1979.) For example, some scientists have suggested that a *critical period* is a period during which a system, such as the visual system, requires specific kinds of experience if normal development is to occur, whereas a *sensitive period* is a period during which normal development is most sensitive to abnormal environmental conditions. Going back to a distinction that was implicit in the different uses of *critical period* in embryology, some have suggested, in the spirit of Spemann, that *critical periods* are periods during which normal development has to be triggered by some stimulus or signal, whereas, in the spirit of Stockard, *sensitive periods* are times during which the animal or organism is most vulnerable to harmful or damaging stimuli (Fox, 1970).

Current developmental neurobiology provides another example of how the terms *sensitive* and *critical* periods are used. For some scientists working in this field a *sensitive period* is the time during development when a specific manipulation or experience changes the developmental trajectory of a system. A *critical period*, in contrast, is the time during development when a change caused by a manipulation or experience can be reversed (P. Levitt, April 28, 1999). On this usage, in the monkey experiment described previously, the period of initial visual deprivation would be the sensitive period, and the period during which reverse closure could assist recovery of function would be the critical period. Of course, on this usage, a sensitive period is certainly *not* a more loosely defined or less rigidly constrained critical period.

Another term one encounters in both the popular and policy literature on brain development is *window of opportunity*. This is not a scientific term. Rather, it is a term introduced into the literature by Patrick Bateson (1979) in a review of the critical or sensitive period concept. In his article, Bateson likened the developing animal to a train traveling from "conception" to a point at which it disappears from the tracks. As he pointed out, a strong view of critical periods would be that the train has all its (opaque) windows closed during the first part of the journey, then has all the windows thrown open to allow the passengers to view the passing scenery. A little later all the windows abruptly shut. A more refined view would see the train as divided into compartments, in which each compartment represents a particular behavioral or brain system, like vision, and in which the windows of different compartments open and close at different times during the journey. A third way to think about critical or sensitive periods, using this analogy, would be to think that the windows on various compartments open at various points in the journey, but never shut, until the train stops running. According to this view, a sensitive period would end not because the windows shut, but because experience changes the occupants of the compartments. Bateson favored this latter analogy because it allows for the known modifiability of critical period effects. It leaves open the possibility of later experiences affecting behavioral systems, if the right experiences can be arranged to appear alongside the tracks.

In the child development literature, we might encounter all of these terms—*critical period*, *sensitive period* or *phase*, and *window of opportunity*. Although *sensitive period* may be the term of choice among scientists, nonetheless, *critical period* remains the term of choice in the early childhood literature. In a database of 564 records that contain material and quotations from the popular, policy, and scholarly work on the brain and early childhood, 66 of the records contain the term *critical period*, whereas only 8 records contain *sensitive period* and 14 records contain *windows of opportunity*. Thus, the popular brain and early childhood literature appears to be at odds with the scientific literature in its preferred usage.

There are at least two nonmutually exclusive explanations for this terminological discrepancy. First, the brain and early childhood literature may rely more on a popular, rather than a scientific, understanding of critical and sensitive periods. This popular understanding appears to be rooted in Lorenz's narrow, rigid understanding of critical periods, windows of opportunity that pop open and slam shut, with permanent irreversible consequences. Second, *critical period* may be the term of choice in this literature exactly because of the charged connotations the term carries—connotations of crisis, of once-in-a-lifetime learning opportunities, and of "use-it-or-lose-it" developmental brinkmanship. It carries the connotation of what Jerome Kagan has called the myth of infant determinism (Bruer, 1999; Kagan, 1998). A *critical period* connotes that as the twig is bent, so inevitably grows the tree. Such deterministic, and possibly dire, connotations and implications are particularly compelling in the policy arena, in which they prompt interest in policy reports, garner media attention, and engender public interest. Qualified talk about ill-defined sensitive periods, with modifiable effects, lack the same emotive and rhetorical force. Nonetheless, if we are committed to basing policy and practice on what the science actually says, the highly qualified sensitive period claims are more likely closer to the scientific truth than are the dramatic window slamming claims of critical periods narrowly construed.

The moral here is that when we attempt to understand what critical or sensitive period research might tell us about early childhood, we have to pay careful attention to how the terms are used and defined in the articles we read. There is no standard usage for these terms. Be particularly cautious of policy recommendations that hang on subtle distinctions between *critical* versus *sensitive periods*. In short, *reader beware!* (From here on, I will only use the term *sensitive period*. Where a particular scientist or author does use *critical period*, I will so indicate.)

TESTING SENSITIVE PERIODS CLAIMS: METHODOLOGICAL ISSUES

Readers interested in sensitive periods also should be aware of methodological issues involved in testing sensitive period hypotheses. The image of developmental windows opening and slamming shut suggests that experimental evidence to establish such effects would be relatively easy to obtain.

However, designing experiments that yield reliable evidence for or against sensitive period hypotheses is not so simple. There are numerous discussions in the review literature about the criteria such experiments must meet and the kinds of evidence they must provide (Bateson, 1979; Bornstein, 1989; Colombo, 1982; Nash, 1978; Sackett et al., 1981).

We can acquire a reasonable grasp of these methodological issues if we return to the core idea underlying sensitive periods. To establish the existence of a sensitive period, a study must show that *an experience (or lack of it) during a given period in development has a more pronounced effect (positive or negative) on the organism than exposure to that same experience at any other time during the organism's development.* Thus, minimally, any experiment cited to support a sensitive period claim must show that a specific experience or experimental manipulation has significantly different effects if experienced at different periods during the organism's development. We have a sensitive period when biological maturation places temporal constraints on how a specific experience affects an organism. This minimal demand places constraints on the kind of experiment a scientist must design and execute to test sensitive period claims. The following four examples, all of which appear as sensitive period claims in the brain and child development literature, although not necessarily advanced as sensitive period claims by the scientists themselves, illustrate experimental features we should keep in mind when we encounter claims about sensitive periods in the early childhood literature.

Example 1: Sensitive Periods in the Visual System: Hubel and Wiesel's Blind Kittens

Hubel and Wiesel's experiments on the development of the cat's visual system figures prominently in scientific policy and popular discussions for very good reason. Although popular and policy presentations of this work may be oversimplified or flawed, the original work is a model of the experimental rigor and care one must observe in testing sensitive period hypotheses.

To determine whether the same experience has different effects at different periods in an animal's development, sensitive period experiments require that the experimenter expose animals to the *same* experience or experimental manipulation at different ages (Colombo, 1982). After exposing the animals to the experience or manipulation, the scientists then observe the animals' subsequent development or behavior and assess the animals' performance using an appropriate outcome measure. If there is a sensitive period, then animals who had the experience at one age, but not animals who had the same experience at other ages, show significantly different performance on the outcome measure. Animals who experience the manipulation outside of the sensitive period should perform like normal, or control, animals on the outcome measure.

In designing an experiment, scientists must honor one important constraint on the experimental manipulation. They must either hold the duration of the manipulation constant for all animals in the experiment or systematically vary the duration of the treatment. If the scientists do not honor this constraint, then they cannot be sure that they have found a sensitive period effect. If they do not honor this constraint, they might only have found a practice effect in which *longer* exposure, not *age* of exposure alone, results in better performance on the outcome measure. Varying the duration of the manipulation also allows scientists to determine if there are periods of higher sensitivity to the intervention or manipulation, periods when even short exposures have substantial effects on the outcome measure, as we will see in Hubel and Wiesel's experiment with the kittens.

So, as we look at the Hubel and Wiesel experiment and the other examples to follow, keep the following questions in mind:

1. What is the experience or experimental manipulation?
2. What is the outcome measure?
3. Did the experimental subjects have the *same* experience at different stages?
4. Did the scientists systematically vary the duration of the experience or did they hold the duration constant?

For Hubel and Wiesel's experiments, we can answer "Yes" to these questions. Figure 1.1 illustrates their experiment design (Hubel & Wiesel, 1970). The experimental subjects were kittens. The experience or experimental manipulation was surgical closure of a kitten's right eye. Thus, Hubel and Wiesel's experiment was a deprivation experiment in which kittens were deprived of normal visual experience. As the solid arrows indicate, the scientists varied both the age at which the kittens first experienced eye closure and the duration of eye closure. After the period of deprivation, the kittens' eyes were opened. At a time subsequent to the opening, the scientists assessed the effects of visual deprivation. As their outcome measure, Hubel and Wiesel used electrophysiological recordings from cells in the left visual area of the kittens' brains. From their recordings, they tabulated how many cells responded when the right, deprived eye was stimulated.

In a study of three normal kittens, which experienced no deprivation, they found that 98% of the cells from which they recorded responded when the kittens' right eyes were stimulated.[1]

---

[1]In discussing this experiment, I introduce one simplification. Hubel and Wiesel's experiment shows that there is a sensitive period for the maintenance of *ocular dominance* columns in the cat visual cortex. Cells in this visual area of the brain are arranged in columns. Hubel and Wiesel found that when they made electro-

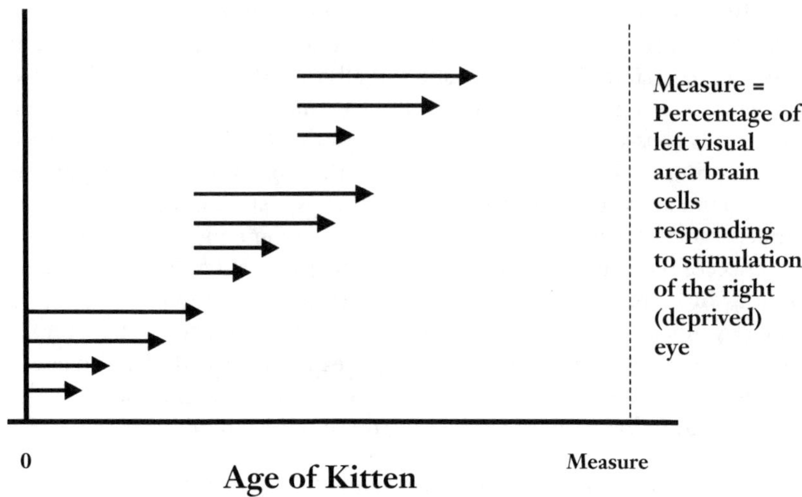

Figure 1.1. Hubel and Wiesel's visual deprivation experiment in kittens. (Key = → Onset and duration of right eye closure.) (From Hubel, D.H., & Wiesel, T.N. [1970]. The period of susceptibility to the physiological effects of unilateral eye closure in kittens. *Journal of Physiology, 206,* 419–436; reprinted by permission.)

Figure 1.2 presents the results of Hubel and Wiesel's recordings from the deprived kittens. It shows the percentage of the recorded brain cells that responded when the right, deprived eye was stimulated. Reading down the columns, you can see how increasing the duration of visual deprivation at a given age early in development disrupts the normal response pattern. Twenty days of visual deprivation starting at age 10 days lowers the response from the normal 98% to 67%. Sixty-five days of deprivation lowers the response to 16%. The area outlined by the dashed line represents what Hubel and Wiesel call the period of susceptibility to single-eye closure in the kitten, or as they call it, the "critical vulnerable period" (Hubel &

physiological recordings of neural activity down the length of a column of cells that these cells responded preferentially to stimulation of one eye or the other. That is, cells tended to be dominated by input to one eye or the other. However, in their recordings, this dominance was not complete. Some cells responded only to stimulation of one eye, some cells responded equally to both, and some cells responded primarily, but not only, to stimulation of one eye. For this reason, Hubel and Wiesel reported their results using seven categories. Cells in category 1 responded only to the right eye. Cells in category 4 responded equally to both eyes. Cells in category 7 responded only to the left eye. Categories 2, 3, 5, and 6 showed "in between" responses. To simplify the discussion, the percentages reported here are the number of cells in categories 1 through 6; all cells show *some* right eye response, divided by the total number of cells from which recordings were made.

Wiesel, 1970, p. 420). Generally, any length of deprivation from the period of birth to 60 days of age has a significant, adverse effect on how nerve cells from the cats' eyes are connected to target cells in their brains.

Because Hubel and Wiesel also systematically varied the duration of the deprivation, they were able to determine when the kitten's visual system is most sensitive to deprivation. The solid line in the diagram outlines this period, a period Hubel and Wiesel call the *sensitive period.* (Note how Hubel and Wiesel use the term.) They found that as little as 3 days of eye closure beginning at age 23 days cut the response from the normal 98% to 50%. Six to nine days of closure experienced between ages 23 and 30 days effectively eliminated cells that responded to the previously deprived right eye. As they concluded, "These experiments show that the sensitive period has a duration of at least several weeks, during which a few days of closure causes marked cortical changes" (Hubel & Wiesel, 1970, p. 425).

Hubel and Wiesel's experiment, which ensured that the experimental subjects received the same experimental manipulation at different ages and for different durations, clearly shows that there is a sensitive period to single-eye closure in the development of the cat's visual system. What they call the period of susceptibility or the critical vulnerable period begins

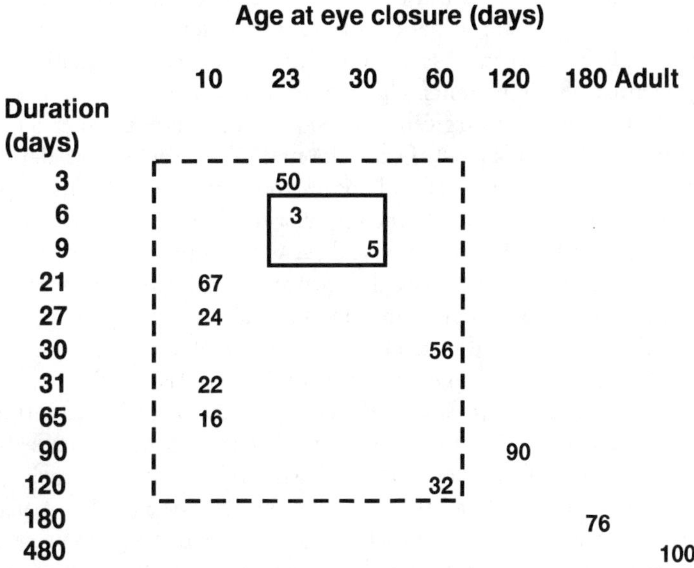

Figure 1.2. Hubel and Wiesel's results: percent cells in left visual area responding to stimulation to right (deprived) eye. Note: The normal response in undeprived kittens is 98%. (From Hubel, D.H., & Wiesel, T.N. [1970]. The period of susceptibility to the physiological effects of unilateral eye closure in kittens. *Journal of Physiology, 206,* 419–436; reprinted by permission.)

shortly after birth and lasts until age 2 months. Within this period there is a time of heightened sensitivity to the experimental manipulation lasting through the fourth and fifth weeks of life. Hubel and Wiesel call this period of heightened sensitivity the *sensitive period.*

As the scientists wrote, "We wished to learn when the susceptibility was greatest, how long it lasted, the duration of the deprivation necessary to produce a severe deficit, and the relation between the timing of the deprivation and ability to recover" (Hubel & Wiesel, 1970, p. 420). Their carefully designed and executed experiment allowed them to learn all these things, launching a monumental neuroscientific research program, involving hundreds of scientists, that continues to this day.

Example 2: A Sensitive Period for Second-Language Learning

One of the benefits of using animal models, as Hubel and Wiesel did, is that scientists can design exacting experiments in which they deprive their experimental subjects of normally occurring experience to study the effects of deprivation. Of course, if we want to study sensitive periods and the effects of deprivation in humans, we cannot deliberately deprive our experimental subjects of normally occurring experiences. To study sensitive periods in humans, scientists must find naturally occurring populations who happen to have had abnormal or different experiences at various times in their lives. For example, to study sensitive periods in the human visual system, scientists study patients who acquired cataracts at different ages and who had the condition surgically corrected at various ages. Such a group of patients would provide a set of experimental subjects who were deprived of visual input at various ages and for various durations. Studying such a group of patients would allow the scientist to identify a sensitive period in the development of the human visual system and to identify the period of optimal sensitivity to such visual deprivation. People who have become deaf at various ages provide another naturally occurring population in which scientists can study the effects of abnormal auditory experience on brain development and language acquisition (see Chapter 8).

A human sensitive period that has received considerable attention from psychologists and psycholinguists, and one that is much discussed in the policy and popular literature, is a sensitive period for second language learning. Jacqueline Johnson and Elissa Newport (1989) designed an experiment to assess such a sensitive period claim. In their study they do use the term *critical period* but use it broadly to describe how maturational changes affect the ability to learn. They intend that their *critical periods* include what other scientists call *sensitive periods.*

The Johnson-Newport experimental design is shown in Figure 1.3. Their subjects were Chinese and Korean immigrants, whose first exposure

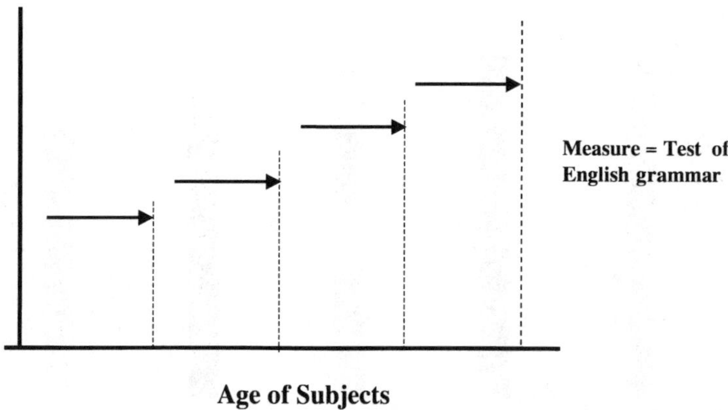

Figure 1.3. Critical period effects in second language learning: Johnson and Newport's natural experiment. (Key = → Onset and length of experience with English as a second language.) (From Johnson, J.S., & Newport, E.L. [1989]. Critical period effects in second language learning. *Cognitive Psychology, 21*[1], 60–99; reprinted by permission from Academic Press.)

to English as a second language occurred when they arrived in the United States. The scientists divided the subjects into four groups: those who arrived between the ages of 3 and 7 years, those who arrived between the ages of 8 and 10 years, those who arrived between the ages of 11 and 15 years, and those who were 17 years or older when they arrived. The experience of interest was exposure to English as a second language. Each of the four groups had this experience beginning at a different point in their lifetimes. However, rather than varying the duration of the experience, in this study Johnson and Newport held the duration of the experience constant. On average, all of their subjects had 10 years experience with English at the time of testing. Holding the duration constant controls for practice effects: All else being equal, we would expect immigrants who had more practice with English to have better grammatical comprehension than those who had less practice, independent of their age of arrival. Thus, we can think of the "experience" in this experiment as 10 years of exposure to English as a second language. The outcome measure was a test of English grammatical understanding.

Johnson and Newport's results appear in Figure 1.4. Just as Hubel and Wiesel reported results on normal kittens, Newport and Johnson reported the average score for a group of native English speakers on the grammar test. The average score for the group of native speakers was 269. After 10 years of exposure to English, children who had arrived in the United States between the ages of 3 and 7 years also achieved a score of 269. Based on the grammar test they were indistinguishable from native English speakers. For the other subjects, however, test performance declined significantly with

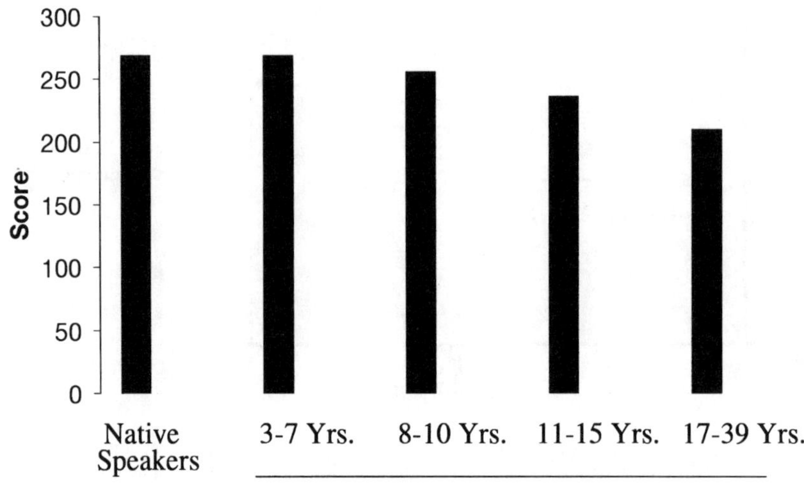

Figure 1.4. Average score on test of English grammar. (From Johnson, J.S., & Newport, E.L. [1989]. Critical period effects in second language learning. *Cognitive Psychology, 21*[1], 60–99; reprinted by permission from Academic Press.)

age. Subjects who had arrived as adults, between the ages of 17 and 39 (after puberty), had an average score of 210 on the grammar test. Johnson and Newport conclude, "This suggests that, if one is immersed in a second language before the age of 7, one is able to achieve native fluency in the language; however immersion even soon after that age results in a decrement in ultimate performance" (Johnson & Newport, 1989, p. 78). Consistent with a sensitive period claim, this result shows that 10 years of experience starting before age 7 results in "normal" native grammatical proficiency, whereas that same experience later in life does not have the same effect.

Does this sensitive period for second language grammar learning end at puberty? Johnson and Newport addressed this question by analyzing their data in a slightly different way. They divided their subjects into two groups: those who arrived before puberty (ages 3–15) and those who arrived after puberty (age 17 and older). In this analysis they found that increasing the age of arrival up to age 15 had a slight negative, linear effect on their subjects' test scores. However, for those subjects first exposed to English after age 17, they found no systematic relationship between age of arrival and English grammatical proficiency. This suggests, they argued, that the window of opportunity for acquiring native fluency in a second language ends around puberty.

The Johnson and Newport study is another excellent example of the kind of experimental design that is required to substantiate or refute sensitive period hypotheses about human behavior. One thing we should note is that their outcome measure is a behavioral task: performance on a grammar test. Thus, the experiment shows a sensitive period for the development of a behavior but says nothing specific about how brain development is involved in this sensitive period. We are still far from being able to link all, or even most, sensitive period effects to brain development.

However, this study also generates some questions critical readers might ask about even such well-designed studies. For example, although the study claims to show a sensitive period effect, some scientists have asked, What would happen if one chose a different age for dividing the subjects into two groups, those arriving before age 15 and those arriving after age 17? When one analyzes the data using different age groups, the sensitive period effect does not appear to be robust (Bialystok & Hakuta, 1994; see also Chapter 2).

Some scientists have asked whether age of arrival in the United States might be confounded with other relevant variables, such as motivation to learn, length of formal educational experience in the United States, and the amount of English spoken. These kinds of variables could certainly have an impact on one's ability to acquire English grammar. Questions like these, in fact, ask a larger question: Is it accurate to assume that 10 years experience with English beginning at age 3 is the *same* experience of 10 years of English beginning at age 17?

Other investigators have asked what would happen if one used a different outcome measure for grammatical or linguistic competence. Is there a critical period for learning all grammatical constructs or only for some? Furthermore, strictly speaking, experiments like these only show that there is a sensitive period for the behavior or condition assessed by the outcome measure. We would have to use different outcome measures to answer the following questions: Are there sensitive periods for phonology or accent? Are there sensitive periods for learning vocabulary? The answers that researchers are finding to questions like these are causing some of them, at least, to reevaluate and refine sensitive periods for second language learning.

Example 3: A Sensitive Period for Music?

In the popular press and in some policy circles, we sometimes see claims that there is a sensitive period for learning to play a musical instrument. In support of this claim, enthusiasts cite a brain recording study. This study was done at the University of Konstanz in Switzerland and published in the scientific journal *Science* (Elbert et al., 1995). This study showed that students who begin to play a string instrument earlier in life had larger areas of their brains devoted to playing the instrument than did students who begin later in life. The experiment's design is shown in Figure 1.5a. The

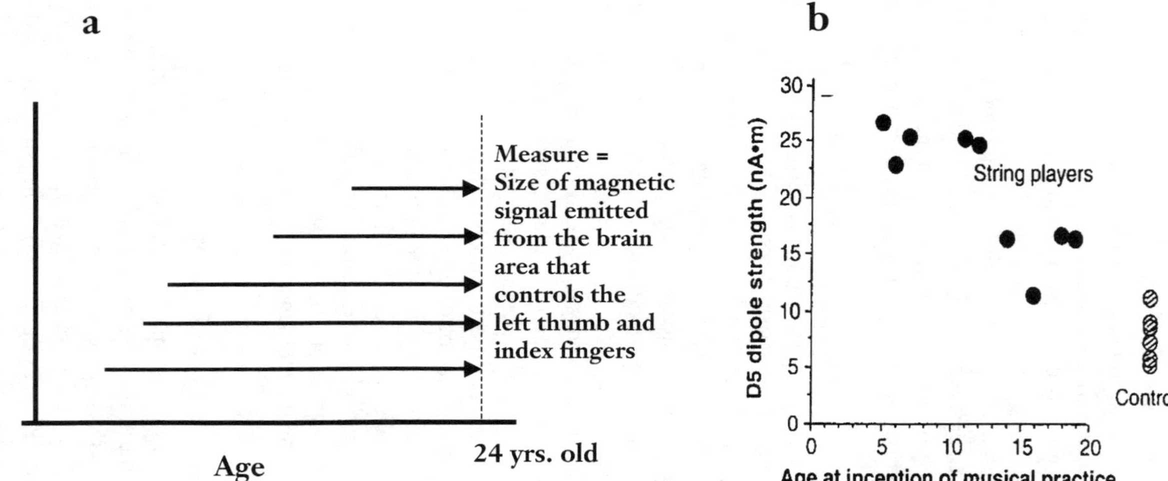

Figure 1.5. A critical period for music? (Key = → Playing a string instrument.) (From Elbert, T., Pantev, C., Wienbruch, C., Rockstroh, B., & Taub, E. [1995]. Increased cortical representation of the fingers of the left hand in string players. *Science, 270,* 305–307; reprinted by permission from the American Association for the Advancement of Science.)

experience or experimental manipulation in this study was playing a string instrument. The subjects in the experiment were young adults (average age: 24 years) who had started playing string instruments at different ages. For their outcome measure, the scientists recorded the strength of the magnetic field on the scalps of their subjects when they moved the fingers of their left hands, the hand a string player would use on the fingerboard of the instrument. Figure 1.5b shows the results. This study also included normal subjects as controls, young adults who had never played a string instrument. It should be no surprise that the size of the brain response in string players (black dots) was significantly larger than the measured brain response in the normal, control subjects (hashed dots). Experience does matter and does have an effect on brain development. Among the string players, the scientists also found that there was a correlation between the age at which a person began playing a string instrument and the size of the person's measured brain response. Generally, they found that the younger the subject was when he or she began playing an instrument, the larger the area of the brain devoted to controlling left-hand finger movements.

However, this experiment does not provide evidence for a sensitive period effect. Although the experience of playing a string instrument did begin at different ages and was of varying duration, this experiment did not systematically vary duration of the experience, nor did it control for duration of the experience. In general, the younger a child is when he or she begins to play an instrument, the longer he or she would have played it by age 24, the average age of the subjects. Thus, this experiment shows, at best, a practice effect, not a sensitive period effect. To show a sensitive period effect, the scientists would have needed an experiment such as Johnson and Newport's. They would have had to look at the effect of, say, 10 years of playing a string instrument in which this experience occurred at different points in their subjects' life spans.

Yet, emphasizing the larger response in earlier beginners appeals to parents anxious about how their children will ever get to Carnegie Hall (or Opryland) as well as to advocates and educators who would like to help the children get there. So, the sensitive period message was the one media treatments emphasized.

Edward Taub, one of the study's authors, told me, "I am definitely not happy with the interpretation and treatment of this article. In fact, I am quite unhappy about it. The interpretation and coverage missed the main point of the work entirely, which was not that you have a greater plasticity in the immature brain than in the mature nervous system, but rather that this plasticity persists, at least in reduced form, into maturity. It is the latter that is contrary to the previously established view in neuroscience and that gives the paper whatever importance it has."

For Taub, what is of neuroscientific interest is that string players who started late, after age 12, also showed significant brain reorganization compared to people who had never played. The important conclusion is that the neural circuitry of our mature brains reorganizes in response to what we do and the experiences we have throughout our lives. What these scientists intended to demonstrate was a practice effect, not a sensitive period effect.

Example 4: A Sensitive Period for Early Childhood Intervention Programs

The North Carolina Abecedarian Project and the Infant Health Program and Development Study are two important studies that are often misinterpreted by well-intentioned advocates and writers (Brooks-Gunn, Gross, Kraemer, Spiker, & Shapiro, 1992; Brooks-Gunn, Klebanov, Liaw, & Spiker, 1993; Brooks-Gunn, Liaw, Klebanov, 1992; Campbell & Ramey, 1994). The popular press and the policy literature often cite these studies as showing that there is a sensitive period from birth to age 3 years during which childhood intervention programs are particularly effective. Such a sensitive period effect is often invoked in popular explanations of why the cognitive gains toddlers make in Head Start disappear by school age (Head Start begins at age 3 years). According to these explanations, age 3 is too late to permanently and irreversibly rewire children's brains. By age 3, the sensitive period has already ended (see, e.g., Begley, 1996). Thus, the argument goes, if we want to permanently change children's intelligence and cognitive abilities, interventions must start before the critical period ends, that is before age 3. The North Carolina Abecedarian study and the Infant Health Program and Development Study have similar experimental designs, so I will use the Abecedarian study as the example.

The Abecedarian Project provided an early childhood program to a small group of economically and culturally deprived North Carolina children. The study design as sketched in Figure 1.6 involved three different enrichment interventions or experiences. Some children participated in a center-based preschool program that began during the children's first year of life and that lasted until entry into kindergarten (solid arrow). Some children received only a home-based program that began after they entered kindergarten and that lasted 3 years (dotted arrow). A third group of children received both the preschool and home-based programs for a total of 8 years (dashed arrow). The outcome measures in the study were age-appropriate standardized IQ tests and standardized school achievement tests administered at ages 5, 8, 12, and 15. Given our current purpose, the results of the study can be easily summarized. The study is most often cited as showing how early childhood interventions have a long-term impact on children's intelligence and school performance. At ages 5, 8, and 15 years

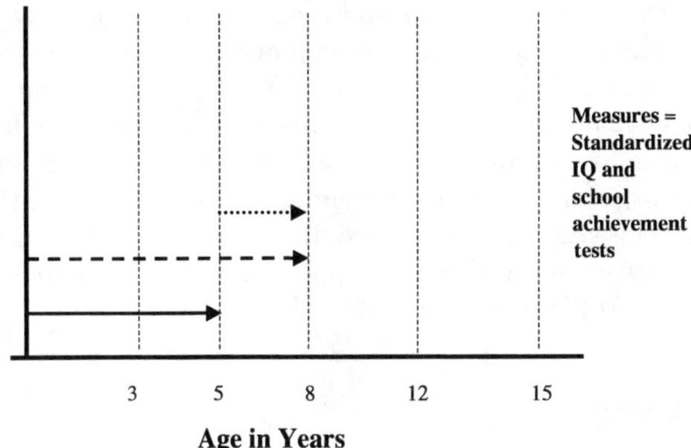

Figure 1.6. Early childhood interventions: The Abecedarian study. (Key = ⟶ Preschool Program; - - ➔ Preschool & In School Program; ····➔ In School Program Only.) (From Ramey, C.T., & Campbell, F.A. [1984]. Preventive education for high-risk children: Cognitive consequences of the Carolina Abecedarian Project. *American Journal on Mental Retardation, 88*[5], 515–523; reprinted by permission of Copyright Clearance Center, Inc.)

children who had been in the preschool program had IQ scores between 4 and 5 points higher than children who had received no enrichment before school entry or during school and had higher test scores in reading and mathematics. From this one can conclude that the preschool experience had a positive impact on these children, although there is debate about whether an increase of 5 IQ points amounts to an educationally significant gain (see Chapter 12).

However, the study does not show that birth to age 3, or any other period in childhood, is a sensitive period. In the Abecedarian study, there are three distinct experimental enrichment activities, all of which begin at different ages and are of different duration. The study cannot answer the sensitive period question, Does the *same* experience at different points in development have different, long-term effects? At best, as its authors point out, this study supports an intensity hypothesis (another name for a practice effect): Longer interventions are better than shorter interventions, and all else being equal, the earlier an intervention begins, the longer it can continue.

The scientists who conducted the studies point to the limitations of their experimental design, noting that the design confounds intervention, duration, and age of exposure (Campbell & Ramey, 1994). As Craig and Sharon Ramey, who have worked extensively on the Abecedarian Project, emphasized, "To date, there are no compelling data to support the notion of an absolute critical period such that educational intervention provided after a certain age cannot be beneficial; rather this is a principal of relative timing effects" (1998, p. 115). Jean Brooks-Gunn, the lead investigator on the Infant Health Program and Development Study, made a similar observation about that study and warned of the dangers of drawing conclusions about sensitive periods from it. "Whether the receipt of services in a different time frame (starting a child care program at 24 or 36 months instead of 12 months) would result in different effects is not known, and it remains a critical unanswered question" (Brooks-Gunn et al., 1993). Until it is answered, we have some evidence to support a duration or intensity claim, but none to support the sensitive period claim.

CONCLUSION

There are other sensitive period claims that we might consider, and indeed many more are presented and discussed in the following chapters. The brief history and the examples presented here should help readers make their own critical appraisals about these and other sensitive period claims. It should help us all take a critical look at critical-sensitive periods.

As you read, keep two questions in mind. First, what do the authors mean by the terms *critical* or *sensitive period*? Be aware of the different senses and meanings these terms can carry. Second, does the experimental evidence show that the *same* experience at *different* stages of development results in significant long-term differences in performance, behavior, or brain structure? Keep Hubel and Wiesel's experimental design in mind as a model.

With these questions in mind, you will be able to give careful consideration to what science does and does not say about sensitive periods and make reasoned judgment about how that knowledge can be best, and most responsibly, used in child development and early childhood education.

As we take this critical look we may find that some of us will have to discard a few of our own pet sensitive period hypotheses. However, this might have a beneficial effect. As Konrad Lorenz pointed out years ago, "It is a good morning exercise for a research scientist to discard a pet hypothesis every day before breakfast. It keeps him young."

REFERENCES

Bateson, P. (1979). How do sensitive periods arise and what are they for? *Animal Behavior, 27*, 470–486.

Bateson, P. (1981). Control of sensitivity to the environment during development. In K. Immelmann, G.W. Barlow, L. Petrinovich, & M. Main (Eds.), *Behavioral development: The Bielefeld Interdisciplinary Project* (pp. 432–453). Cambridge, England: Cambridge University Press.

Bateson, P. (1983). Sensitive periods in behavioral development. *Archives of Disease in Childhood, 58*(2), 85–86.

Begley, S. (1996, February 19). Your child's brain. *Newsweek*, 55–62.

Bialystok, E., & Hakuta, K. (1994). *In other words: The science and psychology of second-language acquisition.* New York: Basic Books.

Bornstein, M.H. (1989). Sensitive periods in development: Structural characteristics and causal interpretations. *Psychological Bulletin, 105*(2), 179–197.

Brooks-Gunn, J., Gross, R.T., Kraemer, H.C., Spiker, D., & Shapiro, S. (1992). Enhancing the cognitive outcomes of low birth weight premature infants: For whom is the intervention most effective. *Pediatrics, 89*(6), 1209–1215.

Brooks-Gunn, J., Klebanov, P.K., Liaw, F., & Spiker, D. (1993). Enhancing the development of low-birthweight, premature infants: Changes in cognition and behavior over first three years. *Child Development, 64,* 736–753.

Brooks-Gunn, J., Liaw, F., & Klebanov, P.K. (1992). Effects of early intervention on cognitive function of low birth weight preterm infants. *Journal of Pediatrics, 120,* 350–359.

Bruer, J.T. (1997). Education and the brain: A bridge too far. *Educational Researcher, 26*(3), 4–16.

Bruer, J.T. (1998). The brain and child development: Time for some critical thinking. *Public Health Reports, 113*(5), 388–397.

Bruer, J.T. (1999). *The myth of the first three years.* New York: Free Press.

Campbell, F.A., & Ramey, C.T. (1994). Effects of early intervention on intellectual and academic achievement: A follow-up study of children from low-income families. *Child Development, 65,* 684–698.

Carnegie Corporation of New York. (1994). *Starting points: Meeting the needs of our youngest children.* New York: Author.

Carnegie Corporation of New York. (1996). *Years of promise: A comprehensive learning strategy for America's children.* New York: Author.

Chow, K.L., & Stewart, D.L. (1972). Reversal of structural and functional effects of long-term visual deprivation in cats. *Experimental Neurobiology, 34,* 409–433.

Colombo, J. (1982). The critical period concept: Research, methodology, and theoretical issues. *Psychological Bulletin, 9*(2), 260–275.

Connolly, K. (1972). Learning and the concept of critical periods. *Developmental Medicine and Child Neurology, 14*(6), 705–714.

Elbert, T., Pantev, C., Wienbruch, C., Rockstroh, B., & Taub, E. (1995). Increased cortical representation of the fingers of the left hand in string players. *Science, 270,* 305–307.

Fox, M.W. (1970). Overview and critique of stages and critical periods in canine development. *Developmental Psychobiology, 4,* 37–54.

Freedman, R.D. (1979). *Developmental neurobiology of vision.* New York: Plenum Press.

Harlow, H.F. (1958). The nature of love. *American Psychiatry, 13,* 673–685.

Harlow, H.F. (1959). Love in infant monkeys. *Scientific American, 200*(6), 68–74.

Harweth, R.S., Smith III, E.L., Crawford, M.L.J., & von Noorden, G.K. (1989). The effects of reverse monocular deprivation in monkeys I. Psychophysical experiments. *Experimental Brain Research, 74,* 327–337.

Hubel, D.H., & Wiesel, T.N. (1970). The period of susceptibility to the physiological effects of unilateral eye closure in kittens. *Journal of Physiology, 206,* 419–436.

Immelmann, K., & Suomi, S.J. (1981). Sensitive phases in development. In K. Immelmann, G.W. Barlow, L. Petrinovich, & M. Main (Eds.), *Behavioral development: The Bielefeld Interdisciplinary Project* (pp. 395–431). Cambridge, England: Cambridge University Press.

Jacobsen, M. (1968). Development of neuronal specificity in retinal ganglion cells of Xenopus. *Developmental Biology, 17,* 202–218.

Johnson, J.S., & Newport, E.L. (1989). Critical period effects in second language learning. *Cognitive Psychology, 21*(1), 60–99.

Kagan, J. (1998). *Three seductive ideas*. Cambridge, MA: Harvard University Press.

Kandel, E.R., & Schwartz, J.H. (1985). *Principles of neural science* (2nd ed.). New York: Elsevier Science.

Kandel, E.R., Schwartz, J.H., & Jessell, T.M. (1991). *Principles of neural science* (3rd ed.). Norwalk, CT: Appleton & Lange.

Konishi, M. (1995). A sensitive period for birdsong learning. In B. Julesz & I. Kovacs (Eds.), *Maturational windows and adult cortical plasticity*. Reading, MA: Addison Wesley Longman.

Lenneberg, E.H. (1967). *Biological foundations of language*. New York: John Wiley & Sons.

Lorenz, K. (1937). The companion in the bird's world. *The Auk, 54*, 245–273.

Nash, J. (1978). *Developmental psychology: A psychobiological approach*. Englewood Cliffs, NJ: Prentice-Hall.

Ramey, C.T., & Ramey, S.L. (1998). Early intervention and early experience. *American Psychologist, 53*(2), 109–120.

Sackett, G.P., Sameroff, A.J., Cairns, R.B., & Suomi, S.J. (1981). Continuity in behavioral development: Theoretical and empirical issues. In K. Immelmann, G.W. Barlow, L. Petrinovich, & M. Main (Eds.), *Behavioral development: The Bielefeld Interdisciplinary Project* (pp. 23–57). Cambridge, England: Cambridge University Press.

Shore, R. (1997). *Rethinking the brain: New insights into early development*. New York: Families and Work Institute.

Sousa, D.A. (1998, December 16). Is the fuss about brain research justified? *Education Week*.

Spemann, H. (1938). *Embryonic development and induction*. New Haven, CT: Yale University Press.

Sperry, R. (1963). Chemo affinity in the orderly growth of nerve fiber patterns and connections. *Proceedings of the National Academy of Science, U.S.A., 5*, 735–743.

Stockard, C.R. (1921). Developmental rate and structural expression: An experimental study of twins, "double monsters," and single deformities and their interaction among embryonic organs during their origins and development. *American Journal of Anatomy, 28*, 115–275.

Wolfe, P., & Brandt, R. (1998). What do we know from brain research? *Educational Leadership, 56*(3), 8–13.

2

Developmental Neurobiology Overview

Synapses, Circuits, and Plasticity

Jeff W. Lichtman

A fundamental tenet of neurobiology is that functions of the nervous system can be reduced to physical processes. This view challenges neuroscientists to discover mechanical explanations for the working of the human brain, which is perhaps the most impenetrable of all known objects. It is a challenge when scientists try to simplify the problem by studying the smaller brains of animals because they also possess nervous systems that, thus far, defy understanding. Nonetheless, conceptual advances have been made, and neuroscience is a burgeoning endeavor with breakthroughs occurring at a rapid rate. Neuroscience has created, in broad outlines, working hypotheses for many brain functions, including the peculiar fact that the brain seems to be sensitive to specific kinds of experiences for only limited periods of life—and those periods by and large occur in young brains.

This chapter aims to familiarize nonneurobiologists with basic principles of brain organization and shows how changes in this organization provide a satisfying, if somewhat incomplete, framework for critical periods.

BRAINS: THE CELLULAR PERSPECTIVE

Brain organization principles can be found at many different levels (Figure 2.1). At a systems level the brain contains regions involved with vision, language, olfaction, and so forth. At a cellular level the brain contains billions of interconnected neurons that fall into hundreds of different categories. At a molecular level the brain can be described as a large bag containing nearly 100,000 different kinds of molecules. Almost every single molecule is distributed in a unique pattern related to its particular functions.

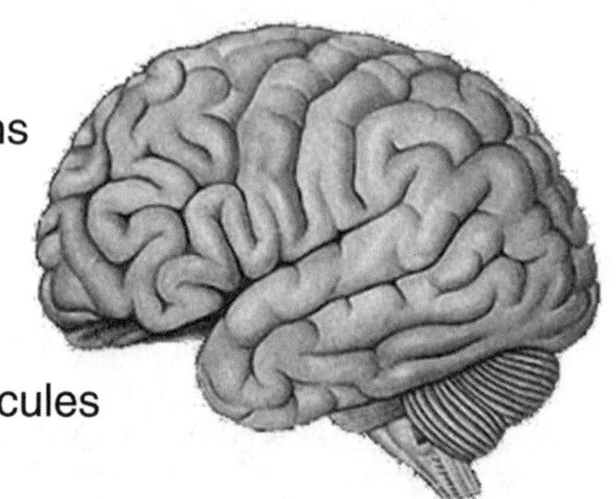

Figure 2.1. The human brain can be described as organized in several different ways: a systems level, a cellular level, and a molecular level.

For example, the visual system, which begins with the retina and progresses to the occipital cortex via a relay in the thalamus, is the major system responsible for receiving and analyzing visual information. The motor system, beginning in the brain and progressing to the spinal cord and ultimately to muscle, is the system that is responsible for the output of the brain that gives rise to action. Modern imaging techniques such as positron emission tomography (PET) and functional magnetic resonance imaging (fMRI) have allowed the flow of information in these regions to be mapped at ever-increasing resolutions.

At the opposite extreme there are principles of brain organization based on the tens of thousands of different *molecules* the brain synthesizes and uses. As the 21st century begins, the human genome is being completely decoded, meaning that eventually the identity and location of many of the genes that are expressed as proteins in the brain will be known.

There is a middle ground, between the system and molecular perspectives, that views the nervous system in terms of the *cells* that comprise it. The cellular perspective is rooted in the fact that the nervous system is actually an interconnected network of billions of cells. Each nerve cell (a *neuron*) is a living semi-autonomous entity surrounded by a membrane and possessing a nucleus. It makes its own proteins, uses oxygen, and stores energy, just like other cells. In addition, neurons have attributes that allow them to receive and send electrical and chemical signals to other cells. The signals allow the nervous system to behave as one complicated electrical circuit. While a full decoding of this circuitry is still in the future, certain fundamental rules of wiring provide a way to get a sense of what the brain is doing.

TRIPARTITE NEURONS

Each neuron, with a few exceptions, divides its functions into three spatially distinct regions: the dendrites, the cell body, and the axon (Figure 2.2). The *dendrites* are the neuron's receivers and are usually highly branched. The signals received by dendrites come from other neurons, but some dendrites are highly specialized to receive particular kinds of sensory stimulation (e.g., light, mechanical vibrations, stretching, temperature, chemo-sensations such as smell and taste). Once information is received by the dendrites it passes electrically to the *cell body* or *soma*, which is where the nucleus resides. The size of the stimulus that reaches the cell body is related to the number of inputs that are signaling the dendrites at the same time. The cell body plays the critical role of deciding whether the signals received from the dendrites are of sufficient importance (i.e., strength) to merit sending them along to other cells. The cell body is a gatekeeper—if the stimuli it receives reaches threshold, it opens a gate and allows the signals to pass onward to the cell's third functional part, the *axon*. The axon's job is disseminating the signals the neuron has received to target cells. The number and location of the axon branches determines how many and which cells will receive the information relayed by the neuron. The axon has an amplifying property that allows it to send signals without any decrement in strength over long distances, and without any weakening at its branch points. The signals that travel along axons usually originate at the cell body and are brief elec-

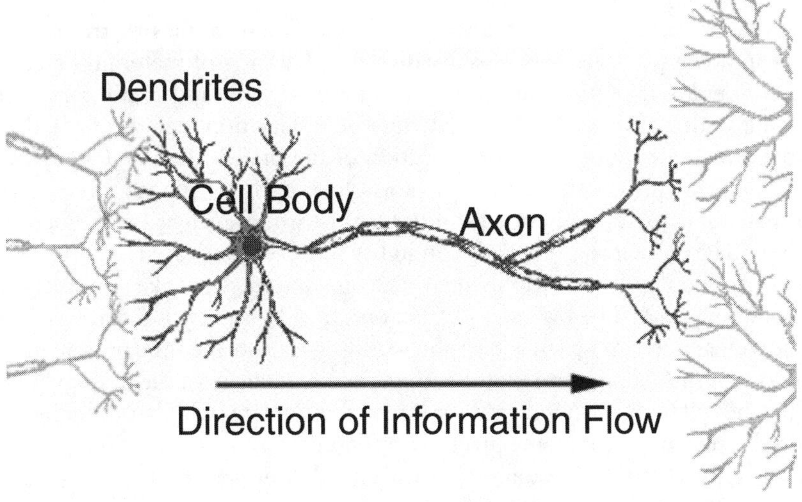

Figure 2.2. Neurons have three functional domains: dendrites, cell body, and axon.

trical fluctuations of about one tenth of a volt, called *action potentials*. The action potentials travel at rapid speeds of up to 120 meters per second, meaning that most signals reach their destinations in units of time measured in milliseconds.

Perhaps the most unusual feature of the nervous system is the highly specialized way action potential signals convey a signal to the sites where the axon meets dendrite branches of target cells. The specialized contact sites between axons and dendrites are called *synapses* (Figure 2.3). Each time an action potential signal enters an axon's synaptic terminal it causes the axon to release a chemical at the synaptic contact site. The released chemical, a *neurotransmitter*, diffuses across a narrow cleft that exists between the axon and the dendrite. When the neurotransmitter reaches the membrane of the dendrites, which takes less than a millisecond, it binds to receptor molecules embedded in the dendrites' outer membrane. The receptor molecules are specifically responsive to the particular neurotransmitter that the axon releases. There are five or six commonly used different neurotransmitters in the brain and many minor neurotransmitters, for each of the specific receptors. Once the neurotransmitter binds to its receptor, it sets up an electrical signal in the dendrite that flows toward the cell body. An axon can establish hundreds or even thousands of synapses with the dendrites of many different neurons. Therefore, the total number of synapses in the brain is in the trillions.

BRAIN CIRCUITS: THE TRIPARTITE BRAIN

Given the vast interconnectedness of billions of neurons making trillions of synaptic connections, it is no surprise that the wiring of the brain exceeds the complexity of any electrical or computer circuit, and is still far from being understood. Nonetheless, certain generalizations can be made that may provide a sense of the organization of the brain's circuits. One organizing principle is that the brain, as a whole, is partitioned into three functional domains. This division is similar to the three-way division of function in individual neurons. Thus, the brain has sensory systems, a receptive side akin to the dendrites of individual neurons designed to take information from the world. The brain also has an output side similar to the axon of an individual neuron, which acts in the world-at-large (called the motor side). Between the sensory and motor systems is the majority of the brain, which like the cell body of an individual neuron contemplates whether to act based on the sensory input at any given time (Figure 2.4).

This tripartite division of labor means that nerve cells belong to sensory pathways, motor pathways, or somewhere in between. The sensory pathways are groups of nerve cells that process the incoming sensory flow in order to extract information. For example, light that enters the eye causes

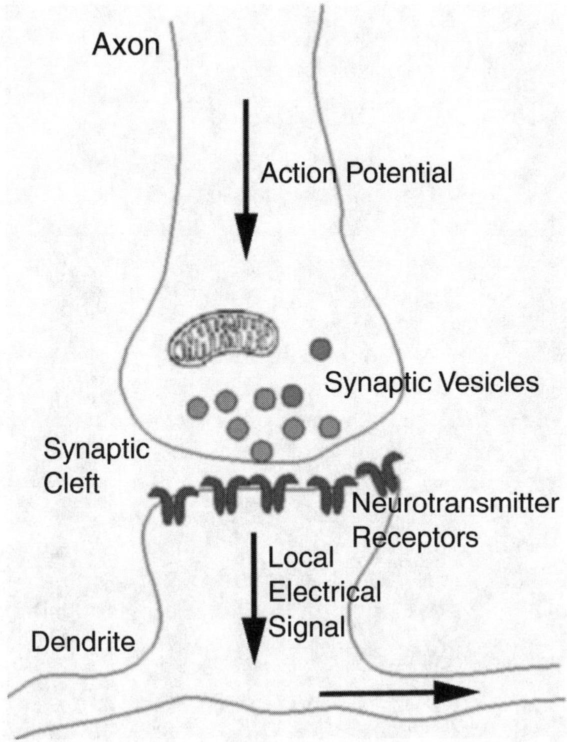

Figure 2.3. Diagram of the synapse: the site where action potentials in one cell conveys a signal via neurotransmitter to the dendrite of another cell.

changes in the electrical properties in the rod and cone cells of the retina. These cells convey the detected signals to other neurons in the retina until activating the final output neuron in the retina known as the retinal ganglion cell that sends light-induced signals along their axons to a relay station called the *thalamus*. Due to interconnections between neurons in the retina and the specific sensitivity of certain retinal cells to particular colors, the retinal signals sent to the thalamus have extracted and enhanced contrast and color information about the light. The axons of the retinal ganglion cells make synapses with cells in the thalamus that serve primarily as a relay. The thalamic neurons send their axons to the occipital cortex to make synapses on the dendrites of cells in the cerebral cortex in a region that is specialized for processing visual sensory information. The cerebral cortex is the layered structure less than an inch thick that resides on the outer surface of the brain. The cortex contains large numbers of cells arranged in intricate, connected circuits with other neurons, near and far away. This is how visual information is processed. This processing allows

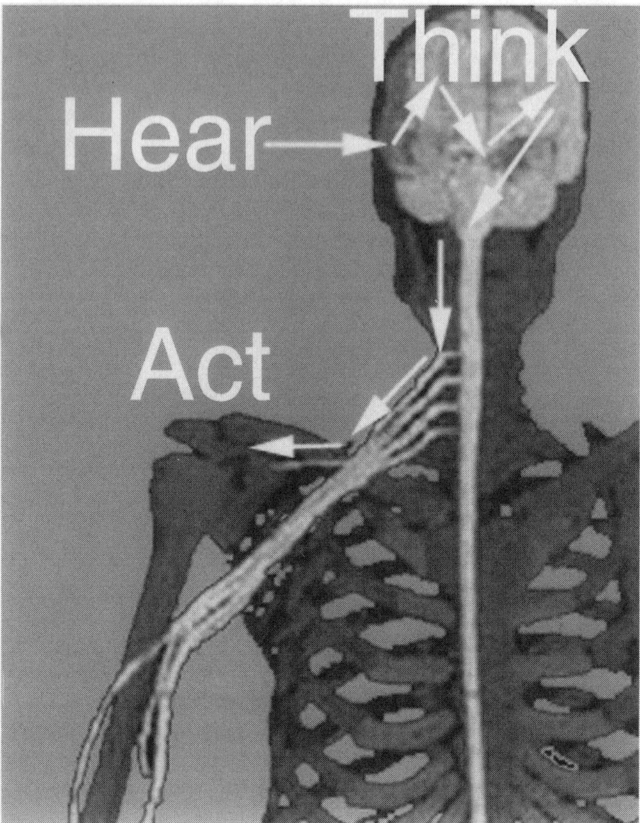

Figure 2.4. The three functional divisions in the brain are sensory input, motor output, and everything in between.

individual neurons in the cortex to respond to progressively more complicated aspects of a visual scene. For example, whereas cells in the retina respond best to spots of light, many cells in the cortex are best stimulated by bars of light and some require that the bar be moving in a particular direction. As visual information passes through one synaptic relay after another, the neurons become tuned to respond ultimately in a way that allows objects to be recognized. The pathway does not stop there. Visual inputs are eventually connected by way of the intervening neuronal synaptic links to the output—the motor pathways of the brain. For example, when driving a person sees a stop sign, the light that enters the eye sets up signals that pass from retina, to thalamus, to visual cortex, and then finally, after many intervening relays, to motor cortex. Here, signals are sent to the spinal cord to activate neurons whose synapses with muscle fibers in the foot release neurotransmitter and cause a person to push the brake pedal. This is a long circuit that passes information from one synaptic relay to another. Simpler circuits, called *reflexes*, also exist and are hard wired into the nervous system.

REFLEXES

Almost every medical checkup includes a test of a synaptic circuit. The tap to the knee cap (or, more accurately, the patellar tendon) with a rubber hammer activates one of the simplest reflexes in the nervous system. This pathway, shown in Figure 2.5, highlights the main features of synaptic circuits. Tapping the tendon to the quadriceps muscle in the thigh causes the muscle to stretch, which activates the dendritic branches of a number of sensory neurons that are embedded in the muscle (1). This causes electrical signals to travel toward the cell bodies of the sensory neurons (2) and beyond the cell body in the axons of these sensory neurons (3). The main synaptic connections of these sensory neurons are with the dendrites of motor neurons (4), which are responsible for movement and have axons (5) that project to muscle fibers. The synapses of sensory axons activate the dendrites of motor neurons, and if the stimulus is strong enough (e.g., if the muscle stretch was brisk enough to activate a sufficient number of the sensory axons) the integrated signal converging on the motor neurons' dendrites will pass threshold and allow the electrical signal (i.e., action potential) to pass down the axon to the synapses of the motor neurons that activate muscle fibers. The synapse between neurons and muscle fibers is called the *neuromuscular junction* (6). Therefore, this circuit begins with a muscle stretch

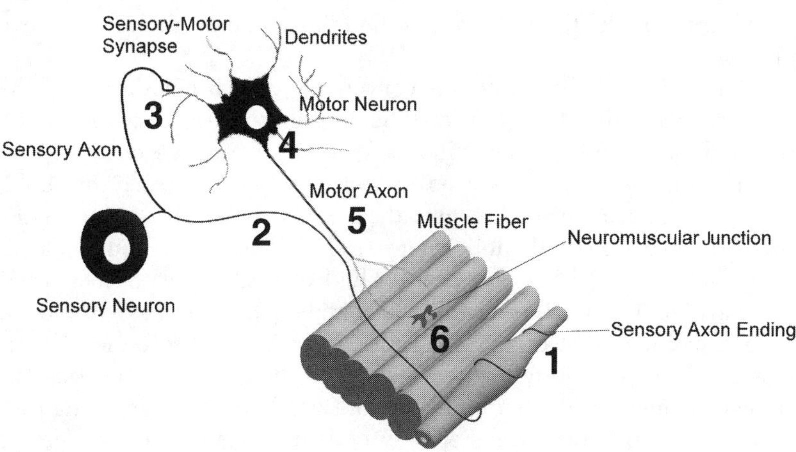

Figure 2.5. The sequential flow of information along a simple reflex.

and ends with a muscle contraction to counteract the stretch. The value of this reflex is that it allows the leg muscles not to buckle when a person suddenly hits the ground. Thus, the brain senses the muscle stretch, deliberates, and then acts to counteract it. This reflex circuit was presumably built into the nervous system through the actions of millions of years of evolution—animals that had such reflexes were at an advantage compared with animals that did not have them. However, what makes this kind of circuit so interesting is that when a teacher asks a class of fourth graders "How many times does 12 go into 60?" the sensory neurons in the students' ears sense the sound, project action potentials to other brain neurons that pass the information along a pathway that deliberates, and, finally, if a brain thinks it knows the answer, neurons send action potentials to motor neurons to cause the right deltoideus muscle to be activated causing the arm to be raised (see Figure 2.4). How is such a reflex-like behavior learned?

DIVERGENCE AND CONVERGENCE

Part of the answer to how a reflex-like behavior is learned may be related to the way the circuits that connect neurons together are arranged. Neurons connect to many different target cells. This divergence allows neurons to communicate with tens or thousands of target cells. Because each synaptic relay adds new neurons as targets, and each of these target neurons connects with other neurons, it is not surprising that the brain is highly interconnected. To get a sense of the power of this divergence, think of the way the body responds to a small pebble in a shoe. That pebble may activate only a single sensory axon in the skin. But if the stimulus is persistent enough, eventually it will cause the entire brain to attend—ultimately causing the arm muscles to reach down to find the irritating speck and remove it (Figure 2.6).

The other side of the coin is convergence. Each neuron also is the recipient of synapses from tens or thousands of other neurons. Although each of these individual connections is weak, the cumulative effect of activation of a number of inputs at nearly the same time can reach threshold, causing the information to be sent to the next neurons in the circuit. To see this aspect in action do the following test: Think of a man. Think of a tall man. Think of a tall man with a beard. Think of a tall man with a beard and a top hat. Think of a tall man with a beard and top hat who was a president. At some point in that exercise Lincoln's name popped to mind. This is because when a person thinks of a man he or she is weakly activating the circuits that underlie the representation of Lincoln in the brain, along with thousands of other men also stored away. With the additional proviso of tall, a smaller number of circuits are still in the running, until only one circuit is strongly activated—the one that makes a person think of Lincoln's

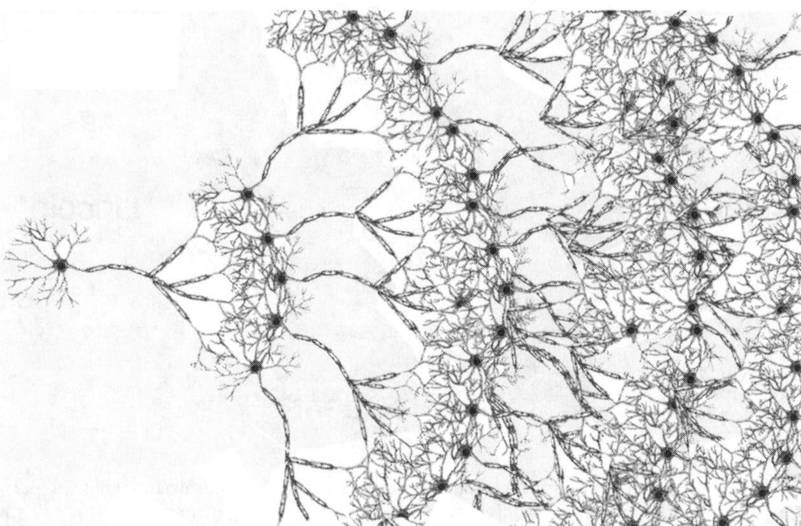

Figure 2.6. Axons branch to contact target neurons and each target cell branch contacts many target cells. This divergence of information allows all parts of the brain to be interconnected.

name. Imagine each of the limiting sentences about Lincoln as causing activation of progressively more of the converging input into the Lincoln circuit until it is finally brought to threshold and awareness (Figure 2.7). Being brought to threshold literally may be the activation of neurons with sufficient strength to pass threshold so that an action potential passes along to the next cell in some chain. Unfortunately, neuroscience has yet to uncover the actual circuitry for thoughts such as the one just elicited in the brain, so this must be taken as a provisional idea. But it raises the question of where such circuitry comes from. How did the ideas of man, tall, beard, top hat, and president get associated synaptically with Lincoln?

SYNAPTIC PLASTICITY

Obviously people were not born with the tendency to raise their hands when asked a question by a teacher, nor to associate bearded men with Lincoln, and yet such circuitry exists in the brain. This means that changes must be occurring because of the experiences during childhood. The consensus is that the changes called *learning* and *memory* are the result of long-lasting alterations in synapses, known by neuroscientists as *plasticity*. In what ways might synapses change to allow new circuitry to be established? Synapses that are present might change their strength. For example, connections that were always present between neurons could now be powerful enough

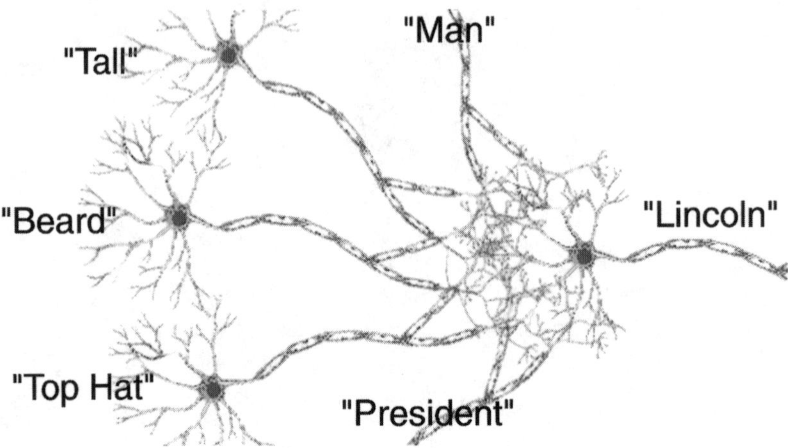

Figure 2.7. Each neuron is a convergence point because its dendritic branches are connected to synaptic input from different axons. Hence, one might imagine that a neuron involved in generating the thought "Lincoln" is only brought to threshold when separate neuronal inputs, each associated with a different attribute, are coactive.

to bring the target cell to threshold, whereas before they were weak. Such increases in synaptic strength do occur. In the *hippocampus*, the part of the brain responsible for the earliest phases of laying down memories, a phenomenon called *long-term potentiation* (LTP) causes synapses that were initially weak to be strengthened in ways that persist for hours. This strengthening is the result of associative activity in which two kinds of inputs to a cell are activated synchronously. By virtue of the synchrony of the activity the weaker input is strengthened. Thus, this kind of change may allow two sensory inputs that are associated in time (e.g., red and rose) to be selectively strengthened when they occur together. The mechanism of this potentiation of synapses is not fully worked out but appears to be due to an increase in the number of neurotransmitter receptors at the potentiated synapse, an increase in the amount of neurotransmitter released by the nerve, or both.

It is not known, and perhaps unlikely, that such strengthening could persist for the decades that learned information is stored. Thus, neurobiologists have looked for more lasting changes at synapses. One idea is that there is a change in the number of synapses, the idea that learning causes new synapses to form and thus establishes connections between neurons to allow for the actual formation of new synaptic circuits. This is a popular idea, but at the moment it is hard to understand how it operates. The particular problem is that generating novel circuitry for each item learned requires action where sets of synchronously active cells seek each other out and grow connections to establish linkages between them. Such connections would take time to develop, yet associations between stimuli (e.g., the color green and the smell of lime) can occur instantly. There is, however, an alternative way learned information might be stored based on changes in circuitry that occur in young brains at the time they are learning.

SYNAPTIC CONNECTIONS ARE ELIMINATED DURING DEVELOPMENT

In the early 1960s, David Hubel and Torsten Wiesel, two research physicians who had clinical experience with vision disorders of childhood, embarked on a landmark series of Nobel Prize–winning experiments (see Chapter 1). Their results suggested that developing brains are rewired by experience, not by establishing new circuits, but instead by selecting to maintain some circuits from a larger initial repertoire. Hubel and Wiesel were interested in the way information from the two eyes is organized in the visual cortex. They were motivated by an interesting and serious clinical problem. Young children who had difficulty seeing out of one eye because of opacities in the lens or because of weak muscle control to one eye that caused crossing or walleye could have their vision surgically corrected without much difficulty. However, the outcomes of these corrections were often dismal—the eye would be returned to normal alignment or clarity but the patient would be nearly blind in the eye that had been deprived of normal visual experiences. This was puzzling because an adult with a cataract in one eye can regain full vision in that eye once the cataract is removed, even if the eye is deprived of vision for years.

Hubel and Wiesel set out to determine what caused the visual deficit in young animals that are deprived of vision. It was clear that the deficit was not due to a change in the eye or retina, nor were these changes explained by alterations in the thalamus, which is the relay station for sensory information. Rather the changes were in the cerebral cortex where visual information is sent. What Hubel and Wiesel found was that the brain organizes the input from the two eyes so that in an adult the input driven by the two eyes is arranged in alternating stripes on the surface of the brain in the same way that zebra stripes are arranged (Figure 2.8). These stripes of eye dominance are called *ocular dominance columns*. Normally, each eye activates about the same amount of territory, just as there is about the same amount of black and white area in a zebra pattern. At the synaptic level they showed that individual neurons in the input layer of the visual cortex were strongly contacted by axons driven by either the right or left eye, but not both.

They found that the pattern of connections was quite different when animals first began using their eyes in postnatal life. If the adult pattern is like a zebra pattern, the neonatal pattern of connections was found to be

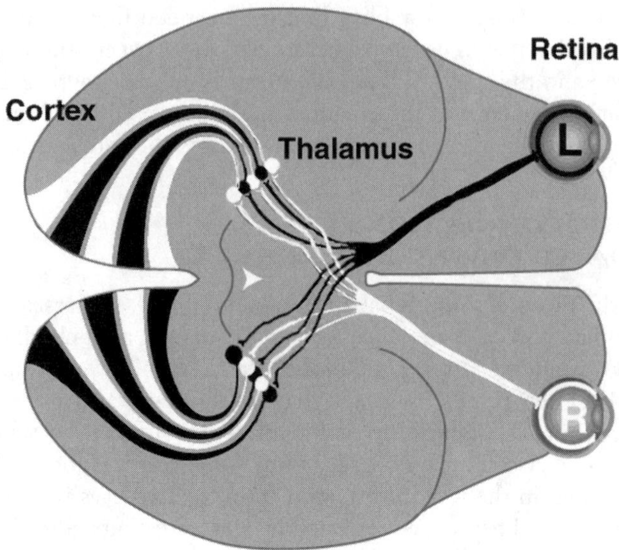

Figure 2.8. This is a view of the brain looking up at it from the bottom. The retinal neurons (e.g., ganglion cells) from the two eyes mix their output as they send axons to both the right and left thalamus.

more akin to a gray pony (Figure 2.9). Rather than being segregated into alternating stripes, the input from the two eyes was interspersed so that the individual cerebral cortex neurons were contacted both by axons driven by the left eye and by the right eye. The emergence of ocular dominance stripes occurred as the inputs driven by the two eyes segregated from each other. Thus, neurons that initially received synapses from both eyes ended up with a skewed distribution that gradually favored one eye or the other. Eventually all trace of input from one of the two eyes disappeared while the remaining input from the other eye became progressively stronger.

SYNAPTIC COMPETITION AND CRITICAL PERIODS

Given the clinical evidence of visual deficits if one is deprived of vision in early life, Hubel and Wiesel asked what happens to the visual cortex if one eye is prevented from experiencing vision during development. The results of monocular deprivation by patching an eye or suturing the lid shut were dramatic (Figure 2.9). Rather than normal ocular dominance segregation in which each eyes loses connection with half the cortical neurons, the inputs driven by the open eye lost none of their connections. Conversely, the deprived eye lost all of its connections. The deprived eye inputs had disconnected from the brain causing the blindness. The effects of monocular deprivation were on both the eye that was not seeing and on the eye that was seeing normally. Hubel and Wiesel argued that this was evidence of competition between the axons that was driven by the two eyes for cortical space. Both eyes begin connected with all the cortical cells, but if one set of axons is more active than the other, then the cells on which they originally converge will remain connected to the more active eye input. If both eyes are active then the cortical cells will choose one eye or the other equally. Indeed, it was found that binocular deprivation did not have nearly as dramatic an effect on ocular dominance column formation as monocular deprivation, suggesting that the relative activity of the two eyes was driving the competition.

These results provided an explanation for the end of the period of susceptibility to monocular deprivation (a critical period). It appeared that the only neurons in the input layer of the visual cortex that were affected by monocular deprivation were neurons that still retained synaptic connections from both eyes. If visual deprivation was begun at birth when no neurons had been captured by one eye or the other, the effect of depriving one eye was that the cortex was no longer partitioned into zebra stripes but was more like a white horse or a black horse, depending on which eye was deprived. But as the input driven by the two eyes began to segregate, the effect of visual deprivation became subtler, making the width of the ocular dominance stripes larger than normal for the open eye and smaller than normal for the closed eye. When the inputs driven by the two eyes were segregated from each other the effect of monocular deprivation was mini-

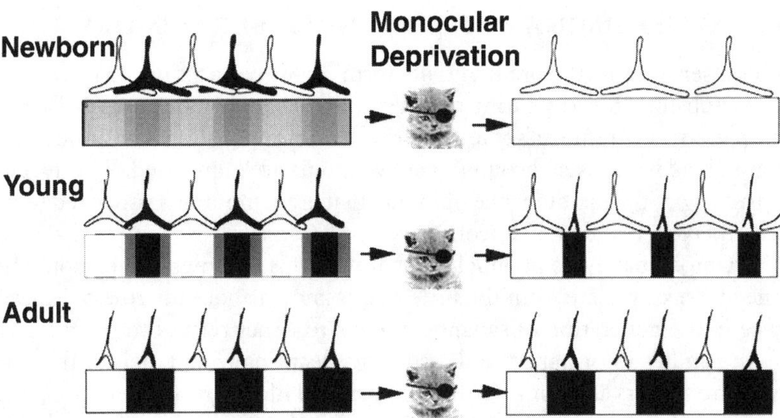

Figure 2.9. The alternating left and right eye dominated stripes emerge normally during development as the inputs from the two eyes segregate from each other (left) but abnormally if one eye is deprived at some point in development (right).

mal (Figure 2.9). Therefore, the effect of visual deprivation was only seen on neurons where the outcome of competition had not yet been decided.

This is a profound result because it indicates that experience shapes synaptic circuits by selection rather than by instruction. Generally, for this idea to be correct it would be necessary that throughout the developing brain axons should be connected to target neurons with which they will lose connections in later life. Indeed, in many parts of the developing nervous system such extra-axonal connections have been seen, including in the cerebellum, autonomic ganglia, and the neuromuscular junction.

The neuromuscular junction has been a useful synapse to study the mechanism of this competition because the synapses are accessible, large, and amenable to detailed study. Similar to what is occurring in the developing visual system, each muscle fiber begins with contacts from many different axons, but in this case all but one are removed. The loss of connections is explained by a trimming back of half the branches axons establish before birth. Results at the neuromuscular junction suggest that the decision as to which axon is maintained and which is removed is made by the target cell, in this case the muscle fiber. The target cell makes this decision much the way a judge does by listening to the synaptic activity of all the competitors and choosing to eliminate all but one input. The way this seems to occur is that the target cell can destabilize axonal connections that are silent when others are active. A target cell may be an intermediary in the competition between inputs by using the activity of one input as a signal to remove inputs that are not active at the same time. This mechanism only allows synchronously active axons to be maintained.

SYNAPSE ELIMINATION AND INDELIBLE MEMORY

This assertion that the brain initially forms many connections that are used as the substrate for generating useful circuits is based on the ability of activity patterns to remove some synapses. Synchronously active inputs are maintained while asynchronously active inputs are eliminated. This mechanism favors the maintenance of inputs that are temporally associated (e.g., red and rose; beard and Lincoln).

Unfortunately, to go much further with this argument there would be a need to extrapolate from the little that is known about the role of experience in the generation of synaptic circuits to issues related to the way the brain handles information and associative learning. Nonetheless, the way synaptic circuits are trimmed during postnatal life suggests the improbable idea that the brain has, from early stages, connections for many, and perhaps even all, of the things we will eventually learn. Through a competitive mechanism, the neural activity generated by some experiences eliminates circuitry that is inconsistent with that experience. In this view, one learns that "b" and "d" are "bee" and "dee" by removing the erroneous connections between the visual input associated with "b" and the sound "dee" and vice versa. Learning by elimination has one advantage—indelibility. Once the inputs for various circuits have segregated, then competition is no longer possible, as competition requires that the inputs interact by activating the same target cell to attempt to destabilize each other. Thus, once a fact is learned it is difficult to unlearn.

This argument may explain why once one has learned to speak one language as a child it is difficult to rid oneself of that accent when one learns another language later on in life. It also may explain why brains that are deprived of some experiences in early life may be unable to respond to those kinds of experiences later in life. Indeed, most of the literature concerning critical periods suggests that the windows of opportunity are not lifelong for many kinds of fundamental learning, including language and vision.

THE CHALLENGE

Understanding the brain is presently one of the largest, if not the largest, research endeavors being tackled worldwide. In the United States alone there are thousands of professional neuroscientists. The amount of new information generated about the brain each day is staggering and far more than any human brain could possibly accommodate. Despite this onslaught, neuroscience as a research field is still in its infancy, and like an infant's brain, many possibilities are still being considered that may eventually be weeded out. At the moment there are two schools of thought concerning the nuts and bolts of learning. One idea is based on the notion that the brain is a machine designed to construct new circuitry. The alternative is that the brain selects circuits from the connections that exist from early life. The latter idea, presented here, brings with it an explanation for developmental critical periods as windows of opportunity for learning certain things or to be without them forever. This debate between the idea that the brain constructs circuits or selects them will not be solved by argument, but rather by further research into the mechanisms underlying brain development. The main challenge for neuroscience is to find ways to make its debates and conclusions accessible to a larger audience.

Given the ability of experience to alter the connections in the brains of children, educators are in essence brain engineers, applied scientists who could, in principle, use the available information as a means of informing their educational practice and policies. This bridge between disciplines is not happening in large part because of the failure of neuroscientists to communicate their conclusions in ways that allow critical scrutiny by nonneuroscientists. In addition, the issues of brain science that are most relevant to humankind concern those aspects of human brain development that are not seen in other animals, such as learning to read. The development of higher human intellectual capacities is out of reach of invasive research. In this instance teachers can provide, but presently do not provide, neuroscience with valuable information about the way the human brain learns.

SUGGESTED READINGS

Changeux, J.P. (1997). *Neuronal man: The biology of mind.* Princeton, NJ: Princeton University Press.

Hubel, D.H. (1995). *Eye, brain, and vision.* San Francisco: W.H. Freeman.

Lichtman, J.W., & Colman, H. (2000). Synapse elimination and indelible memory. *Neuron, 25,* 269–278.

Lichtman, J.W., & Purves, D. (1985). *Principles of neural development.* Sunderland, MA: Sinauer Press.

II

Critical Periods in Basic Sensory Systems

3

Critical Periods in the Development of the Visual System

Jonathan C. Horton

The phrase *nature versus nurture* captures in three words the essence of a debate central to the study of human development: How does the interplay between genetic influences and environmental factors result in a normal, healthy child? This issue has engendered controversy for centuries among both scientists and philosophers. In 1694 the empiricist philosopher William Molyneux wrote a letter to John Locke posing a hypothetical question about a man born blind, but whose sight was restored miraculously: Would the man be able to identify by sight a cube or sphere, known previously only by touch (Wade, 1998)? In his reply, published in the *Essay Concerning Human Understanding*, Locke responded that the blind man would not be able, with certainty, to distinguish between the cube and the sphere. His answer was predicated on the belief that experience is required for the brain to learn how to interpret visual images. He reasoned that an adult with sight suddenly restored would see no better than a newborn child. In fact, we know today that the vision of such an adult would be even worse than that of a newborn child, because of a disease called amblyopia.

Amblyopia is defined as a disorder caused by abnormal visual experience during early childhood, which results in a unilateral decrease in acuity that cannot be explained by pathology within the eye itself. For example, if a child is born with a dense cataract in one eye, the retina will be deprived of visual stimulation. When the child grows up, the visual acuity in the affected eye will be poor—even if the cataract is removed later by surgery and replaced by a clear lens with the appropriate refractive power. Without an ocular explanation for the permanent loss of vision caused by visual deprivation, investigators have long suspected that amblyopia is caused by anomalous wiring of the eye's central connections in the brain. This view has been confirmed by experiments suturing closed the lids of one eye in kittens or monkeys at an early age to mimic a cataract (von Noorden, Dowling, & Ferguson, 1970; Wiesel & Hubel, 1963, 1965; see Chapters 1 and 2). It is important to note that amblyopia develops only in the young, when the visual system is still immature and vulnerable to the effects of sensory deprivation. This brief interval of early vulnerability is called the *critical period*.

Amblyopia usually results in a *unilateral* decrease in visual acuity. However, under special circumstances, amblyopia can be *bilateral*: If a baby is born with cataracts in both eyes, both eyes may develop amblyopia. Under these circumstances the parents are likely to realize that their child cannot see, and the cataracts will be diagnosed promptly and removed before any permanent damage ensues. For this reason, cases of bilateral amblyopia have become rare. In the 17th century, however, the prognosis for individuals with congenital cataracts was bleak. Cataract removal was accomplished by using a sharp instrument to push the opaque lens into the vitreous cavity, a procedure called couching. This operation seldom resulted in restoration of good vision. Not surprisingly, those with blindness in both eyes from congenital cataracts were quite common. Molyneux and Locke probably had such people in mind when they exchanged their famous letters. They believed that if sight could be restored to individuals with congenital blindness, one could answer the nature versus nurture riddle. They did not count, however, on the confounding problem of amblyopia.

Although bilateral amblyopia is rare today, thanks to modern cataract surgery, unilateral amblyopia is still quite prevalent, occurring in 1%–2% of Americans. Children rarely complain or betray any symptoms when vision is poor in one eye only. As a result, a unilateral cataract often goes undetected until formal vision screening is conducted sometime in later childhood. At this point it may be too late to save the child's vision. Devising reliable and economical ways to screen young children for amblyopia is an important public health challenge.

OCULAR DOMINANCE COLUMNS

Before delving any further into the biology of amblyopia, it is worth reviewing the anatomy and physiology of the visual system. In the back of the eye, a light-sensitive membrane called the *retina* captures images and converts them to electrical signals. These signals ultimately converge onto a class of neurons called *retinal ganglion cells*. The axons of ganglion cells project from the eye to the brain along the optic nerve. The two optic nerves meet in the midline to form a structure called the optic chiasm. Here, ganglion cell axons that originate from the nasal half of each retina cross into the contralateral optic tract. As a result of this partial crossing, the visual pathway on each side of the brain beyond the optic chiasm contains a representation of the contralateral hemifield of vision (Figure 3.1).

The optic tracts terminate in a thalamic relay station called the lateral geniculate body. In the lateral geniculate body, cells that receive retinal input project, in turn, to the primary visual cortex. The primary visual cortex is often called the striate cortex, referring to a prominent myelinated stria in layer IV discovered in 1776 by an Italian medical student named Francisci Gennari. Early in the 20th century, Korbinian Brodmann parceled the cerebral cortex into 47 different regions based on subtle distinctions in cortical histology. He assigned the arbitrary label of area 17 to the primary visual cortex. In recent years other visual areas have been discovered in the cortex surrounding the primary visual cortex. The primary visual cortex has received the prosaic designation of V1 (visual area 1) and the adjacent association visual cortical areas have been named V2, V3, V4, V5, and so forth. Primary visual cortex, striate cortex, area 17, and V1 are all synonyms for the same piece of tissue. According to the traditional view, striate cortex performs an initial analysis of incoming visual information, extracts a critical essence required for perception, and transmits it to the surrounding visual association cortex. It is thought that this extrastriate visual associa-

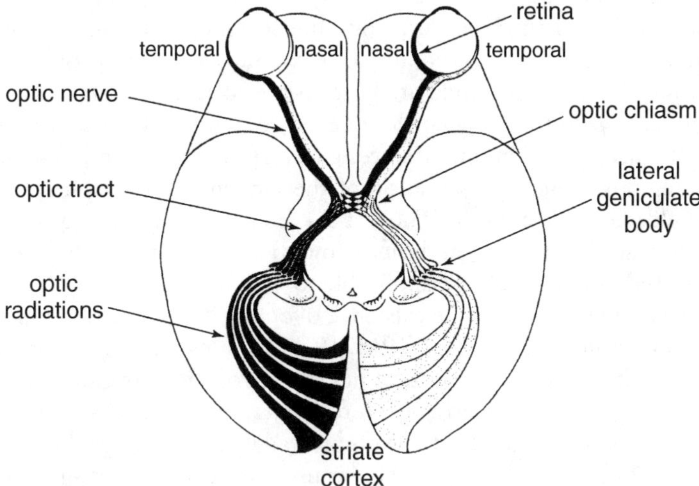

Figure 3.1. Diagram of the human brain, viewed from underneath, showing the visual pathway from the eyes to the cortex. Fibers (axons) of ganglion cells in the retina pass via the optic nerve, optic chiasm, and optic tract to make connections (synapses) with neurons in a thalamic relay nucleus, called the lateral geniculate body. Neurons in the lateral geniculate body project to striate (primary visual) cortex. Note that fibers from the nasal retinae cross at the optic chiasm, so that the contralateral hemifield of vision is represented in striate cortex of each hemisphere. (From Polyak, S. [1957]. *The vertebrate visual system* [p. 289]. Chicago: University of Chicago Press; adapted by permission.)

tion cortex is where actual comprehension or interpretation of visual scenes takes place.

Axon projections from cells of the lateral geniculate body serving either the right eye or the left eye are not randomly distributed in striate cortex, but are segregated into a system of alternating parallel stripes called ocular dominance columns (Figure 3.2a). These columns can be labeled by injecting a radioactive tracer, [^{3}H]proline, into one eye of a monkey (Wiesel, Husel, & Lam, 1974). After passing across a synapse in the lateral geniculate body, the radioactive tracer is transported to striate cortex. It can be visualized by coating brain sections with an emulsion sensitive to radioactive particles. When the emulsion is developed to prepare an image called an autoradiograph, bright silver grains are concentrated over cortex containing the greatest radioactivity. This technique reveals the ocular dominance columns as bands about 0.5 millimeters (mm) wide in layer IV of striate cortex (Figure 3.2b). The dark gaps between the labeled bands represent the ocular dominance columns of the uninjected eye.

In humans the ocular dominance column can be labeled in specimens of striate cortex obtained from individuals with a history of monocular visual loss prior to death. The cortical tissue is stained for cytochrome oxidase, a mitochondrial enzyme involved in supplying energy to cells. After the loss of one eye, physiological activity is reduced in columns formerly supplied by the missing eye. As a consequence, levels of cytochrome oxidase fall, revealing the ocular dominance columns as a mosaic of light and dark bands. By unfolding and flattening striate cortex, one can reconstruct the complete pattern of ocular dominance columns in the human striate cortex (Figure 3.3). Columns are present everywhere, except in two monocular regions—the representation of the far temporal periphery of the visual field and the blind spot. The fact that humans have ocular dominance columns, just like monkeys and cats, shows that data obtained from experimental studies in animals are applicable to humans.

The first evidence for the existence of ocular dominance columns was obtained by Hubel and Wiesel (1965, 1977) from electrophysiological recordings. When they made vertical microelectrode penetrations from the cortical surface to the underlying white matter, they found that all cells in any given penetration tended to be dominated by the same eye. When they made long oblique penetrations, ocular preference would swing back and forth gradually between the two eyes (Figure 3.4). Most cells in striate cortex were binocular (i.e., they would respond by firing spikes when stimulated via either eye), although they usually displayed a stronger response to one eye. The only exception was found in layer IV, which receives the major geniculate input to the cortex. At this first stage of cortical processing, ocular inputs are kept segregated and cellular responses are purely monocular. Projections from monocular cells in layer IV generate binocu-

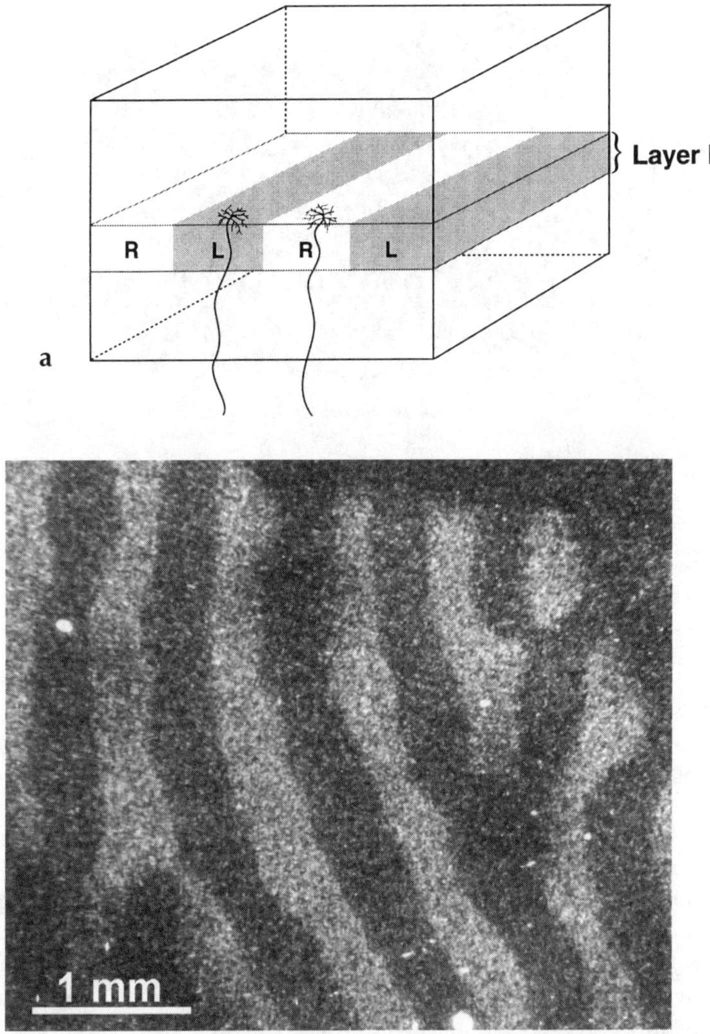

Figure 3.2. a) Diagram showing a small piece of striate cortex containing two sets of ocular columns. They appear as parallel slabs (R = right eye, L = left eye) in layer IV. This layer receives input from the eyes via neurons situated in the lateral geniculate body. The inputs are drawn schematically as single axons with a spray of fine branches at their ends (axon terminals) which make synapses onto cells in layer IV. b) An autoradiograph, prepared from a single section cut through layer IV, in a plane parallel to the columns shown in Figure 3.2a. A radioactive tracer, [^{3}H]proline, was injected into one eye and transported only to those axon terminals located in the injected eye's ocular dominance columns. Under darkfield illumination the tracer appears bright, giving rise to a pattern of alternating light columns interrupted by dark columns, which correspond to the unlabeled columns of the other eye.

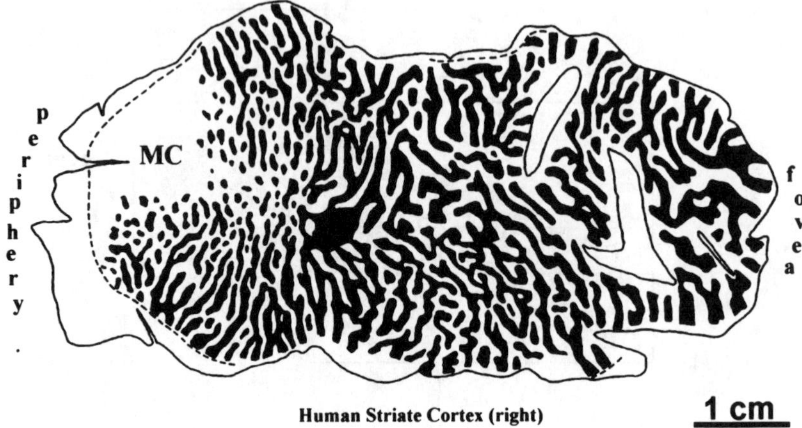

Figure 3.3. Drawing of the ocular dominance columns in human striate cortex from a man who went blind in his left eye a few months before death. The reconstruction was prepared from serial sections processed for cytochrome oxidase. The dark columns correspond to the ocular dominance columns of the remaining right eye, which contained greater metabolic activity. The dark oval represents the blind spot region of the left eye and MC denotes the monocular crescent representation.

lar cells in other layers, which have more elaborate properties. The binocular cells outside layer IV are thought to mediate depth perception.

To characterize the ocular dominance of individual cells, Hubel and Wiesel devised a seven-point scale based on the relative effectiveness of each eye at driving a response. A typical ocular dominance profile compiled from recordings in normal kittens, ages 3–4 weeks old, is shown in Figure 3.5. Cells in Category 1 are monocular, responding only to stimulation of the contralateral eye. Cells in Category 7 also are monocular, responding only to stimulation of the ipsilateral eye. Most cells are binocular and therefore distributed in Categories 2 through 6, depending on whether they favor one eye or the other. Cells that respond equally to both eyes are assigned to Category 4.

EARLY VISUAL DEPRIVATION

Newborn human infants have a visual acuity of approximately 20/400 in each eye (Boothe, Dobson, & Teller, 1985; Teller, 1997). Acuity increases rapidly after birth, reaching an adult level by age 1 year. From these observations, one can infer that visual function is partially innate, but considerable improvement occurs postnatally. In a child born with dense bilateral cataracts, this postnatal refinement of vision fails to occur, and, in fact, visual function deteriorates to a level far below 20/400. To learn why, Hubel and

Wiesel (1965) raised kittens with both eyes sutured (see Chapter 1). When the animals were 3 months old, they made physiological recordings from striate cortex (Figure 3.6). In normal animals, cells in the cortex have a low rate of spontaneous discharge. For each cell there is an area in the visual field—called the cell's receptive field—where appropriate visual stimulation will elicit a burst of electrical discharges. In kittens raised with bilateral visual deprivation, many cortical cells lacked a receptive field (i.e., they became unresponsive to visual stimulation). Their presence was revealed only because they fired occasional spontaneous spikes. Such cells were encountered rarely in normal animals.

In bilaterally deprived kittens, even those cells that were still responsive often had abnormal properties. In normal animals cells display an important receptive field property called orientation specificity. The best response from single cells is evoked by a slit or bar of light held at the correct orientation (e.g., horizontal, vertical, oblique). Orientation specificity is thought to be crucial for visual perception because it allows cells to encode information about image contours. Recordings in newborn animals have shown that oriented cells are present at birth, although the accuracy of orientation tuning increases over the first postnatal months (Chino, Smith, Hatta, & Cheng, 1997; Wiesel & Hubel, 1974). In kittens raised with both

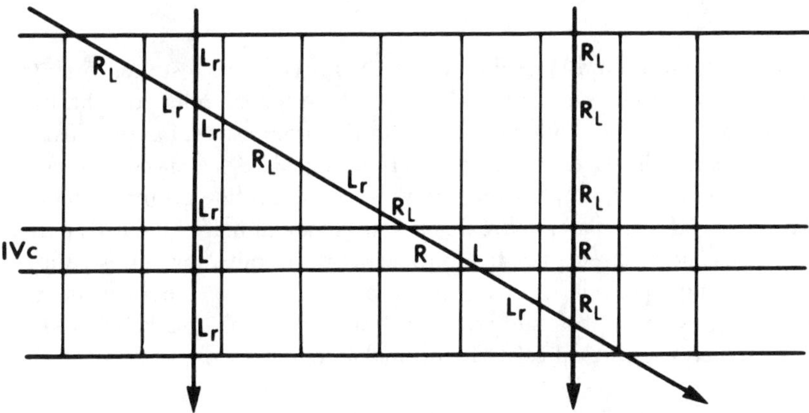

Figure 3.4. Schematic section through the visual cortex, showing two vertical electrode penetrations and a single oblique one. The surface of the cortex is at the top and the white matter lies at the bottom. The vertical lines represent the ocular dominance columns, which are seen here in cross-section rather than in tangential section, as in Figures 3.2 and 3.3. Note that the vertical penetrations stay within a single ocular dominance column so cells tend to be dominated by the same eye (L = left, R = right). The oblique penetration crosses from one ocular dominance column to another so the ocular preference of cells shifts accordingly. (From Hubel, D.H., & Wiesel, T.N. [1977]. Functional architecture of macaque monkey visual cortex. *Proceedings of the Royal Society of London [Biology], 198,* 1–59; reprinted by permission.)

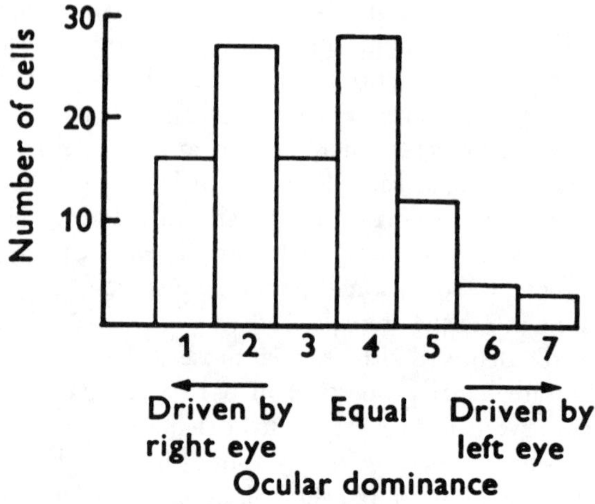

Figure 3.5. Ocular dominance histogram showing the relative ability of the right eye versus the left eye at driving cells in striate cortex of two kittens at age 3–4 weeks. Recordings were made in the left visual cortex, so Category 1 corresponds to complete dominance by the contralateral eye and Category 7 to complete dominance by the ipsilateral eye. Note that cells are found in all categories, although the contralateral eye has slightly more influence. (From Hubel, D.H., & Wiesel, T.N. [1970]. The period of susceptibility to the physiological effects of unilateral eye closure in kittens. *Journal of Physiology* [*London*], *206,* 419–436; reprinted by permission.)

lids closed, Hubel and Wiesel found that many cells had lost their orientation tuning (Figure 3.6). Although these cells still responded to light, they could no longer signal information about the orientation of a stimulus.

These landmark experiments by Hubel and Wiesel showed that visual stimulation is required after birth to preserve and refine normal function. After 3 months of bilateral visual deprivation, about half of the cells in the cortex lose normal receptive field properties or become unresponsive altogether. Longer periods of visual deprivation have more severe consequences and result in more profound blindness. Bilateral amblyopia is believed to develop because cortical cells lose normal receptive field properties.

THE CRITICAL PERIOD

For comparison, Hubel and Wiesel (1963, 1965, 1970) also raised kittens with unilateral eyelid suture. After closure of one eye from birth to age 1 month, cells in the visual cortex showed a mild bias in favor of the open eye (Figure 3.7a). When the deprivation lasted a week longer, to Day 37, a radical shift occurred in ocular preference (Figure 3.7b). Virtually all the cells in the cortex responded exclusively to the open eye. Comparing Figures 3.6 and 3.7b one can appreciate that unilateral and bilateral eye closure produce quite different effects. With bilateral closure many cells develop abnormal receptive field properties but both eyes retain equal influence. With unilateral closure most cells respond normally but the open eye becomes dominant. It continues to develop normal acuity, while the closed eye becomes amblyopic.

Hubel and Wiesel (1977) suggested that geniculocortical axon terminals serving each eye compete for synaptic connections onto cells in layer IV of the developing visual cortex. When one eye is closed, loss of visually driven activity places it at a disadvantage and it loses inputs onto cortical cells. Blindness ensues because the eye becomes partially disconnected from the cortical circuits required for processing and interpreting the visual input

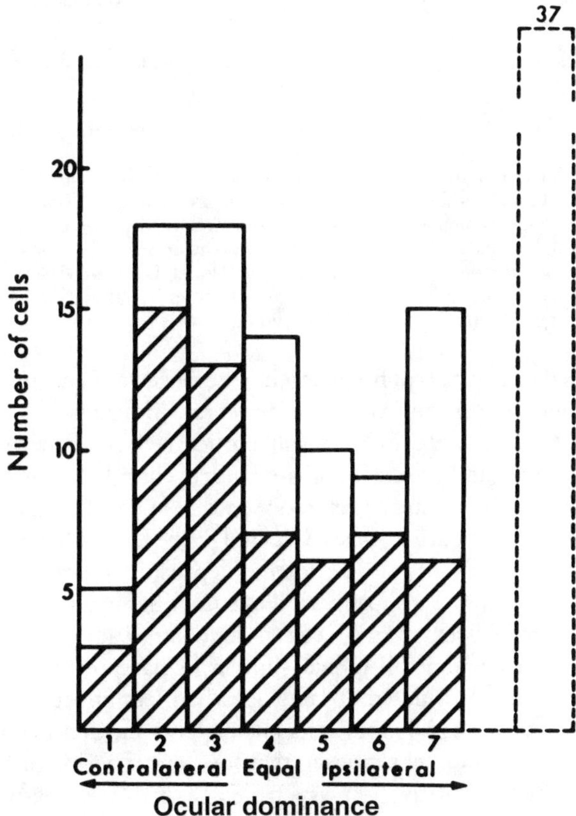

Figure 3.6. Ocular dominance histogram showing responses of 126 cells recorded in four kittens raised from birth to age 3 months with bilateral eyelid suture. Although the profile of ocular dominance is unchanged from control animals (Figure 3.5), many cells have become unresponsive or unoriented. (Key = ▨ Normal; ▭ No orientation; ⬚ No response.) (From Hubel, D.H., & Wiesel, T.N. [1965]. Binocular interaction in striate cortex of kittens reared with artificial squint. *Journal of Neurophysiology, 28,* 1041–1059; reprinted by permission.)

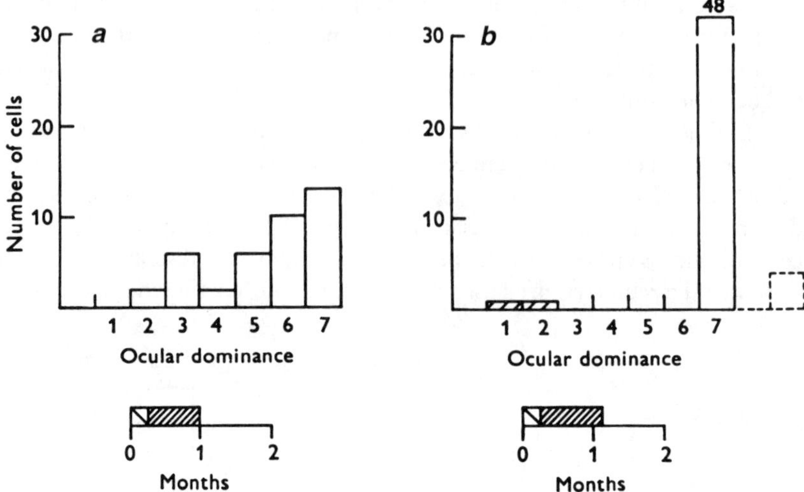

Figure 3.7. a) Ocular dominance histogram from a single kitten, deprived by suture of the right eye until age 1 month. There is a modest shift in the profile of cells toward the open eye (Category 7). b) Ocular dominance histogram from a littermate, deprived until Day 37. Note that including a fifth week of deprivation induces a dramatic effect: Almost all cells have shifted allegiance to the open eye (Category 7). (From Hubel, D.H., & Wiesel, T.N. [1970]. The period of susceptibility to the physiological effects of unilateral eye closure in kittens. *Journal of Physiology* [*London*], *206,* 419–436; reprinted by permission.)

it provides. As the terminals of fibers serving the closed eye become reduced, those of the open eye sprout to make extra connections onto cortical cells abandoned by the deprived eye. As a result, cortical cells retain normal receptive field properties but become dominated nearly entirely by the open eye.

The radical shift in ocular preference caused by extending monocular suture to Day 37 (compare Figures 3.7a and 3.7b) led Hubel and Wiesel (1970) to test the effects of brief periods of deprivation starting at various ages. Figure 3.8 compares a short period of suture before, at, and after age 1 month. Remarkably, less than a week of deprivation at 4–5 weeks of age was enough to produce a full-blown shift in ocular preference. Longer periods of deprivation initiated at later ages had less effect (Figure 3.9). Deprivation starting at age 4 months had no effect, even after many months of suture. Hubel and Wiesel proposed that the critical period of sensitivity to the effects of visual deprivation lasts from ages 3 to 12 weeks in the kitten, with a peak in sensitivity at ages 4–5 weeks.

DEVELOPMENT OF OCULAR DOMINANCE COLUMNS

Hubel and Wiesel's initial discoveries regarding the critical period were based on electrophysiological recordings from single cells in kitten visual cortex. A technique to label the cortical projections serving the two eyes came later, with the introduction of [^{3}H]proline autoradiography. In 2-week-old kittens, eye injections of [^{3}H]proline tracer showed a continuous distribution of label in layer IVc (LeVay, Stryker, & Shatz, 1978). With eye injections at later ages, columns of label began to emerge in layer IVc (Figure 3.10). These experiments showed that geniculocortical afferents serving each eye are intermixed during fetal life and then begin to segregate into ocular dominance columns after birth. The process of column segregation can be prevented by injecting each eye with tetrodotoxin, a toxin that prevents the propagation of electrical impulses by blocking sodium channels (Stryker & Harris, 1986). This result indicates that electrical activity in the afferent visual pathway is essential for development of ocular dominance columns. The fact that electrical activity is required for the development of ocular dominance columns raises the question of whether spontaneous discharges are sufficient or whether visual experience is necessary. A role for visual experience is implied by the fact that the segregation of ocular dominance columns in kittens begins only after the opening of the eyes 7–10 days after birth. Swindale (1981) has claimed that ocular dominance columns are absent in cats raised in the dark, indicating that visual experience (or at least light exposure) is vital for catalyzing their formation.

Rakic (1977) studied the development of ocular dominance columns in monkeys by making [^{3}H]proline eye injections in fetal animals. At Embryonic Day 144 (E144) he found continuous label in layer IVc, indicating that geniculocortical inputs serving each eye are intermingled 3 weeks before birth. However, silver grain counts showed a slight fluctuation in den-

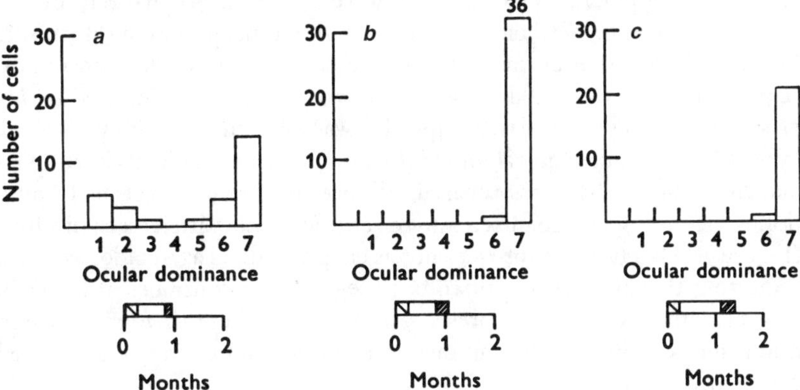

Figure 3.8. Ocular dominance histograms showing the effects in three kittens of less than a week of deprivation a) before, b) around, and c) after 1 month of age. A nearly maximal effect is achieved by just a week of deprivation during ages 25–39 days. This time represents the peak of the critical period for susceptibility to the effects of visual deprivation in kittens. (From Hubel, D.H., & Wiesel, T.N. [1970]. The period of susceptibility to the physiological effects of unilateral eye closure in kittens. *Journal of Physiology* [*London*], *206*, 419–436; reprinted by permission.)

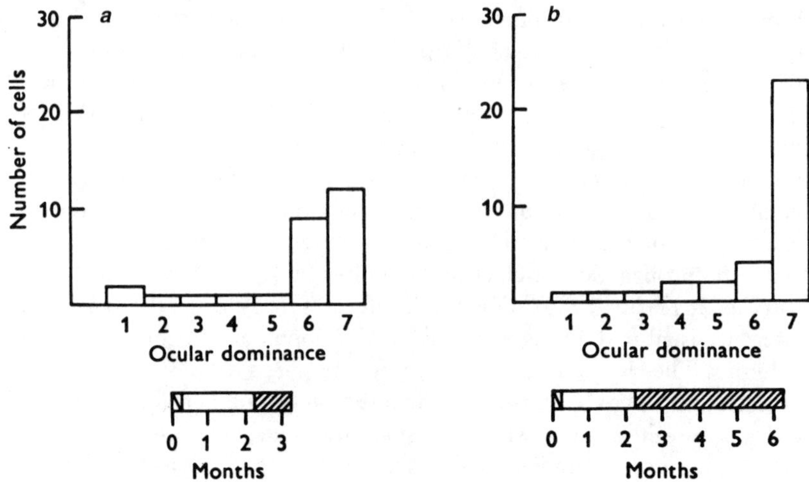

Figure 3.9. a) Ocular dominance histogram from a kitten deprived after age 2 months. The shift in ocular preference of cortical cells is less marked than following earlier deprivation (compare with Figure 3.8). b) Ocular dominance histogram of another kitten, deprived for 4 months, starting after age 2 months. Despite the long period of deprivation, the effects are less striking than after deprivation for only 1 week at age 1 month. (From Hubel, D.H., & Wiesel, T.N. [1970]. The period of susceptibility to the physiological effects of unilateral eye closure in kittens. *Journal of Physiology* [*London*], *206,* 419–436; reprinted by permission.)

sity, hinting that formation of columns was already underway. To settle the question of whether visual experience or light exposure is required for column development, fetal monkeys were delivered prematurely by cesarean section at E157, 8 days before the end of usual gestation (Horton & Hocking, 1996). To prevent light exposure, the cesarean section and all subsequent procedures were done in absolute darkness, using infrared night-vision goggles. The next day, [^{3}H]proline was injected into one eye. A week later at E165/P0, the equivalent of full-term pregnancy, animals were killed and autoradiographs were prepared. All three newborn animals had ocular dominance columns, organized into the characteristic pattern seen in adults (Figure 3.11). The columns were not as crisply defined as in older animals, indicating that the process of column segregation continues after birth. However, they were clearly present, proving that the formation of ocular dominance columns is programmed innately and not contingent on visual experience.

ANATOMICAL EFFECTS OF VISUAL DEPRIVATION

[^{3}H]proline autoradiography also has been used to show the anatomical effects of monocular eyelid suture on the ocular dominance columns in striate cortex (Horton & Hocking, 1997; Hubel & Wiesel, 1977; Shatz & Stryker, 1978; Swindale, Vital-Durand, & Blakemore, 1981). Figure 3.12 shows the ocular dominance columns in a monkey raised with suture of the right eye from age 1 week. The radioactive tracer was injected into the deprived right eye. Its ocular dominance columns appear severely shrunken and fragmented. Instead of filling half the cortex, their net area amounts to only 16% of layer IV.

Although deprivation causes shrinkage of the ocular dominance columns belonging to the closed eye, it does not affect their basic periodicity. Instead, the columns of the open eye expand so that the width of a column set (deprived plus open) remains unchanged. Figure 3.13 shows the ocular dominance columns from another animal also raised with suture of the right eye from age 1 week. In this case the radioactive label was placed into the

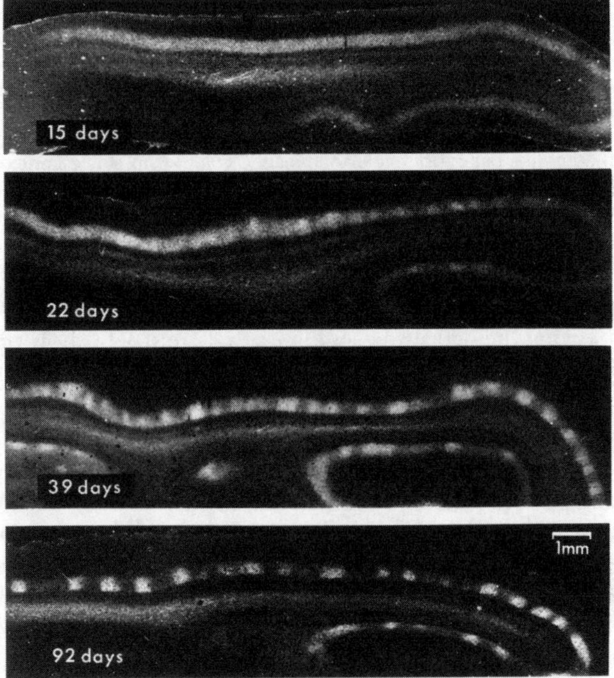

Figure 3.10. Segregation of ocular dominance columns in kitten visual cortex, shown in autoradiographs prepared from four different kittens at the indicated ages. The columns are shown in cross-section, as in Figure 3.4, rather than in tangential section. At age 15 days the ocular dominance columns have just started to form, so radioactive label appears as a nearly continuous band in layer IV. The columns emerge gradually over the first few months of life, giving rise to clumps of label, separated by gaps corresponding to the other eye's inputs. (From LeVay, S., & Stryker, M.P. [1979]. The development of ocular dominance columns in the cat. *Society for Neuroscience, 4,* 32–98; reprinted by permission from Wiley-Liss, Inc., a subsidiary of John Wiley & Sons, Inc.)

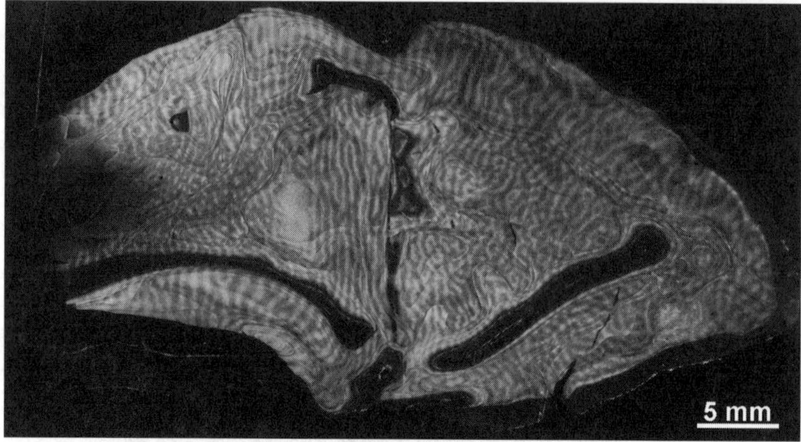

Figure 3.11. Autoradiographic montage of the right striate cortex from a monkey studied at E165/P0 that received an injection of [^{3}H]proline in the right eye at E158. Although the animal never received any light exposure, the ocular dominance columns are well formed and organized into an adult-like pattern, indicating that visual stimulation is not required for the formation of ocular dominance columns. (From Horton, J.C., & Hocking, D.R. [1996]. An adult-like pattern of ocular dominance columns in striate cortex of newborn monkeys prior to visual experience. *Journal of Neuroscience, 16,* 1791–1807; reprinted by permission from the Society for Neuroscience.)

normal left eye. The entire cortex is filled with [^{3}H]proline, except for narrow, fragmented gaps corresponding to the shrunken ocular dominance columns serving the deprived eye. Figures 3.12 and 3.13 show that shrinkage of the deprived eye's columns is accompanied by expansion of the open eye's columns.

The degree of column shrinkage is less marked when eyelid suture is performed at later ages in monkeys. Figure 3.14 shows the visual cortex from a monkey sutured at age 3 weeks. The dark ocular dominance columns of the closed eye are shrunken, but less severely than lid suture at age 1 week (compare Figures 3.13 and 3.14). In monkeys, the critical period for susceptibility to column shrinkage from eyelid suture lasts until 12–14 weeks. Beyond this age, eyelid suture has no affect on the appearance of the ocular dominance columns.

Previously in this chapter it was emphasized that the critical period in kittens does not begin until age 3 weeks. In macaque monkeys the critical period begins sooner, as one can infer by noting that eyelid suture at age 1 week produces more column shrinkage than suture at age 3 weeks. Why is the timing of the critical period different in cats and monkeys? The answer lies with the relative maturity of visual function in these two species at birth. In kittens the eyes do not open until 7–10 days after birth. After they open the optics are cloudy and vision is poor. By contrast, monkeys are born with their eyes open and begin immediately to explore their environment visually. The earlier timing of the critical period in the monkey simply reflects the fact that the kitten lags behind a month in relative visual maturity. The timing of critical periods for different brain regions is linked to their relative state of maturation and varies widely by species and function.

Injecting the eye with [^{3}H]proline is a useful technique for showing the distribution of thousands of labeled geniculate afferents in striate cortex. It provides no information, however, about input to the cortex from single fibers. In recent years it has proven possible to reconstruct the terminal arbors of single axons by making small injections of a tracer (Phaseolus lectin) into the lateral geniculate body. Figure 3.15 shows examples of single fibers serving the normal eye and the sutured eye from kittens that underwent a month of deprivation after the time of normal eye opening (Antonini & Stryker, 1996). The arbors serving the normal eye contain more branches and axon terminals than those serving the deprived eye. These morphological differences reflect the greater number of synaptic connections made onto cortical cells by arbors of the normal eye. This finding explains an old observation made by Hubel and Wiesel (1963) who noticed shrinkage of cell bodies in layers of the lateral geniculate nucleus supplied by the deprived eye in kittens raised with monocular eyelid suture. The geniculate cell bodies become smaller because their cortical arbors are reduced in size and complexity.

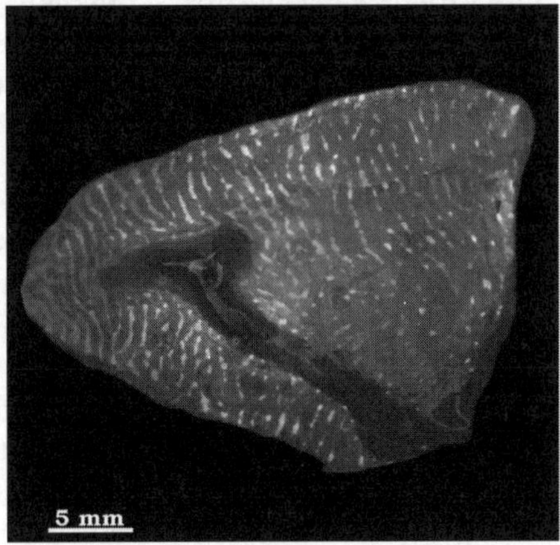

Figure 3.12. Autoradiographic montage of the ocular dominance columns in a macaque raised with suture of the right eye starting at age 1 week. After injection of radioactive label into the deprived eye, its ocular dominance columns appear as shrunken, fragmented islands amid a dark sea belonging to the open, normal eye. (From Horton, J.C., & Hocking, D.R. [1997]. Timing of the critical period for plasticity of ocular dominance columns in macaque striate cortex. *Journal of Neuroscience, 17,* 3684–3709; reprinted by permission from the Society for Neuroscience.)

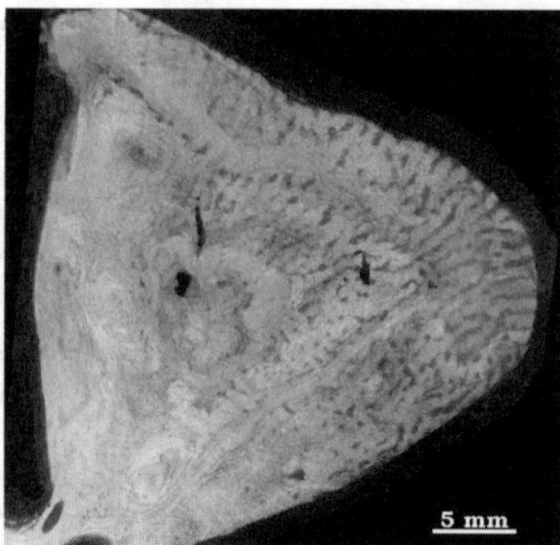

Figure 3.13. Another macaque raised with suture of the right eye from age 1 week, showing the appearance of the ocular dominance columns after injection of the radioactive tracer into the open eye. The cortex is filled with label, except for thin gaps representing the shrunken columns of the deprived eye. (From Horton, J.C., & Hocking, D.R. [1997]. Timing of the critical period for plasticity of ocular dominance columns in macaque striate cortex. *Journal of Neuroscience, 17,* 3684–3709; reprinted by permission from the Society for Neuroscience.)

Figure 3.16 shows schematically how visual deprivation affects the geniculocortical projections serving each eye. At birth, the ocular dominance columns in monkeys are well formed and equal in width (Figure 3.11). Along column borders, geniculocortical afferents serving each eye are in immediate proximity and may synapse onto the same cells in layer IV. When one eye is deprived the frequency of electrical activity is reduced in its geniculocortical afferents. This drop in activity leads to loss of synaptic connections with cells in layer IV. The loss of synapses is greatest along column borders, where geniculocortical afferents serving the closed eye are locked in direct competition with those of the open eye. As a result, the terminal arbors serving the deprived eye begin to retract, abandoning their cortical territory. Their retreat is followed by sprouting of geniculocortical afferents driven by the open eye. As this process continues, the open eye's ocular dominance columns become abnormally wide and the deprived eye's ocular dominance columns become shrunken (Figure 3.16).

Suturing the eyelids closed in a baby monkey causes no harm to the eye. Nonetheless, depriving the retina of patterned visual stimulation dramatically alters the balance of thalamic inputs to the cortex. It is remarkable that sensory deprivation alone is sufficient to affect the normal anatomy of the visual cortex. The shrinkage of ocular dominance columns induced by eyelid closure remains one of the most striking examples of how brain anatomy can be influenced by rearing conditions. It seems likely that other areas of the cerebral cortex in the developing primate, areas that have nothing to do with vision, also may depend upon sensory stimulation to form the proper anatomic circuits required for normal adult function. Few other areas, however, have lent themselves for easy demonstration of such clear-cut effects, and it remains unclear how widely one can extrapolate from the visual cortex to other regions of the brain.

CRITICAL PERIOD VERSUS SENSITIVE PERIOD

The visual system has provided an excellent proving ground for testing philosophers' ideas about how the brain works and responds to experimental manipulations. It offers many features for the scientist seeking to probe how nature and nurture contribute to neural development. One advantage is that visual function can be measured easily and precisely (Kiorpes & Movshon, 1990). For example, with relatively little effort, one can test visual acuity or determine whether depth perception is present or absent. As any investigator can attest, being able to measure accurately the outcome of an experiment is half the battle. Research on child development often is limited by disagreement over how results should be assessed or recorded.

In the visual system deprivation can be induced simply by suturing closed the lid of one eye. This procedure allows one to isolate the effects of pure sensory deprivation because no lesion is made. The visual system also has the advantage that function is neatly dichotomized into separate chan-

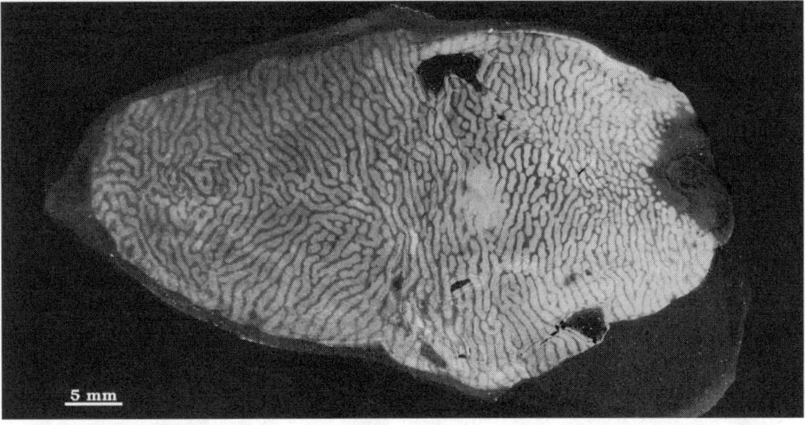

Figure 3.14. Montage of columns in a macaque raised from age 3 weeks with suture of the right eye. The [^{3}H]proline tracer was placed into the normal left eye. Note that the ocular dominance columns are less shrunken than after earlier suture at age 1 week (compare with Figure 3.13). (From Horton, J.C., & Hocking, D.R. [1997]. Timing of the critical period for plasticity of ocular dominance columns in macaque striate cortex. *Journal of Neuroscience, 17,* 3684–3709; reprinted by permission from the Society for Neuroscience.)

nels: the left eye and the right eye. After depriving only one eye, one can compare and contrast the effects on each eye. Finally, the psychophysics, anatomy, and physiology of the visual system were studied intensively during the 20th century. Although much remains to be learned, it is probably the best understood of all neural systems, making it relatively easy for the scientist to design experiments.

It is not surprising, given these attributes, that many insights into neural development have come from studies involving the visual system. It has been found that certain properties of the visual system develop *in utero*, without any need for light or visual stimulation, according to an innate program. Ocular dominance columns, orientation columns, receptive field properties, and a retinotopic map are all present in primate visual cortex at birth. However, they require refinement after birth to achieve a normal adult level of function. Deprivation during the critical period can interfere with maturation of the visual system, resulting in amblyopia.

In their original discussion of the critical period, Hubel and Wiesel (1970) invoked the work of Konrad Lorenz (1935) on imprinting behavior in birds. Lorenz learned that goslings can be trained to follow human decoys after hatching. Their affinity for imprinting upon a maternal target—whether a goose or human—peaked about 17 hours after hatching. According to Lorenz, they would not engage in this behavior before 12 hours or after 24 hours. Hubel and Wiesel saw an analogy with their kitten experiments because the susceptibility to eyelid closure began suddenly near the start of the fourth postnatal week and then declined a month later. They presumed that in both the goose and the kitten the critical period was linked to a period of transient plasticity in the brain region governing the behavior in question.

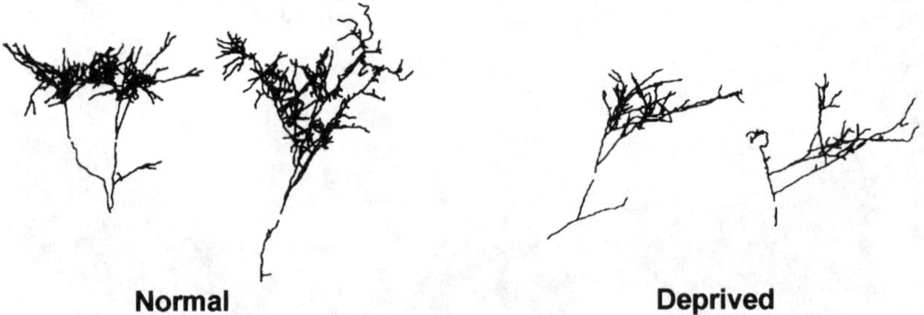

Figure 3.15. Four examples of single geniculocortical afferents in kittens raised with monocular eyelid suture, labeled by injection of the tracer Phaseolus lectin. The fibers serving the deprived eye have simpler terminal arbors with less branch points and synaptic terminals. They make fewer synaptic connections in striate cortex and project to shrunken ocular dominance columns. (From Antonini, A., & Stryker, M.P. [1996]. Plasticity of geniculocortical afferents following brief or prolonged monocular occlusion in the cat. *Journal of Comparative Neurology, 369,* 64–82; reprinted by permission from Wiley-Liss, Inc., a subsidiary of John Wiley & Sons, Inc.)

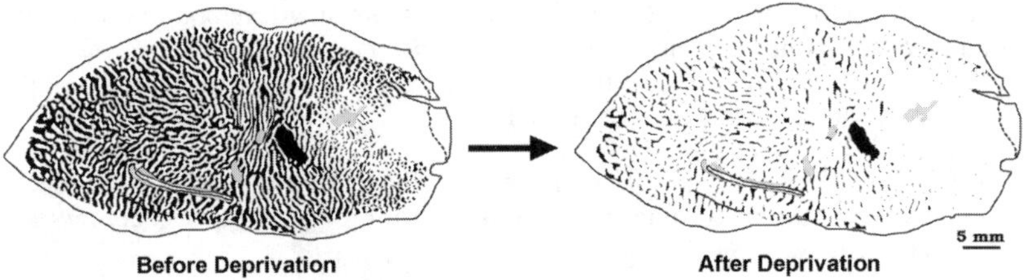

Figure 3.16. Diagram showing how visual deprivation causes shrinkage of the deprived eye's ocular dominance columns and expansion of those serving the normal eye. Note that the process begins at the boundaries of the ocular dominance columns and extends into the column cores, sparing only the eroded centers of the deprived eye's columns. (From Horton, J.C., & Hocking, D.R. [1997]. Timing of the critical period for plasticity of ocular dominance columns in macaque striate cortex. *Journal of Neuroscience, 17,* 3684–3709; reprinted by permission from the Society for Neuroscience.)

Although Lorenz emphasized the brevity of the critical period in waterfowl, it actually extends over a period of days, rather than hours, and has a more gradual beginning and end than he acknowledged. For this reason the term *sensitive period* is preferable to *critical period*, although it lacks the same cachet. The same point should be made regarding the duration of the critical period in the visual system. In primates, sensitivity to the effects of visual deprivation begins at birth and lasts for years. Although shrinkage of ocular dominance columns can be produced by monocular suture in monkeys only until age 3 months, shifts in the ocular preference of cells (without actual changes in column boundaries) can be induced for up to a year after birth. In humans, amblyopia from form deprivation, strabismus, or refractive error can occur up to age 10. It is a mistake, therefore, to conceive of the critical period as a single phenomenon or a brief moment in development. Confusion over this point has led some investigators to deny the existence of critical periods or to question the relevance of studies on visual development. The complexity of higher cortical functions, especially those vital to scholastic performance, almost guarantees that critical periods will take a more subtle form in other regions of the brain. The principles derived from experiments on the visual system deserve careful attention because they demonstrate the vital impact of normal sensory stimulation on brain development and underscore the importance of providing children with an adequate and healthy sensory environment during their earliest years.

REFERENCES

Antonini, A., & Stryker, M.P. (1996). Plasticity of geniculocortical afferents following brief or prolonged monocular occlusion in the cat. *Journal of Comparative Neurology, 369,* 64–82.

Boothe, R.G., Dobson, V., & Teller, D.Y. (1985). Postnatal development of vision in human and nonhuman primates. *Annual Review of Neuroscience, 8,* 495–545.

Chino, Y.M., Smith III, E.L., Hatta, S., & Cheng, H. (1997). Postnatal development of binocular disparity sensitivity in neurons of the primate visual cortex. *Journal of Neuroscience, 17,* 296–307.

Horton, J.C., & Hocking, D.R. (1996). An adult-like pattern of ocular dominance columns in striate cortex of newborn monkeys prior to visual experience. *Journal of Neuroscience, 16,* 1791–1807.

Horton, J.C., & Hocking, D.R. (1997). Timing of the critical period for plasticity of ocular dominance columns in macaque striate cortex. *Journal of Neuroscience, 17,* 3684–3709.

Hubel, D.H., & Wiesel, T.N. (1965). Binocular interaction in striate cortex of kittens reared with artificial squint. *Journal of Neurophysiology, 28,* 1041–1059.

Hubel, D.H., & Wiesel, T.N. (1970). The period of susceptibility to the physiological effects of unilateral eye closure in kittens. *Journal of Physiology (London), 206,* 419–436.

Hubel, D.H., & Wiesel, T.N. (1977). Functional architecture of macaque monkey visual cortex. *Proceedings of the Royal Society of London (Biology), 198,* 1–59.

Hubel, D.H., Wiesel, T.N., & LeVay, S. (1977). Plasticity of ocular dominance columns in monkey striate cortex. *Philosophical Transactions of the Royal Society of London (Biology), 278,* 377–409.

Kiorpes, L., & Movshon, J.A. (1990). Behavioral analysis of visual development. In J.R. Coleman (Ed.), *Development of sensory systems in mammals* (pp. 125–154). New York: John Wiley & Sons, Inc.

LeVay, S., & Stryker, M.P. (1979). The development of ocular dominance columns in the cat. *Society for Neuroscience, 4,* 32–98.

LeVay, S., Stryker, M.P., & Shatz, C.J. (1978). Ocular dominance columns and their development in layer IV of the cat's visual cortex: A quantitative study. *Journal of Comparative Neurology, 179,* 223–244.

Lorenz, K.Z. (1935). Der kumpan in der umwelt des vogels; die artgenossen als auslösendes moment sozialer verhaltensweisen. *Journal für Ornithologie, 83,* 137–213.

Polyak, S. (1957). *The vertebrate visual system* (p. 289). University of Chicago Press.

Rakic, P. (1977). Prenatal development of the visual system in rhesus monkey. *Philosophical Transactions of the Royal Society of London (Biology), 278,* 245–260.

Shatz, C.J., & Stryker, M.P. (1978). Ocular dominance in layer IV of the cat's visual cortex and the effects of monocular deprivation. *Journal of Physiology (London), 281,* 267–283.

Stryker, M.P., & Harris, W.A. (1986). Binocular impulse blockade prevents the formation of ocular dominance columns in cat visual cortex. *Journal of Neuroscience, 6,* 2117–2133.

Swindale, N.V. (1981). Absence of ocular dominance patches in dark-reared cats. *Nature, 290,* 332–333.

Swindale, N.V., Vital-Durand, F., & Blakemore, C. (1981). Recovery from monocular deprivation in the monkey III. Reversal of anatomical effects in the visual cortex. *Proceedings of the Royal Society of London (Biology), 213,* 435–450.

Teller, D.Y. (1997). First glances: The vision of infants. *Investigative Ophthalmology and Visual Science, 38,* 2183–2203.

von Noorden, G.K., Dowling, J.E., & Ferguson, D.C. (1970). Experimental amblyopia in monkeys I. Behavioral studies of stimulus deprivation amblyopia. *Archives of Ophthalmology, 84,* 206–214.

Wade, N.J. (1998). *A natural history of vision*. Cambridge, MA: The MIT Press.

Wiesel, T.N., & Hubel, D.H. (1963). Single-cell responses in striate cortex of kittens deprived of vision in one eye. *Journal of Neurophysiology, 26*, 1003–1017.

Wiesel, T.N., & Hubel, D.H. (1965). Comparison of the effects of unilateral and bilateral eye closure on cortical unit responses in kittens. *Journal of Neurophysiology, 28*, 1029–1040.

Wiesel, T.N., & Hubel, D.H. (1974). Ordered arrangement of orientation columns in monkeys lacking visual experience. *Journal of Comparative Neurology, 158*, 307–318.

Wiesel, T.N., Hubel, D.H., & Lam, D.M.K. (1974). Autoradiographic demonstration of ocular-dominance columns in the monkey striate cortex by means of transneuronal transport. *Brain Research, 79*, 273–279.

4

Critical Periods for Development of Visual Acuity, Depth Perception, and Eye Tracking

Lawrence Tychsen

The previous chapter discusses the results of experiments on animals in which an eyelid is sewn shut to deprive the animal of visual experience early in life. The deprivation causes the growth of the visual brain to be stunted permanently. This chapter extends these findings to human beings by discussing common problems of visual development in children. The clinical studies of children convey a clear message: The basic wiring of the visual system is innate, but the brain needs proper early visual experience to refine the connections and achieve adult levels of performance. There are two major requirements for proper early visual experience: 1) that the eyes form clear images and 2) that both eyes are stably aligned so that they are pointed at the same target in space and send nearly identical, nonconflicting images to the brain. If the eye does not form a clear image, the critical period for development of acute vision is severely disrupted. If the eyes are not properly aligned, the critical periods for depth perception, eye tracking, and motion vision are disrupted.

This study was supported by National Institutes of Health Grant No. R01 EY 10214 and an unrestricted grant to the Department of Ophthalmology and Visual Sciences at the Washington University School of Medicine.

RAPID DEVELOPMENT IN INFANCY

The critical period for development of acute vision in children has two phases: an early phase of rapid development spanning birth to approximately age 10 months and a later phase of slower development spanning age 10 months to approximately age 10 years (Norcia & Tyler, 1985; Orel-Bixler, 1989). The development is shown in the bottom graph of Figure 4.1 with the Y axis indicating increasing visual acuity and the X axis indicating age after birth. The acuity is measured by recording the strength of electrical activity over visual regions of the brain using the evoked potential

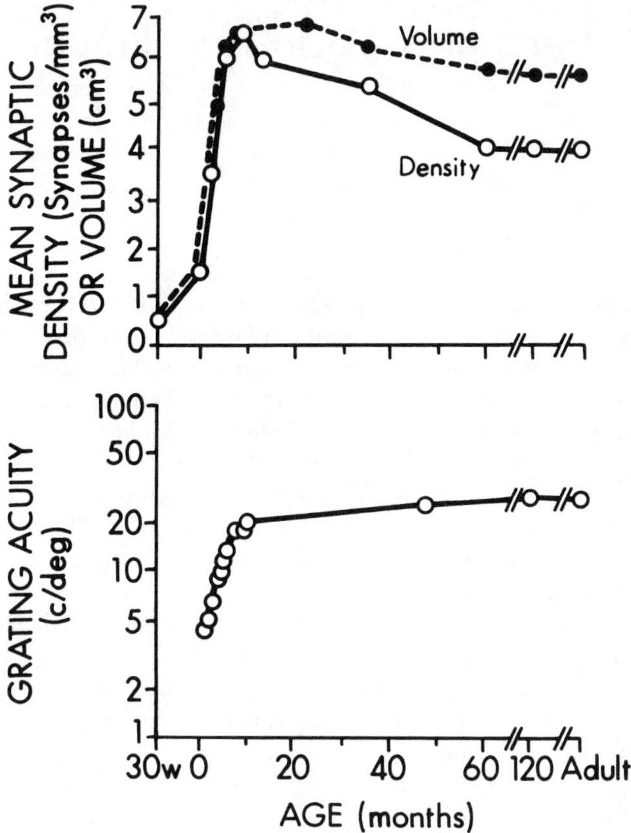

Figure 4.1. Two phases in the critical period for development of primary visual cortex and visual acuity in humans. *Upper panel*: Synaptic density and cortical volume rapidly increase from birth to age 10 months and then slowly decline to reach adult levels by age 9. *Lower panel*: Two phases of development of visual acuity as measured using the grating spatial-sweep visually evoked potential (VEP) technique; a rapid increase occurs in the first 10 months of life followed by a gradual increase in acuity from age 10 months to 10 years. (Data courtesy of Anthony Norcia and Deborah Bixler, Smith Kettlewell Institute, San Francisco.)

technique (Norcia, 1994). Patterns that the infant brain can resolve produce strong voltages, and patterns that are too fine to be resolved produce little or no voltage. The rise of visual acuity after birth in this graph cannot be explained by focusing limitations of the eyeball itself (the front end of the visual system), because the retina and lens are well developed in full-term infants at birth (Hendrickson, 1993). A back end (e.g., brain) explanation for the rise is appealing because the rise in acuity in the first months of life closely matches the rapid increase in the development of neuronal connections and cerebral cortex volume (Figure 4.1, top graph) as measured from autopsies of infants' brains (Huttenlocher, 1987; Huttenlocher, de Courten, Garey, & Van der Loos, 1982).

MONOCULAR DEPRIVATION IN THE FIRST WEEKS OF ACUITY DEVELOPMENT

From clinical studies of infants born with a cataract, it is known that the most serious damage to acute vision results from persistent deprivation during the earliest phase of rapid development. *Cataract* is a clouding of the lens that degrades the image formed on the retina. The cataract acts as a filter, stopping sharp, detailed (high spatial frequency) images and transmitting only the blurriest, crudest (low spatial frequency) images. The blurred image of the deprived eye produces weak signals from the eye to the visual cortex (LeVay, Wiesel, & Hubel, 1980). What happens to the visual circuitry of the infant's cortex if the monocular deprivation persists?

The answer is shown in Figure 4.2, which plots the visual acuity of monocularly deprived children when tested at age 5 years using standard letter targets. Each square represents an individual child (Birch & Stager, 1996). If the monocular deprivation was corrected by combined cataract surgery, optical correction, and patching therapy by age 7 weeks, the child was able to develop good to excellent vision. If the identical therapy was delayed beyond this interval, the visual acuity fell systematically, such that the best acuity attained even for surgery in late infancy was no better than the level of legal blindness (approximately 20/200 vision).

INFANT DEPTH PERCEPTION AND EYE MISALIGNMENT

In addition to a critical period for sharp vision in one eye (monocular acuity), there is a critical period for visual functions that requires use of the two eyes together—the binocular function of depth perception. Figure 4.3 shows binocular depth perception in the form of three-dimensional (3-D) vision (i.e., stereopsis) is not present at birth. It develops abruptly in typical infants between ages 3 and 5 months as it reaches adult-like levels of performance. The data shown in the graph were gathered by testing more than 50 infants

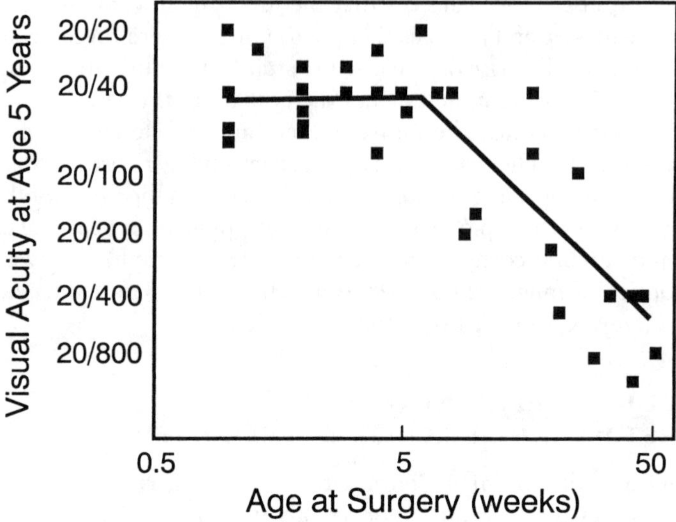

Figure 4.2. Children who had monocular deprivation at birth: Visual acuity in children 5 years after combined surgery and patching therapy for monocular congenital cataract. Infants who had surgical repair by age 6 weeks developed good vision in the involved eye. Delay of repair beyond age 6 weeks produced a predictable (bilinear) and permanent decrease in vision, often to the levels of legal blindness (20/200 or worse). (Data courtesy of Eileen Birch and David Stager, Southwest Research Institute, Dallas, Texas, and Lawrence Tychsen.)

using the preferential looking method (Figure 4.4; Birch, Shimojo, & Held, 1985; Birch & Stager, 1985). The method is based on the principle that when faced with the choice of viewing a simple or a complex stimulus, infants choose to gaze at a complex stimulus and tend to ignore a simple stimulus (Teller, 1979). The infant wears goggles containing polarizing lenses and is shown stimuli that are correspondingly polarized[1] so that when viewed with the goggles, the stimuli, otherwise indistinguishable, appear either as flat (simple) or as 3-D (e.g., complex, in depth, stereoscopic). The position of the 3-D stimulus is randomized from trial to trial, and if the position to which the infant shifts gaze correlates significantly with the position of the 3-D stimulus one can reliably infer the development of depth perception.

Stereoscopic depth perception requires that the brain compare precisely the image received from the right eye to that received from the left eye (Tychsen, 1992). If the eyes are pointed at different targets in space—

[1]Polarizing lenses consist of a transparent material containing embedded crystals that allow images conveyed to the two eyes to be separated entirely, so that the right eye and the left eye can see slightly different views of a flat scene, recreating a sense of real depth or natural perspective.

if they are misaligned—the precise comparison is impossible. The ophthalmic term for pathologic eye misalignment is *strabismus*, from the Greek root meaning "to look at crooked." Convergent (turned in to the nose or esotropic) eye misalignment (Figure 4.5) begins to appear in infants with strabismus between ages 2 and 6 months and is 50 times more common than infant cataract (von Noorden, 1996; Wright, 1995). The typical infant with crossed eyes retains good acuity in both eyes and will switch viewing from eye to eye depending on the location of the target of momentary interest. In most instances, the misalignment is not due to weak or structurally abnormal eye muscles. Rather, the eye muscles appear to receive the wrong

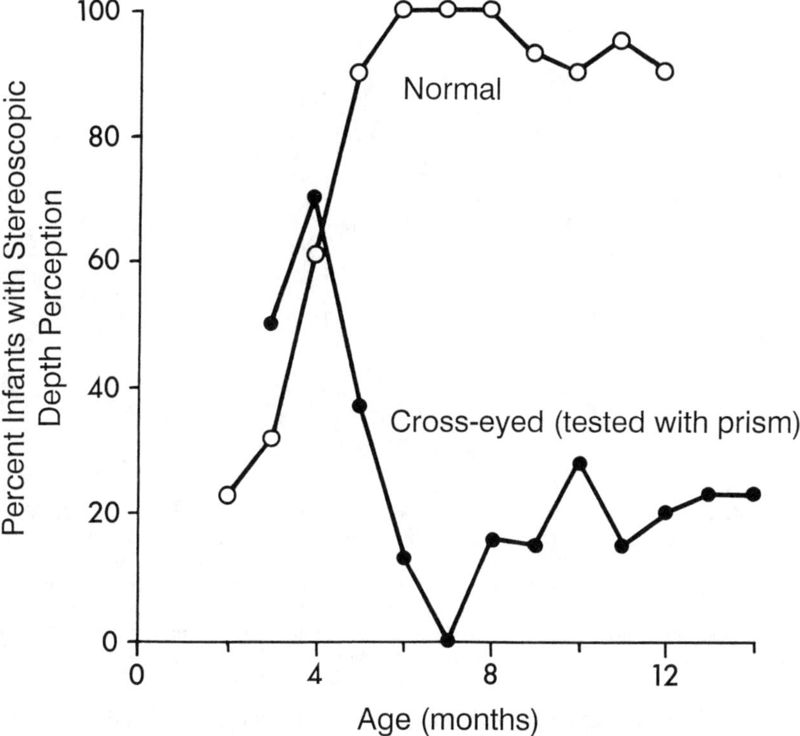

Figure 4.3. Criticial period for depth perception: Development of stereoscopic (e.g., 3-D) depth perception in normal (and strabismic) human infants with crossed eyes using the preferential looking behavioral method of testing. Normal infants show onset of stereopsis abruptly at ages 2–4 months. Infants with crossed eyes were tested by optically realigning their eyes temporarily in the testing laboratory using goggles fitted with prisms. The infants with crossed eyes initially showed a capacity for stereopsis that deteriorated abruptly after age 4 months. Approximately 50 infants composed each testing group (e.g., normal versus strabismic). The infants with crossed eyes tested after age 4 months represent late detection of the strabismus and late referrals to the pediatric ophthalmologist.

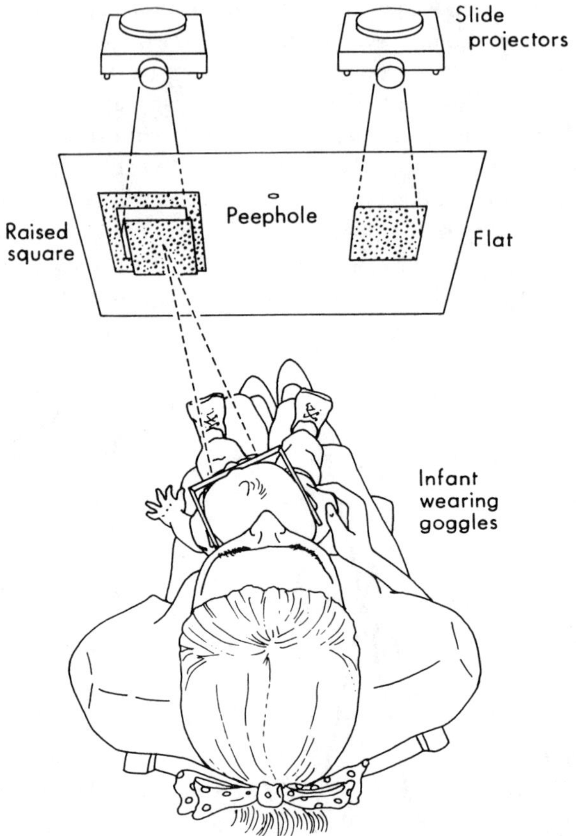

Figure 4.4. Preferential looking method used to measure stereoacuity (or visual acuity) in infant human and monkey. The infant, wearing polaroid goggles, shifts eye and head position in the direction of the more compelling of two polaroid random-dot targets. In the trial shown, only the left stimulus contains a center region of binocular 3-D disparity. Stimuli are randomized left-right from trial to trial. Gratings can be substituted (without goggles) for testing of visual acuity, and printed card stimuli (e.g., Teller acuity cards) or video monitor images can be substituted for the projectors and slides.

commands from maldeveloped brain circuits that should calibrate eye position (Tychsen, 1999).

If the misalignment (strabismus) is constant and persists longer than 60 days during the first 9 months of life, the development of 3-D depth perception in human infants is permanently damaged (Figure 4.6; Birch, Stager, & Everett, 1995). If the strabismus is corrected by eye muscle microsurgery before 60 days of constant misalignment, the development of stereoscopic 3-D vision can be restored (Birch, Fawcett, & Stager, 2000; Wright, Edelman, McVey, Terry, & Lin, 1994). Delay in surgical repair beyond this 60-day period produces good motor alignment of the eyes in the majority of children, but restoration of robust 3-D stereoscopic perception is unlikely.

DEVELOPMENT OF EYE TRACKING (PURSUIT) AND MOTION VISION

Smooth eye tracking, like stereoscopic depth perception, is not present at birth but matures rapidly in the first year of life (Tychsen, 1994). Vision is degraded by inaccurate (e.g., jerky, too slow) eye tracking, and the direction of tracking that is most inaccurate at birth is that required to follow targets that move from the nose toward the ear when viewing with either eye. Tracking is measured clinically by making the infant view with one eye while the examiner moves a small target horizontally, first to the right and

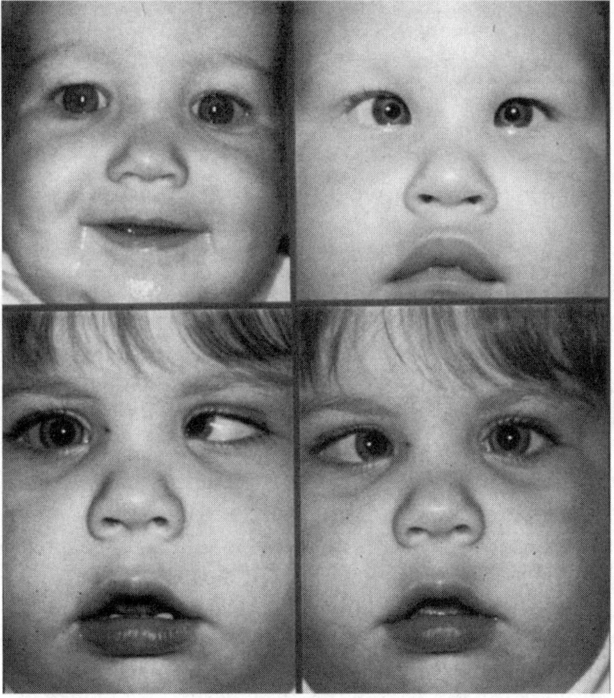

Figure 4.5. One normal infant (top left) and two infants who had eye crossing (strabismus) in the first 4 months of life. *Top right:* infant who prefers to look with left eye and has convergent strabismus of right eye. If the unilateral strabismus persists, the brain will suppress the columns of the visual cortex driven by the misaligned right eye (causing amblyopia). The infant also will have abnormal depth perception and poor eye tracking and motion vision. *Bottom panels:* infant with alternating strabismus who will look at any given moment with the right or left eye (alternating fixation). Input from each eye is therefore suppressed 50% of the time, causing loss of depth perception and poor eye tracking and motion vision but normal visual acuity (no amblyopia).

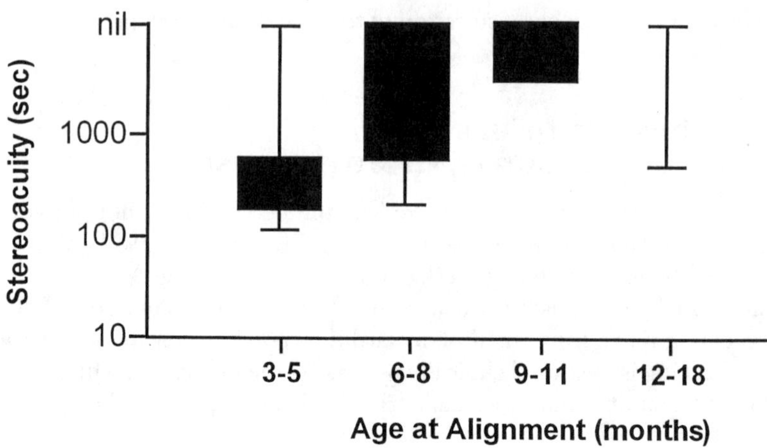

Figure 4.6. Quality of stereopsis 5 years after surgery: Quality of stereoscopic depth perception in children who had crossed eyes in infancy and surgical repair at different ages. Infants repaired (realigned) by age 3–5 months regained good stereopsis. Infants who had repair delayed beyond age 1 year had very poor-to-absent stereopsis (e.g., stereo-blindness).

then to the left, at a steady speed (Figure 4.7). The visual brain connections required to smoothly track targets that move inside to out (e.g., naso-temporal smooth pursuit) are not present at birth but develop in normal infants by age 6 months (for low speed targets) (Tychsen, 1992, 1994). The development of these connections requires normal binocular experience in early infancy. If binocular experience is disturbed (e.g., by eye misalignment during the first 6 months of life) the cerebral connections necessary to smoothly track and hold the eye stable are impaired permanently (Tychsen & Lisberger, 1986). The impairment is evident as 1) asymmetric pursuit of moving targets (temporal-to-nasal tracking is smooth, but nasal-to-temporal tracking is inaccurate) and 2) eye drifting when attempting to view stationary targets (i.e., nystagmus) (Tychsen, Hurtig, & Scott, 1985; Tychsen & Lisberger, 1986). The impairment also is evident in perception of object motion. Children who have eye tracking deficits not only pursue inaccurately but also fail to accurately judge the direction of target motion. Using evoked brain potentials or psychophysical tests in adults who have eye misalignment dating from early infancy, it is known that perceptual abnormalities persist permanently (Norcia, 1996; Tychsen & Lisberger, 1986; Tychsen, Rastelli, Steinman, & Steinman, 1996).

MALDEVELOPMENT OF NEURONAL CONNECTIONS IN THE VISUAL CORTEX

To reveal neural mechanisms for the abnormalities of binocular vision described previously, behavioral and anatomic experiments were carried out on a special group of macaque monkeys who, like their human counterparts, had onset of eye crossing in infancy (Boothe, Kiorpes, & Carlson, 1985; Kiorpes & Boothe, 1981). The monkey experiments allowed examination of the cerebral circuitry at a level of detail not possible in studies of human infants (Tychsen & Burkhalter, 1995, 1997; Tychsen, Burkhalter, & Boothe, 1996). To verify that the animals had the same behavioral impairments as children whose eyes were crossed, they were trained first to per-

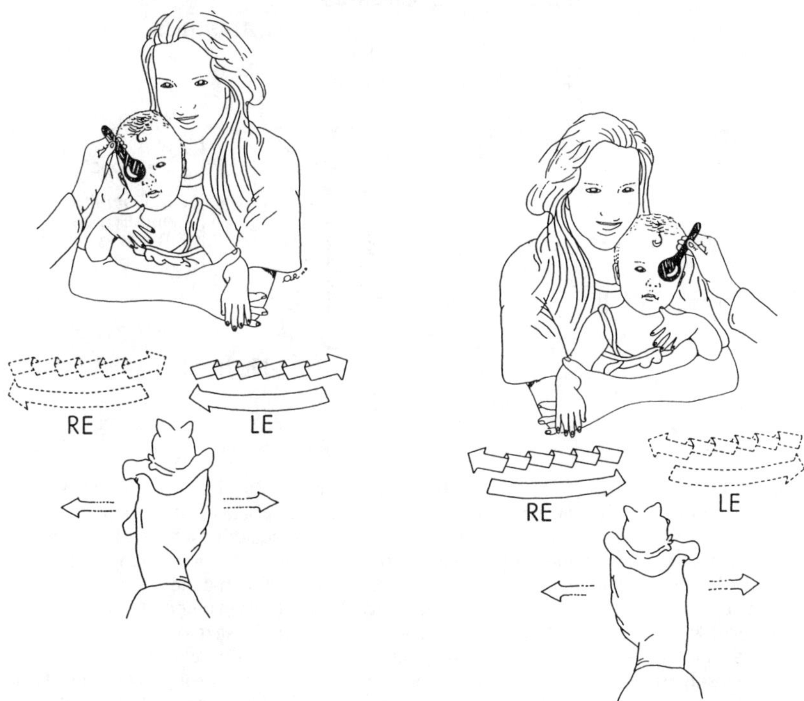

Figure 4.7. Asymmetry of horizontal smooth pursuit evident during monocular viewing. When a handheld toy is moved from a temporal-to-nasal position before the fixating eye, pursuit is smooth. Pursuit is absent or cogwheel when the target moves nasal-to-temporal. The movements of the two eyes are conjugate, and the direction of the asymmetry reverses instantaneously with a change of fixating eye so that the direction of robust pursuit is always for nasally directed targets in the visual field. The asymmetry is seen best by moving the target at a brisk pace. The asymmetry indicates immaturity of binocular eye tracking and vision motion connections in visual cortex. *Dashed lines:* conjugate movements of the eye under the cover.

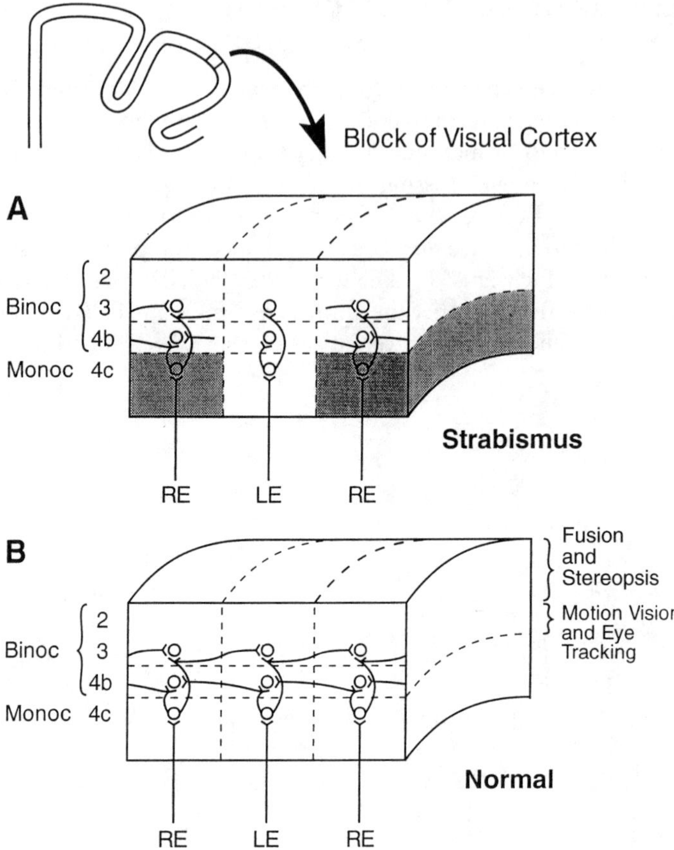

Figure 4.8. Neuroanatomic abnormalities found in primary visual cortex of monkeys with strabismus esotropia who alternated fixation and had normal visual acuity in both eyes: lack of binocular connections and nasotemporal inequalities of metabolic activity. *Upper panel:* Strabismic monkey has a paucity of horizontal connections for binocular vision; neurons are connected within individual ocular dominance columns (ODCs), but there are few connections to neighboring ODCs of the opposite ocularity. Connections to other ODCs of the same ocularity (e.g., right eye to right eye ODCs) are not shown for the sake of clarity. Layer 4c of right eye ODCs in the left visual cortex (e.g., contralateral eye or nasal retina ODCs) stains more intensely (dark shading) for cytochrome oxidase activity, indicating higher metabolic activity in nasal ODCs and suppression of temporal ODCs. *Lower panel:* In normal monkeys, neurons in layers 2 and 3 form part of the parvo-interblob pathway, which plays a major role in fine (random-dot) stereopsis. Neurons in layer 4b form part of the magno pathway, which plays a major role in motion perception and pursuit eye movement.

form visual acuity, depth perception, and eye tracking tasks for a fruit juice reward. Under anesthesia, the monkey's visual cortex was injected with tracer substances that label individual neurons and their connecting branches.

The animals were euthanized and the brains removed and anatomically sectioned for analysis.

The schematic of the visual cerebral cortex shown in Figure 4.8 summarizes the key findings from these experiments. The cortex is organized as columns of neurons, half of which are dominated by input from the right eye and half from the left eye so that every other column in the cortex is driven by a different eye (Hubel & Wiesel, 1977). In animals who have normal eye alignment, the eyes are pointed at the same target in space and send nearly identical signals to the columns. The columns in this case have equal levels of activity and are interconnected by horizontal fibers to facilitate a sharing of information between right and left eye neurons (Tychsen & Burkhalter, 1995). In animals with crossed eyes, each eye points at a different target, and the two eyes send markedly different signals to their respective columns in the cortex. Hence, the activity in the right and left eye columns conflicts. The cortex in this case resolves the conflict by partially shutting off the columns from one eye (i.e., one set of columns in each cerebral hemisphere dominates and begins to suppress the activity in the neighboring columns, as depicted by the dark shading in Figure 4.8) (Horton, Hocking, & Adams, 1999; Tychsen & Burkhalter, 1997). If the conflicting activity and suppression persist for more than a few months in infancy, communicating fibers (binocular connections) between the right and left eye columns are permanently lost (Tychsen, 1999; Tychsen & Burkhalter, 1995). The behavioral correlates of the anatomic loss of binocular connections are loss of depth perception, inability to fuse together images to the two eyes, inaccurate (asymmetric) pursuit eye tracking, and unstable gaze (fixation nystagmus).

The development of binocular vision and ocular dominance column interconnections can be viewed metaphorically from the perspective of a good and a bad marriage. In a good marriage (normal cortex), two unique individuals (strong right and left eye dominance columns) with separate talents and duties subjugate their egos in service to the other, ensuring that neither profits at the expense of the other. The balance of the egos is complemented by strong communication (interconnections) to work toward common goals. From this unified front of cooperation and communication come good offspring (proper downstream signals from primary to secondary visual cortex) in the form of normal depth perception, stable eye fixation, and smooth eye tracking. A bad marriage (the maldeveloped visual cortex in eye crossing) is the opposite: two warring egos (right and left eye columns driven by eyes pointed in different directions) are engaged in a tug-of-war (switching fixation from one eye, exclusively, to the other), begetting offspring (impaired depth perception and unstable, asymmetric eye tracking) warped by the conflict and lack of unified goals.

WHAT WE KNOW, THINK WE KNOW, AND NEED TO KNOW

In order to rescue visual acuity, there must be intervention to correct severe monocular deprivation in human infants within the first 2 months of life. To rescue robust depth perception and normal eye tracking, a corrective procedure must be done within 2–3 months of onset of eye misalignment.

The ability to perceive complex form and motion images lags behind the development of the functions described here, and there is evidence that these complex functions are able to be repaired in impaired children well beyond infancy. A minor, but substantial, fraction of children who have monocular deprivation or crossed eyes have disappointing outcomes despite early therapy, as shown by the graphs in this chapter. Innate differences in brain plasticity may account for the failure to correct maldevelopments in these cases.

It is difficult to gather information about visual impairments in children. First, there is a need to better understand the impact of binocular visuomotor disorders on children's learning. The current dearth of hard clinical and neuropsychological facts in this area has been filled by pseudoscience and psychobabble, particularly with regard to vision training and learning disabilities. Good information could be gathered by small, well-designed studies conducted in the next 5 years. Second, the earlier children with visual impairments are seen by a pediatric ophthalmologist, the better the chances of restoring normal function. But, every infant cannot and should not be seen by an ophthalmologist. Pediatricians and nurse practitioners are capable of screening infants, but they need better tools. The screening methods now in use are quick and inexpensive but not accurate, and there are more sophisticated methods used in university labs that are accurate but not quick or inexpensive (Tychsen, 1992). An inexpensive and accurate electronic-digital device that will verify normal eye alignment and clear focusing of both eyes needs to be in the hands of lay screeners, nurses, and therapists. With sufficient attention, this biomedical engineering goal could be achieved in the next 5 years.

As for more ambitious and longer term goals, there always will be children who, for one reason or another, show up in the ophthalmologist's office after the critical periods. For these children, we need a "magic pharmacologic bullet" (an injection or pill) that would restore visual cortex plasticity and make delayed surgical repair efficacious. The challenge is to do this without perturbing development of other normal brain circuits. Neuroscientists have shown that this is possible using simple animal models (Berardi & Maffei, 1999), but it is estimated that it will take decades to achieve this goal in humans.

REFERENCES

Berardi, N., & Maffei, L. (1999). From visual experience to visual function: Roles of neurotrophins. *Journal of Neurobiology, 41*, 119–126.

Birch, E.E., Fawcett, S., & Stager, D.R. (2000). Why does early surgical alignment improve stereopsis outcomes in infantile esotropia? *Journal of the American Association of Pediatric Ophthalmology and Strabismus, 4*, 10–14.

Birch, E.E., Shimojo, S., & Held, R. (1985). Preferential-looking assessment of fusion and stereopsis in infants ages 1 to 6 months. *Investigative Ophthalmology & Visual Science, 26*, 366–370.

Birch, E.E., & Stager, D.R. (1985). Monocular acuity and stereopsis in infantile esotropia. *Investigative Ophthalmology & Visual Science, 26*, 1624–1630.

Birch, E.E., & Stager, D.R. (1996). The critical period for surgical treatment of dense congenital unilateral cataract. *Investigative Ophthalmology & Visual Science, 37*, 1532–1538.

Birch, E.E., Stager, D.R., & Everett, M.E. (1995). Random dot stereoacuity following surgical correction of infantile esotropia. *Journal of the American Association of Pediatric Ophthalmology and Strabismus, 32*, 231–235.

Boothe, R.G., Kiorpes, L., & Carlson, M.R. (1985). Studies of strabismus and amblyopia in infant monkeys. *Journal of the American Association of Pediatric Ophthalmology and Strabismus, 22*, 206–212.

Hendrickson, A. (1993). Development of the primate retina. In K. Simons (Ed.), *Early visual development: Normal and abnormal* (pp. 287–295). New York: Oxford University Press.

Horton, J.C., Hocking, D.R., & Adams, D.L. (1999). Metabolic mapping of suppression scotomas in striate cortex of macaques with experimental strabismus. *Journal of Neuroscience, 19*, 7111–7129.

Hubel, D.H., & Wiesel, T.N. (1977). Functional architecture of macaque monkey visual cortex. *Proceedings of the Royal Society of London (Biology), 198*, 1–59.

Huttenlocher, P.R. (1987). The development of synapses in striate cortex of man. *Human Neurobiology, 6*, 208.

Huttenlocher, P.R., de Courten, C., Garey, L., & Van der Loos, H. (1982). Synaptogenesis in human visual cortex: Evidence for synapse elimination during normal development. *Neuroscience Letters, 33*, 247–252.

Kiorpes, L., & Boothe, R.G. (1981). Naturally occurring strabismus in monkeys (Macaca nemestrina). *Investigative Ophthalmology & Visual Science, 20*, 257–263.

LeVay, S., Wiesel, T.N., & Hubel, D.H. (1980). The development of ocular dominance columns in normal and visually deprived monkeys. *Journal of Comparative Neurology, 191*, 1–51.

Norcia, A.M. (1994). Vision testing by visual evoked potential techniques. In S.J. Isenberg (Ed.), *The eye in infancy* (2nd ed., pp. 157–173). St. Louis: Mosby.

Norcia, A.M. (1996). Abnormal motion processing and binocularity: Infantile esotropia as a model system for effects of early interruptions of binocularity. *Eye, 10*, 259–265.

Norcia, A.M., & Tyler, C. (1985). Spatial frequency sweep VEP: Visual acuity during the first year of life. *Vision Research, 25*, 1399–1408.

Orel-Bixler, D.A. (1989). Unpublished doctoral dissertation. University of California at Berkeley.

Teller, D. (1979). The forced-choice preferential looking procedure: A psychophysical technique for use with human infants. *Infant Behavior and Development, 2*, 135–153.

Tychsen, L. (1992). Binocular vision. In W.M. Hart (Ed.), *Adler's physiology of the eye: Clinical applications* (9th ed., pp. 773–853). St. Louis: Mosby.

Tychsen, L. (1994). Development of vision. In S. Isenberg (Ed.), *The eye in infancy* (2nd ed., pp. 121–130). St. Louis: Mosby.

Tychsen, L. (1999). Infantile esotropia: Current neurophysiologic concepts. In A.L. Rosenbaum & A.P. Santiago (Eds.), *Clinical strabismus management* (pp. 117–138). Philadelphia: W. B. Saunders Company.

Tychsen, L., & Burkhalter, A. (1995). Neuroanatomic abnormalities of primary visual cortex in macaque monkeys with infantile esotropia: Preliminary results. *Journal of the American Association of Pediatric Ophthalmology and Strabismus, 32*, 323–328.

Tychsen, L., & Burkhalter, A. (1997). Nasotemporal asymmetries in V1: Ocular dominance columns in infant, adult, and strabismic macaque monkeys. *Journal of Comparative Neurology, 388*, 32–46.

Tychsen, L., Burkhalter, A., & Boothe, R.G. (1996). Functional and structural abnormalities of visual cortex in infantile strabismus. *Klinische Monatsblatter fur Augenheilkunde, 208*, 18–22.

Tychsen, L., Burkhalter, A., & Boothe, R.G. (1996). Neural mechanisms in infantile esotropia: What goes wrong? *American Orthoptic Journal, 46*, 18–28.

Tychsen, L., Hurtig, R.R., & Scott, W.E. (1985). Pursuit is impaired but the vestibulo-ocular reflex is normal in infantile strabismus. *Archives of Ophthalmology, 103*, 536–539.

Tychsen, L., & Lisberger, S.G. (1986). Maldevelopment of visual motion processing in humans who had strabismus with onset in infancy. *Journal of Neuroscience, 6*, 2495–2508.

Tychsen, L., Rastelli, A., Steinman, S., & Steinman, B. (1996). Biases of motion perception revealed by reversing gratings in humans who had infantile-onset strabismus. *Developmental Medicine and Child Neurology, 38*, 408–422.

von Noorden, G.K. (1996). *Binocular vision and ocular motility.* St. Louis: Mosby.

Wright, K.W. (1995). *Pediatric ophthalmology and strabismus.* St. Louis: Mosby.

Wright, K.W., Edelman, P.M., McVey, J.H., Terry, A.P., & Lin, M. (1994). High-grade stereo acuity after early surgery for congenital esotropia. *Archives of Ophthalmology, 112*, 913–919.

III

Critical Periods in Social and Emotional Development

5

Sensitive Periods in Attachment?

Ross A. Thompson

A baby's first relationship provides a foundation for later relationships. The amount of security and trust experienced in the initial human bond will be anticipated in future relationships. As a result, the quality of the first relationship has a formative effect on the young child, shaping that child's capacities to develop close, intimate ties to others in later years.

The idea of the enduring importance of the first relationship has deep roots in Western culture and psychological theory. This view has philosophical origins dating back to the 17th- and 18th-century writings of John Locke and Jean-Jacques Rousseau that emphasized formative early influences on the child, as well as the 19th-century Victorian romantic era portrayal of the mother–infant bond. This view also is reflected in Sigmund Freud's famous dictum that the mother–infant relationship is "unique, without parallel, established unalterably for a whole lifetime as the first and strongest love-object and as the prototype for all later love-relations" (1940, p. 45). Since Freud's days, an emphasis on the formative influence of the first attachment relationship has been echoed by other psychological theorists. For example, Erikson (1963) portrayed the mother–infant relationship as the initial forum for addressing the lifelong psychosocial challenge of establishing basic trust versus mistrust. Based initially on the quality of the child's bond to the mother, Erikson believed the world at large would be regarded either as a safe and trustworthy environment or as a place with hidden dangers and threats. Likewise, Bowlby initially believed that good mothering "is

The conference on which this chapter is based was a stimulating and thought-provoking exchange of ideas, and this chapter benefited considerably from discussions with other conference participants who also were interested in questions of early experience, social relationships, and critical periods.

almost useless if delayed until after the age of 2½ years. In actual fact this upper age limit for most babies is probably before 12 months" (1951, p. 49).

How important is the first attachment to a child's later capacity for relationships? Do infants and toddlers derive lifelong lessons from the experience of security—or its absence—that they experience in their first relationship with a caregiver? How are the enduring effects of early relationships enfolded into a young child's developing capacities for social understanding and relating? If infants and young children are denied the opportunity to form a close, loving relationship with a consistent caregiver, are their capacities to establish intimacy with another person later in life forever impaired?

These questions are theoretically and practically important, motivating considerable research during the latter part of the 20th century. Much of this inquiry has been guided by the formulations of attachment theory, which describes how infants develop their first attachments to caregivers and the immediate and long-term significance of these relationships (Ainsworth, 1973; Ainsworth, Blehar, Waters, & Wall, 1978; Bowlby, 1969/1982, 1973; Thompson, 1998). Some of this research has examined the effects of the deprivation of attachment that can occur in aberrant conditions of institutional child care or in experimental studies of maternal absence in primates. These studies provide initial answers to the question of whether sensitive periods exist for human attachment, and if so, what are their defining characteristics.

The purpose of this chapter is to summarize this research and its implications for current thinking about the importance of early attachment relationships and for sensitive periods in development. The chapter opens with a brief analysis of sensitive periods and why these are difficult to identify in socioemotional and personality development. Next, two sides to human attachment are distinguished. The first concerns *the opportunity to form an initial attachment to a caregiver*, and the second concerns *the quality or security of the initial attachment relationship*. The importance of distinguishing between the *formation* and the *security* of attachment relationships is discussed, and then research evidence concerning the existence of sensitive periods relevant to each of these facets of attachment is summarized. The chapter closes with a reconsideration of the usefulness of sensitive period concepts and introduces formulations from the field of developmental psychopathology as additional conceptual tools for thinking about the enduring influences of early experiences.

SENSITIVE PERIODS IN SOCIAL AND PERSONALITY DEVELOPMENT

Developmental psychologists have explored whether sensitive periods exist in social and personality development, which is consistent with our culture's long-standing belief in the importance of early care experiences. *Sensitive periods* can be defined as unique episodes in development when specific structures or functions become especially susceptible to particular experiences in ways that alter their future structure or function (Bornstein, 1989).

In developmental psychology generally, and especially in the study of social and personality development, the term *sensitive periods* is preferred to *critical periods* because it implies less rigidity in the nature of the formative early experiences, their developmental timing, and their developmental outcomes (Immelmann & Suomi, 1981). Although critical periods have been identified in research in the developmental neurosciences, as well as in ethology and embryology (from which this concept is borrowed), the multidetermination and complexity of early socioemotional growth processes make the identification of such critical periods particularly challenging. Consequently, the focus has shifted to the equally important but conceptually broader concept of sensitive periods. Sensitive periods, like critical periods, imply two important features about early development. First, certain early experiences uniquely prepare young children for the future by establishing certain capabilities at a time when development is most plastic and responsive to stimulation. Second, the child is highly vulnerable to the *absence* of these critical experiences, and the result may be permanent risk or dysfunction, such as an enduring deficit in physical ability.

One effort to identify sensitive periods in socioemotional development focused on the bonding that may occur between mother and infant immediately after birth. Based on comparative animal studies indicating that the initial moments after birth are important for maternal identification and acceptance of the young in certain animal species, Klaus and Kennell (1976, 1982) proposed that a similar postpartum sensitive period may exist for the establishment of adult emotional attachments to their newborns. Based partly on their views, perinatal hospital practices changed nationwide to permit a period of physical contact and focused interaction between newborn infants and their parents immediately after birth. However, research evidence did not support the view that the early postpartum period is a sensitive one for mother–infant bonding because few reliable, enduring consequences of the amount or quality of early contact could be determined (Eyer, 1992; Lamb & Hwang, 1982; Myers, 1984). Moreover, developmental researchers noted that many factors contribute to the strength of the mother–child bond besides the amount of context they share immediately after birth.

Sensitive periods in early social and personality development can be difficult to identify. Although the concept of sensitive periods is intuitively meaningful, scientific study of sensitive periods requires clarity about the timing, mechanisms, consequences, and modifiability of hypothesized periods of sensitive influence so they can be studied carefully and insightfully.

Bornstein (1989) has identified a variety of structural characteristics that define sensitive periods (see also Immelmann & Suomi, 1981; Knudsen, 1999). With respect to their *timing*, for example, Bornstein argues that developmental scientists must be able to identify

- Developmental dating: when the sensitive period occurs in the life course
- Onset and offset functions: the speed with which sensitivity to critical experiences increases (onset) and declines in sensitivity after the maximum level is achieved (offset); many critical periods are characterized by a rapid onset, but a subsequent gradual decline occurs in sensitivity after the peak is achieved (Knudsen, 1999)
- Duration of sensitivity: how long the individual remains sensitive to critical experiences
- Asymptote: changes or fluctuations in sensitivity to critical experiences during the sensitive period

Additional structural characteristics of sensitive periods concern the mechanisms by which behavior changes, including

- Experience: the specific qualities, duration, and intensity of the experiences triggering changes in the individual
- Outcome: the specific ways that an individual is changed through exposure to the critical experiences, when these changes occur in development, and the duration of these changes
- Mechanisms: the processes by which change occurs (e.g., hormonal, neural, anatomical)

Finally, some parameters of sensitive periods concern the flexibility of this developmental process, including

- Variability: the range and causes of variation, both within and among species, in the timing, quality, and outcome of critical experiences during a sensitive period
- Modifiability: the extent to which the timing and quality of critical experiences in a sensitive period can be changed (often experimentally) and the extent to which the behavioral changes deriving from critical experiences can be subsequently altered

Not surprisingly, few accounts of sensitive periods in development are capable of specifying many of these defining parameters. In many cases, systematic experimental investigations are necessary, while in other instances the relevant studies are ethically impermissible. Generalizing conclusions about sensitive periods across species can be hazardous. This makes the scientific study of sensitive periods a challenging task, even when developmental processes are studied at the most basic, intracellular level.

Additional challenges are encountered when sensitive period concepts are applied to early human socioemotional and personality development. This is because the growth of social and personality processes consists of the development, integration, and coordination of many complex behavioral systems, each with their own specific developmental timetables, activation and inhibitory influences, and interconnections to related behavioral processes. Complex systems that are encompassed within straightforward processes such as attachment and bonding include, for example, the coordination of multiple neural processes related to perception, memory, emotion, and other behavioral systems that also are associated with other complex psychological processes (e.g., mediating self-awareness, sociability with unfamiliar adults, exploration of the environment). Moreover, emerging socioemotional and personality capacities also develop transactionally over time through cumulative interactions between the young child and the environment in ways that alter both the child and the social world in which he or she lives (Thompson & Nelson, 2001). Thus, early personality and social growth can be regarded as complexly constructive, transactional, and emergent over time (Laible & Thompson, 2000).

For these reasons, while the metaphor of critical periods in the organization of neural systems in the visual cortex or of imprinting in lower species may offer an attractive heuristic to students of human development, the complexity of the behavioral systems to which these concepts are applied in young children makes it difficult, if not impossible, to identify the parameters of sensitive periods with appropriate specificity. This is particularly true of social and personality processes, like attachment, because of the complexity, integration, and intercoordination of the behavioral systems that constitute attachment.

UNDERSTANDING AND STUDYING HUMAN ATTACHMENT

Just as it is important to achieve a clear understanding of the meaning of sensitive period as it is applied to human development, it also is important to understand the meaning of attachment in infants and young children. Generally, *attachment* can be defined as the development of an affectionate relationship between a child and a specific caregiver that endures over time and place (Ainsworth, 1973). Infants typically begin to develop emotional ties to regular caregivers between 6 and 12 months of age as they are gradually constructing expectations for the behavior of other people (Gekoski, Rovee-Collier, & Carulli-Rabinowitz, 1983; Lamb & Malkin, 1986), becoming more socially competent (Fogel, 1993), and acquiring a dawning awareness of the psychological qualities of other people (Stern, 1985; Tomasello, Kruger, & Ratner, 1993). By the end of the first year, infants are clearly attached to one or more of their regular caregivers. Within this broad conceptualization, however, *attachment* can describe two facets of this developmental process: 1) the opportunity to initially create an affectional relationship to a caregiver, and 2) the quality of the affectional relationship that results, commonly portrayed as secure or insecure.

The distinction between these two facets of attachment is crucial. On one hand, virtually all infants in typical circumstances develop attachments to one or more caregivers. The incentives appear to be so deeply rooted in humans that, given the opportunity to interact regularly with even a modestly responsive caregiver, infants will develop emotional ties, especially if that person is the only available attachment figure. Only in aberrant conditions of care, such as extreme neglect or institutional deprivation, are young children denied the opportunity to form an attachment to anyone. On the other hand, once an attachment has developed, it can be secure or insecure in quality. Not all infants develop secure attachments to their caregivers. Some develop insecure attachments, characterized by avoidant uncertainty in the caregiver's responsiveness or angry resistance to that person (Ainsworth et al., 1978). Thus, young children vary considerably in the trust and confidence inspired by their attachments to their caregivers. *An insecure attachment is not, however, equivalent to no attachment at all.* Even though a young child may be uncertain—even doubtful—about the caregiver's nurturance and responsiveness, that child still derives important emotional support from the caregiver's presence that would not be derived from the company of someone to whom the child had no attachment at all (Ainsworth, 1967).

The distinction between the opportunity to develop an initial attachment relationship, and the security of that attachment, is important in considering sensitive periods in attachment. Different questions concerning critical early experiences are pertinent to each facet of attachment. For example, with respect to forming an initial attachment, one might inquire whether children who have been deprived of any opportunity to become attached in the early year(s) of life become incapable of developing close relationships with people at all. If the opportunity to develop an initial attachment relationship is significantly delayed, does this impair the quality of later relationships or other aspects of psychosocial functioning? If so, can later experiences help to ameliorate these difficulties? With respect to the security or insecurity of attachment, other questions might be posed. Once a young child has become securely attached to a caregiver, does that relationship remain secure in the years that follow? Does the security of a young child's initial attachment increase the probability that subsequent close relationships with other partners also will be trusting and secure?

Does early security or insecurity of attachment influence other aspects of psychosocial growth?

These questions are at the heart of understanding the importance of early experiences—and of relationships—to healthy early socioemotional growth. Because of this, there has been considerable research devoted to understanding the immediate and long-term effects of variations in the security of attachment in the early years of life. Researchers have developed and validated laboratory and parent-report measures to assess the security of early attachment relationships. On the basis of these measures, a large research literature concerning the consistency, correlates, and outcomes of secure or insecure attachments between young children and their caregivers has been generated (see Thompson, 1998, for a recent review; see also Cassidy & Shaver, 1999; Colin, 1996; Lamb, Thompson, Gardner, & Charnov, 1985). General conclusions concerning whether there are early sensitive periods, during which the development of secure or insecure attachment relationships has enduring consequences for psychological development, are reviewed in this chapter. Because attachments are typically developed by the end of the first year, it would be reasonable to expect that the experience of security (or insecurity) at that time has a formative influence on the child's capacities to develop close, secure relationships with others in the years to come.

By contrast, much less is known about young children who are denied any opportunity to create attachment relationships early in life. This is not surprising because such children are likely to be found in conditions of disadvantage and neglect in which their healthy psychosocial development is undermined by hazards other than relational deprivation. As a consequence, the conclusions of studies of children in neglect and institutional deprivation must be viewed in the context of other studies that experimentally deprive animals of the opportunity to form attachments to conspecifics. On the basis of these studies, it is possible to derive provisional conclusions about the importance of the formation of these attachments to healthy psychosocial growth.

BECOMING ATTACHED

Why is attachment important? To young children, an attachment figure inspires confidence that they are not alone in coping with the challenges of early experience. Even when the attachment is insecure, an attachment figure offers assistance in relief from distress, protection from unanticipated hazards while exploring, support when negotiating interactions with other people, responsiveness to the child's intentions and signals, the satisfaction of basic physical needs, and the opportunity for mutual affection. Thus, it is not surprising that attachment is related to many aspects of psychological growth, including exploration, self-concept, emotion regulation, and sociability with others (Colin, 1996; Lamb et al., 1985; Thompson, 1998).

Attachment also is important from the wider view of the human species. As Bowlby (1969/1982) initially theorized, and as later writers have elucidated (Belsky, Steinberg, & Draper, 1991; Chisholm, 1996, 1999; Lamb et al., 1985; Thompson, 1998), mother–infant attachment is a motivational system that ensures close contact between dependent human young and adult caregivers who can protect, nurture, and guide their development. It has functioned this way throughout the long history of human beings. Even when attachments are insecure, attachment relationships have helped to ensure the survival of infants and young children who might otherwise have been lost to predation, abandoned, or wandered away. Thus, attachment is an essential species-typical behavioral system for group-living mammals such as humans and other primates. To some theorists, early attachment relationships also provide significant environmental cues that influence subsequent development, including the timing of sexual maturity, pair bonding, and mature reproductive strategy (Belsky et al., 1991; Chisholm, 1999).

From these perspectives, there are good reasons to expect that the opportunity to develop an attachment relationship is an essential feature of early development for which a sensitive period might exist. Because sensitive (and critical) periods are meant to ensure that essential developmental accomplishments are achieved early in life, natural selection may have organized initial attachment formation as a behavioral system resembling a sensitive period. Such a system has a rapid developmental onset at 6–12 months of age during which the component cognitive and motor skills required for attachment are acquired (Ainsworth, 1973). By a child's first birthday, he or she is a highly motivated, animated social partner who responds preferentially to familiar caregivers (Thompson & Limber, 1990). This is when attachment relationships typically develop through a baby's regular interaction with a responsive, supportive caregiver. The emergence of a period of attachment-in-the-making during the last half of the first year of life is reflected in adoption studies that show that infants exhibit few adjustment difficulties if they are adopted before 6 months of age, but considerable stress results if adoption occurs after the first birthday (Yarrow & Goodwin, 1973). Although toddlers subsequently form additional new attachments to regular caregivers, the development of this initial attachment ensures that the essential protective, nurturant, and socializing functions of an attachment relationship are in place, and the child's capacities to socialize effectively with the caregiver and with other people are on track. In this sense, a young child who has formed an initial attachment relationship in infancy is fundamentally different from a child denied this opportunity.

This portrayal of the process of becoming attached is consistent with current research on early socioemotional growth (Thompson, 1998), but, fortunately, there is little research that would enable scholars to further test this quasi-sensitive period formulation. Such research must include young children who had been denied the opportunity to form an attachment relationship in the early years to identify the immediate and long-term consequences of this deprivation. Such studies also would enable researchers to understand whether infancy is a particularly crucial period for forming initial attachments or whether attachment relationships can develop later in childhood and, if so, whether they are developmentally adequate. Fortunately, it is rare to find human infants raised in conditions that prevent forming attachments—such child-rearing conditions are markedly species-*atypical* for humans—and when these conditions occur, young children are usually deprived of adequate nutrition, environmental stimulation, health care, and other necessities of adequate growth. It is difficult to determine whether the significant and enduring psychosocial difficulties children exhibit in these conditions can be attributed primarily to early relational deprivation. The effects of these conditions on subsequent attachment have not been systematically assessed (Rutter, 1981, 1995).

Two comprehensive longitudinal studies may, however, offer better insight into the consequences of early relational deprivation. In one study, a large sample of children who had been cared for in a residential nursery in their early years were studied at subsequent ages as the children were adopted, placed in foster care, or returned to their original biological parents (Tizard & Hodges, 1978; Tizard & Rees, 1975; Tizard & Tizard, 1971). The quality of care in the residential nurseries was excellent, but staff turnover and institutional policies, which discouraged discriminating relationships between caregivers and children, undermined the opportunity for close attachments to develop. By 2 years of age, for example, young children had been cared for by an average of 24 different adults, and by age 4, the average was 50 different caregivers. Based on this, it appears that opportunities to form attachments were limited, if not impossible.

Early follow-up studies of these children found that their social relationships were problematic. At age 2, for example, children in residential care tended to form broad emotional ties to a large number of adults (even some whom they had just met), and by age 4, children were characterized by indiscriminately friendly, attention-seeking behavior with adults and little wariness of strangers. Conduct and behavior problems also were apparent at ages 4 and 8. Even so, children who were adopted into warm, loving homes in childhood formed close attachments to their adoptive parents. By the time of the most recent follow-up at age 16, close attachments to substitute parents were true of the large majority of institution-reared children placed into adoptive homes, although continuing psychosocial difficulties (particularly concerning peer relationships) remained (Hodges & Tizard, 1989a, 1989b). In sum, the relational deprivation of early institutional care did not appear to impair the capacity of these children to develop close attachments to adults who were warm and responsive to them, even though some enduring psychosocial difficulties remained for these children.

These results suggest that a rather long period for the creation of initial attachments may exist for children who are denied the typical relational experiences of early care, but they are difficult to interpret in light of the quality of early care that children received in these British institutions. In fact, the children in the residential nurseries may have had opportunities to form early attachment relationships: Half of the children were visited regularly by their mothers, for example, and others had special relationships with particular caregivers at the residential nurseries who took a special interest in them (Tizard & Tizard, 1971). These young children also showed differential preferences for specific caregivers in the institutions, which is one of the hallmarks of an attachment relationship. Thus, it is unclear the extent to which relational deprivation—to the extent necessary to prevent early attachment relationships from developing—truly characterized young children's psychological experience in the residential nurseries.

This interpretive caution does not seem to apply to a second group of children who also have been studied longitudinally. With the overthrow of the Ceaucescu regime late in 1989, the plight of thousands of infants and young children in deplorable state-run orphanages in Romania elicited world attention, and concerted efforts were made to find adoptive homes for these children among families in the West. In the orphanages, child-to-caregiver ratios ranged from 10 to 1 for infants to as high as 20 to 1 for children older than age 3; children spent as many as 20 hours daily in their cribs; and custodial practices, as well as the attitudes of caregivers, further undermined the children's capacities to form emotional attachments to the adults who cared for them (Chisholm, Carter, Ames, & Morison, 1995; Rutter & the English and Romanian Adoptees Study Team, 1998). These children were raised in institutions of relational deprivation, as well as many other forms of neglect (see Chapter 7).

Fortunately, some of these children were adopted into supportive families in Canada, Great Britain, and other countries. Ames, Chisholm, and their colleagues have conducted follow-up investigations of children adopted to Canadian families 1–2 years following their adoption and again at 3 years after adoption (Chisholm, 1998; Chisholm et al., 1995). Based on parent-report measures and an observational procedure, each designed to measure parent–child attachment, these researchers sought to determine whether Romanian adoptees were capable of forming attachment relationships to their adoptive parents after early relational neglect and deprivation. Remarkably, no adoptees were discovered to be unattached to their adoptive parents, despite (for some) prolonged residence in the state-run orphanage. However, the quality of their attachment relationships varied significantly depending, in part, on the length of their orphanage residence. For a group of Romanian children who had been adopted early (i.e., before 4 months of age), the majority were able to develop secure attachments to their adoptive parents. For children who had been adopted after their first birthday or later, following a more prolonged period in the orphanage, the majority of attachments were insecure. Although some of the latter children were capable of warm, secure attachment relationships with their adoptive parents, one third of the late-adopted group exhibited attachment relationships characterized by atypical, sometimes bizarre and disorganized, insecurity.

What can account for these individual differences in the quality of attachment relationships among later-adopted children? Among other correlates, attachment security was associated with measures of parenting stress: Among the later-adopted children, parents reporting greater stress tended to have insecure relationships with their adopted children. Although the direction of effects is unclear, this finding suggests, consistent with the Tizard findings, that a secure attachment was more likely to occur when adoptive parents could offer children a warm, responsively supportive relationship (see Chapter 7). The duration of institutional deprivation that children experienced also was a predictor of their psychosocial difficulties (Fisher, Ames, Chisholm, & Savoie, 1997). Similar findings have been reported by other investigators studying the long-term outcomes of Romanian adoptees (Marcovitch et al., 1997; Rutter et al., 1998).

The research by Tizard, and Ames and Chisholm, indicated that there is certain flexibility to the attachment behavioral system in early development. Contrary to earlier studies indicating that early institutionalized children were incapable of developing attachments with substitute parents (Goldfarb, 1945a, 1945b; Spitz, 1945), these longitudinal studies each suggest that if children are deprived of developmentally appropriate early opportunities to form attachments in infancy, they remain capable of forming attachments when opportunities arise later in childhood. To be sure, they remain at considerable risk for insecure attachments, and these children also are vulnerable to other enduring behavior problems, as well as difficulties in peer relationships (Fisher et al., 1997). They also may require especially nurturant, responsive adoptive caregivers if they are to establish relational security later in childhood. But, the expanded window of opportunity for the creation of initial attachment relationships reflects, it seems, an adaptation of the attachment behavioral system to atypical rearing conditions, ensuring that children can benefit from whatever relational possibilities are offered them later in childhood. It is unknown how long this adaptive capability endures.

Experimental studies of attachment in nonhuman primates, which examine the consequences of far more deprived rearing conditions than those explored in the human studies, complement the findings of the adoption research. Beginning with the work of Harlow in the 1950s, comparative psychologists have conducted carefully designed investigations into the immediate and long-term effects of maternal deprivation and social isolation on the psychosocial functioning of primate infants and whether the consequences of relational deprivation can be later ameliorated (Suomi, 1982, 1991, 1999; see Chapter 6). Taken together, these studies show that isolation has devastating effects on social functioning that persist throughout adulthood, especially when isolation begins early in life and persists for at least 6 months. Even when infant monkeys are raised in conditions of substitute care, such as with peers, they still exhibit enduring difficulties in social functioning, show extreme stress responses to novel or challenging events, and are deficient in caring for their own offspring later in life. Remarkably, however, this research also indicates that the psychosocial damage of early relational deprivation can be reduced through carefully constructed regimens of social contact and species-typical social stimulation, although, despite these interventions, some enduring deficits in stress management remain. Thus, the psychosocial deficits of early deprivation need not necessarily endure, although concerted efforts are necessary to rehabilitate deprived monkeys to species-typical social functioning, and some lingering problems remain.

What can we conclude from these studies about the existence of a sensitive period for initial human attachment? By contrast with its reliable, rapid onset in infancy, the length of time during which young children are capable of developing a first attachment relationship is quite variable depending on the opportunities that exist for forming such a bond. Although infants normally consolidate their first attachment relationships by the first birthday, in atypical rearing conditions this period of attachment formation may be quite extended—at least to 4 or 5 years of age—when young children are deprived of early opportunities to become attached. Thus, the period of attachment-in-the-making (Bowlby, 1969/1982) has a rapid onset but a duration that can be extended when early relational deprivation occurs. This is consistent with sensitive periods for language, visual organization, and other neurodevelopmental processes that are extended in duration when individuals are deprived of crucial stimulation, although, as with attachment formation, enduring deficits may remain (Bornstein, 1989; Knudsen, 1999). Moreover, just as enhanced stimulation may be necessary to restore language functioning if it is acquired later than normal, unusually nurturant and supportive parental care may be necessary for young children to develop satisfactory first attachments after infancy. But the fact that attachment can develop at all after such a delay attests to the adaptability of this behavioral system. The attachment behavioral system resembles what Greenough and colleagues describe as experience-expectant brain development that is crucial to species-typical functioning and requires critical stimulation (e.g., responsive, supportive social contact) that is typically ubiquitous in early human experience (Greenough & Black, 1992; Greenough, Black, & Wallace, 1987). Natural selection appears to have made it possible for the first attachment to develop outside of the species-typical period in which it typically emerges.

But extending the sensitive period exacts a cost. Because initial attachments are important for other early developmental processes—including the growth of social competence, self-representation, exploratory motivation, self-regulation, and other capabilities—a significant delay in attachment formation causes allied processes of psychosocial development to be delayed or to develop in atypical or aberrant ways. Over time, a cumulation of psychosocial deficits in emotion regulation, self-concept, and other facets of psychological growth is likely because of the cumulative, transactional quality of early development. These deficits may endure even when the young child is eventually provided the opportunity to develop an initial attachment relationship and are likely to occur if the conditions contributing to early relational deprivation are associated with other risks to healthy psychosocial development (as is true of the orphanage studies). Moreover, the quality of the attachment relationship itself may be impaired by the compounding psychosocial problems that accompany its delayed development. This means that although a capacity to form an attachment endures, healthy psychological growth is imperiled because many features of early psychosocial development depend on the developmentally appropriate timing of the formation of an attachment relationship. This, too, is consistent with sensitive period formulations that indicate that, although early deprivation of critical stimulation can extend the period of sensitivity, enduring deficits may nevertheless remain.

This is a speculative account of how initial attachment formation may resemble, in some respects, a sensitive period for human development. It fails to specify many of the parameters required for sensitive period formulations described previously in the chapter, and many gaps remain in understanding the nature of the specific social experiences required to form an attachment, how the child is changed as a result of becoming attached, and the underlying (e.g., neural, hormonal) mechanisms by which these changes occur. Perhaps most important, there is no reliable research indicating when the period of potential attachment-in-the-making ever closes, which is necessary to understand if the development of attachment resembles a sensitive period. Even so, this formulation may have useful applications to how practitioners and researchers think about early attachment in conditions of deprivation and disadvantage for young children. For example, clinically relevant disorders of attachment in infancy and early childhood may be related not only to the delay or deprivation in the opportunity to form an attachment but to the variety of allied psychological capacities that are altered in the absence of an early attachment relationship (Lieberman & Zeanah, 1995; Zeanah, Mammen, & Lieberman, 1993). Moreover, the quality of care necessary for the development of satisfactory attachment relationships in infancy may be inadequate for fostering secure attachment at later ages. First attachments formed later in childhood may require unusually sensitive, responsive parenting if they are to be developmentally adequate. Thus, the portrayal of attachment formation as resembling a quasi-sensitive period sheds new light on early psychosocial growth and raises many important questions that are catalysts for future research inquiry.

SECURITY OF ATTACHMENT

The studies of children in residential nurseries or Romanian orphanages, or rhesus monkeys raised in isolation, suggest additional reasons why attachment is central to healthy psychological functioning. There are at least two important contributions that an attachment relationship offers to psychological growth.

First, an attachment figure reduces a young child's fear or anxiety in novel or challenging situations through social contact, soothing, or other interventions and thus promotes the child's confidence in exploring the environment (what is commonly described as "secure base behavior"). Attachment contributes to exploratory self-confidence and the growth of stress management, perhaps as the relationship buffers the developing brain against the potentially deleterious effects of stress hormones on developing neural tissue (Gunnar, Broderson, Nachmias, Buss, & Rigatuso, 1996). This is the *emotion regulation* function of attachment relationships.

Second, by responding promptly and appropriately to the child's intentions, signals, and needs, the attachment figure strengthens a young child's sense of competence and efficacy. A caregiver's responsiveness contributes to the delight of social interaction, and it also contributes to relieving distress and reducing anxiety. In each case, the caregiver's behavior strengthens a child's sense of confidence in the responsiveness of another to the child's signals. This is the *self-efficacy* function of attachment relationships.

This view of attachment relationships suggests that the critical social experiences required for the development of an attachment relationship must include 1) a young child's regular interaction with a discriminated person, 2) experiences of positive social reciprocity with that person, and 3) that person's efficacy in managing the child's fear or anxiety in difficult circumstances. These experiences are lost in social isolation and also in the perfunctory caregiving activities of the adults in the Romanian orphanages and, quite possibly, in the residential nurseries.

Caregivers vary in how well they manage a young child's distress, reciprocate a child's social initiatives, and respond appropriately to the child's signals. Many factors influence their behavior (e.g., social stress, personality, competing demands), but from the child's perspective the adult's reliable support inspires confidence in the caregiver's future assistance, while inconsistent or poor responsiveness reduces this sense of security. According to attachment theorists, the adult's sensitivity inspires a secure attachment, while insensitivity contributes to the development of an insecure attachment relationship (Ainsworth, 1973; Ainsworth et al., 1978; Bowlby, 1969/1982; Isabella, 1995; Thompson, 1998).

How important is the security of early attachment for a child's later social and personality functioning? Does an attachment relationship tend to remain secure or insecure over time? Does the security of the initial attachment relationship render the child more likely to trust others in close relationships? These questions reveal another manner in which sensitive period formulations can be applied to human attachment. In contrast to asking whether there is a sensitive period for the *formation* of an initial attachment relationship, these questions ask whether there is a sensitive period for the *quality* of initial attachment such that early security or insecurity has enduring consequences for psychosocial development.

Because infants typically become attached to their caregivers, it has been much easier to study these questions than those concerned with the effects of early relational deprivation. There is broad research literature concerned with two questions that are central to understanding the enduring effects of early secure or insecure attachments. First, once an attachment relationship is secure or insecure in quality, does it tend to remain that way over time? If a sensitive period governs the security of initial attachment, a securely attached child should remain that way with the same caregiver over time. Second, does a secure or insecure attachment predict other important features of a child's psychological growth? If a sensitive period governs early attachment security, then securely attached children should be fundamentally different from insecurely attached children in other psychosocial outcomes, such as their capacities for forming close relationships or getting along with other people.

CONSISTENCY AND CHANGE IN THE SECURITY OF ATTACHMENT

Many research studies have been designed to examine whether securely or insecurely attached children tend to remain that way with the same partner over time, using well-validated procedures that assess the security of attachment through laboratory observations, parent-report measures, or (with older children and adults) self-report instruments. A review of this research concluded that there is no normative level of consistency in the security of attachment (Thompson, 1998, 2000). In other words, sometimes a child's attachment security endures over time and sometimes it changes.

The changes, as well as the consistencies, in attachment security can be striking. For example, for 2 decades developmental researchers have examined the short-term consistency in the security of attachment of infants observed in the Strange Situation, a well-validated laboratory procedure designed to assess attachment relationships in infants and toddlers (Ainsworth et al., 1978). They were inspired by an initial report by Waters (1978) that when 50 infants were observed in this procedure at 12 and 18 months of age, 96% were consistently either securely or insecurely attached at each age. But the most recent report using this procedure found that only about half the infants observed over the same 6-month period were consistent in their attachment security at each age (Belsky, Campbell, Cohn, & Moore, 1996). Over longer periods of time, the same variability in the consistency of attachment security is apparent (Main & Cassidy, 1988; Wartner, Grossmann, Fremmer-Bombik, & Suess, 1994; Zimmermann, Fremmer-Bombik, Spangler, & Grossmann, 1997).

What determines whether the security of attachment remains consistent over time or changes? Because a secure attachment denotes the quality of a parent–child relationship, factors that change how parents and children interact with each other can influence attachment security (Thompson, 1998). These can include typical family events, such as changes in parents' employment commitments, altered child care arrangements, the birth of a sibling, or moving to a new home. They can include more atypical family events, such as marital separation or divorce. Parent–child relationships also can change in response to developmental changes in the child, such as how a toddler's insistence on "doing it myself" or a young preschooler's self-assertion can impose different demands on parental sensitivity than what was required when the child was an infant. Sometimes the influences on attachment security can be complex and multifaceted. In one study, for example, Teti, Sakin, Kucera, Corns, and Das Eiden (1996) found that attachment security in first-born preschoolers decreased following the birth of a new sibling, but the children whose security dropped most dramatically had mothers with significantly greater depression or anger compared with other mothers.

There are other influences associated with whether initial security is maintained over time. There is research indicating that children from disadvantaged circumstances are likely to carry the effects of relational security into their later years. Children who initially are securely attached are more likely than insecurely attached children to remain consistent in later assessments. Unfortunately, however, there is little systematic research into the causes and correlates of changes in attachment in the early years. It has become increasingly clear that although some young children maintain early relational influences into their later years while others change significantly, better understanding of these influences on attachment security is essential.

SECURITY OF ATTACHMENT AND LATER BEHAVIOR

A secure or insecure attachment is important not only as an indicator of the early parent–child relationship, but it is believed to influence emergent self-representation, social skills and dispositions, personality development, and self-regulation. The influences of attachment security increasingly characterize the child, not just the relationship with the parent. Consequently, as children mature it is appropriate to consider whether securely attached children differ from insecurely attached children in their psychosocial characteristics. In this regard, researchers have inquired whether early attachment security has a formative effect on other aspects of socioemotional and personality functioning. If a sensitive period governs early security of attachment, it would be reasonable to expect that it does.

Because of the importance of these questions, there have been many studies examining the correlates and consequences of attachment security in infancy or early childhood. Comprehensive reviews of this research literature have reached several conclusions (Thompson, 1998, 1999, 2000). First, the associations between attachment and other behavior measured at the *same age* are much stronger than are the associations between attachment and *subsequent* behavior. Attachment security has been associated with concurrent measures of self-concept, emotional understanding, peer relations, and personality, although attachment security is a much less reliable predictor of these characteristics in the future. This is not surprising as longitudinal relations between attachment and later behavior may be altered by the influences of intervening events and new developmental challenges for the child. But correlational, concurrent associations between attachment security and other behavior cannot, of course, establish causal pathways. Studies of the correlates of attachment security provide little insight into whether a secure attachment has a formative influence on the development of other features of psychosocial growth.

Second, a secure attachment best foreshadows a more positive parent–child relationship in the years that follow, and securely attached children also may be more successful in other close relationships. In a sense, a secure attachment relationship inaugurates what Maccoby (1983, 1984) has called a "mutual interpersonal orientation of positive reciprocity" between parent and child that heightens the child's receptiveness to the parent's socialization incentives in the years that follow (Kochanska & Thompson, 1997; Waters, Kondo-Ikemura, Posada, & Richters, 1991). Securely attached children also appear to develop more positive, supportive relationships with teachers, friends, camp counselors, and others whom they come to know later in life. Although there is some evidence that securely attached children also interact more positively with unfamiliar partners, it is in the context of close relationships that children most clearly exhibit the positive relational expectations that are inspired by a secure parent–child relationship or, in the case of insecurely attached children, their relational distrust or ambivalence. Research has, however, revealed few reliable personality characteristics that are predicted by an early secure or insecure attachment. Although some studies reveal that a secure attachment is associated with features like ego resiliency and insecure attachment with behavior problems, others have failed to replicate these associations.

Third, the consequences of attachment security appear to wane over time. The evidence that a secure attachment foreshadows a more positive later parent–child relationship is strongest, for example, in follow-up assessments 1 or 2 years following the attachment assessment, and there is little prediction to parent–child relationships several years later. Thus, the influence of attachment security diminishes over time as intervening events also influence developmental pathways. To be certain, some longitudinal studies find that attachment in infancy modestly predicts much later behavior, even after the influence of intervening events is considered (Sroufe, Egeland, & Kreutzer, 1990). The weight of the evidence suggests, however, that the infant–parent relationship has more significant immediate and short-term effects than it does long-term consequences for psychosocial functioning.

These conclusions indicate that early attachment security is developmentally important, but in a more circumscribed manner than traditional formulations have suggested (Thompson, 1998, 1999, 2000). The early experiences of sensitive parental care leading to a secure attachment are significant influences in psychosocial growth, but so are later experiences that also shape socioemotional and personality development. Social dispositions, personality features like ego resiliency, and the emergence of behavior problems in childhood are influenced not only by the security of early attachment relationships but also by a variety of other developmental influences as the child matures (Sroufe, Carlson, Levy, & Egeland, 1999). Moreover, while some characteristics of the child (e.g., sociability) may be shaped by the early influence of a secure or insecure attachment, others (e.g., self-image) may be guided primarily by developmental influences that emerge after the first attachment develops. In this respect, the early experiences contributing to attachment security may be a foundation for certain social and personality competencies, but not others that require more sophisticated mental representations and self-understanding (Caspi, 1998; Thompson, 1998). Finally, it is important to remember early childhood is characterized by many relationships within and outside the family, including attachments to regular baby sitters, child care teachers, and extended family. Each of these attachment relationships may influence a child's psychosocial growth in specific ways, and multiple attachments are likely to have influences that are sometimes overlapping or conflicting, depending on a child's specific experiences with each partner. Developmental researchers have the important challenge of understanding how these diverse relational influences are integrated as they influence a young child's psychosocial functioning.

As a result of these studies, the central questions of attachment research have shifted from a concern with formative early influences to an interest in the integration of attachment with other developing influences on a child's life (Sroufe et al., 1999). Instead of asking, "Does the security of early attachment have long-term consequences?" developmental scientists are instead inquiring, "In what circumstances do the effects of early attachment relationships endure, and in what conditions are they more transient?"

What can we conclude about the existence of a sensitive period for the security of initial attachment relationships? It is doubtful that early attachment security or insecurity influences subsequent development in a manner resembling a sensitive period. Although the development of a secure or insecure parent–child relationship is clearly important, its broader consequences for psychosocial growth are provisional, contingent on many other influences on psychosocial growth as well as continuity or change in the parent–child relationship itself. Fortunately, a child whose initial attachment is insecure is not destined for later psychosocial difficulty because of the multidetermination of developmental outcomes. Equally important, an initial secure attachment does not buffer the young child against the challenges and stresses that also are part of human growth. In each case, the initial attachment provides a provisional foundation for the growth of later psychosocial competencies in the years to come. Subsequent experiences may build on, or alter, this initial developmental pathway. The first attachment relationship may constitute a prototype for close relationships for a few years but not for a lifetime.

FUTURE DIRECTIONS

Inevitably, the complexity of the issue of sensitive periods in attachment relationships has highlighted many new questions requiring much-needed research. With respect to the formation of an initial attachment relationship, it remains unclear how long children remain capable of developing their first attachment if they are initially deprived of an opportunity to do so and how the delay in attachment formation has detrimental effects on other aspects of sociopersonality functioning. With respect to the security or insecurity of attachment, it is unclear why changes occur in attachment relationships, why greater continuity exists for some children than for others, and the ways that attachment interacts with other developmental influences to shape psychosocial growth. While much is known about attachment development, there is a significant agenda for future research.

It appears clear, however, that although the security of attachment is developmentally important, it does not influence psychosocial growth as a sensitive period. Moreover, it is still unclear whether a sensitive period governs the formation of initial attachment relationships. The uncertainty in applying sensitive period formulations to the process of attachment development underscores the complexity of socioemotional and personality development. It also underscores the value of considering less deterministic models of early developmental influences that emphasize the probabilistic and predispositional, rather than formative, effects of early experiences.

Alternative approaches to understanding the influences of early experiences can be found in the field of developmental psychopathology (Cicchetti, 1990; Cicchetti & Cohen, 1995; Sroufe & Rutter, 1984). Because they view children at psychological risk as developing persons, developmental psychopathologists are especially interested in understanding the enduring impact of early experiences and the prediction of long-term developmental outcomes in children. Contrary to deterministic models of early influences, however, they tend to emphasize the effects of *cumulative and transactional risks* that have a progressive influence on psychosocial growth over time. Developmental psychopathologists argue that single risk factors or disadvantages occurring early in life are rarely determinative of later problems, but risks are important as they inaugurate processes by which disadvantages cumulate for the developing child. Developmental psychopathologists also emphasize understanding *risks in relation to protections*, recognizing that protective factors may exist within the child (e.g., temperamental resiliency) or in the child's ecology (e.g., social support) that can buffer the influence of risk factors. The principle of *equifinality* notes that multiple pathways can lead to any psychological problem and the complementary principle of *multifinality* underscores that any particular risk factor can lead to diverse outcomes in developing children (Cicchetti & Rogosch, 1997). Finally, developmental psychopathologists underscore the *plurality of developmental influences* within and surrounding the child and the importance of considering their direct and indirect effects on psychosocial growth.

Understanding the growth of attachment relationships seems better informed by developmental models that emphasize the probabilistic and predispositional rather than deterministic influences of early experiences. Such approaches to development show that psychosocial development is rarely the result of critical, single turning points early in life, but rather the cumulative effects of multiple influences on the young child.

REFERENCES

Ainsworth, M.D.S. (1967). *Infancy in Uganda: Infant care and the growth of love*. Baltimore: Johns Hopkins University Press.

Ainsworth, M.D.S. (1973). The development of infant-mother attachment. In B. Caldwell & H. Ricciuti (Eds.), *Review of child development research, 3,* 1–94. Chicago: University of Chicago Press.

Ainsworth, M.D.S., Blehar, M.C., Waters, E., & Wall, S. (1978). *Patterns of attachment*. Mahwah, NJ: Lawrence Erlbaum Associates.

Belsky, J., Campbell, S.B., Cohn, J.F., & Moore, G. (1996). Instability of infant-parent attachment security. *Developmental Psychology, 32,* 921–924.

Belsky, J., Steinberg, L., & Draper, P. (1991). Childhood experience, interpersonal development, and reproductive strategy: An evolutionary theory of socialization. *Child Development, 62,* 647–670.

Bornstein, M.H. (1989). Sensitive periods in development: Structural characteristics and causal interpretations. *Psychological Bulletin, 105,* 179–197.

Bowlby, J. (1951). Maternal care and mental health. *World Health Organization Monograph Series, 2,* 49. Geneva, Switzerland: World Health Organization.

Bowlby, J. (1973). *Attachment and loss: Vol. 2. Separation*. New York: Basic Books.

Bowlby, J. (1982). *Attachment and loss: Vol. 1. Attachment* (2nd ed.). New York: Basic Books. (Originally published in 1969)

Caspi, A. (1998). Personality development across the life course. In W. Damon (Ed.) & N. Eisenberg (Vol. Ed.), *Handbook of child psychology: Vol. 3. Social, emotional, and personality development* (5th ed., pp. 311–388). New York: John Wiley & Sons.

Cassidy, J., & Shaver, P. (1999). *Handbook of attachment: Theory, research, and clinical applications*. New York: The Guilford Press.

Chisholm, J.S. (1996). The evolutionary ecology of attachment organization. *Human Nature, 1,* 1–37.

Chisholm, J.S. (1999). *Death, hope, and sex: Steps to an evolutionary ecology of mind and morality*. New York: Cambridge University Press.

Chisholm, K. (1998). A three year follow-up of attachment and indiscriminate friendliness in children adopted from Romanian orphanages. *Child Development,* 69, 1092–1106.

Chisholm, K., Carter, M.C., Ames, E.W., & Morison, S.J. (1995). Attachment security and indiscriminately friendly behavior in children adopted from Romanian orphanages. *Development and Psychopathology,* 7, 283–294.

Cicchetti, D. (1990). The organization and coherence of socioemotional, cognitive, and representational development: Illustrations through a developmental psychopathology perspective on Down syndrome and child maltreatment. In R. Thompson (Ed.), *Socioemotional development. Nebraska Symposium on Motivation, 36,* 259–336. Lincoln: University of Nebraska Press.

Cicchetti, D., & Cohen, D.J. (1995). Perspectives on developmental psychopathology. In D. Cicchetti & D.J. Cohen (Eds.), *Developmental psychopathology. Vol. 1. Theory and methods* (pp. 3–20). New York: John Wiley & Sons.

Cicchetti, D., & Rogosh, F.A. (1997). Equifinality and multifinality in developmental psychopathology. *Development and Psychopathology, 8*, 597–600.

Colin, V.L. (1996). *Human attachment*. New York: McGraw-Hill.

Erikson, E.H. (1963). *Childhood and society* (2nd ed.). New York: Norton.

Eyer, D. (1992). *Maternal-infant bonding: A scientific fiction*. New Haven: Yale University Press.

Fisher, L., Ames, E.W., Chisholm, K., & Savoie, L. (1997). Problems reported by parents of Romanian orphans adopted to British Columbia. *International Journal of Behavioral Development, 20*, 67–82.

Fogel, A. (1993). *Developing through relationships*. Chicago: University of Chicago Press.

Freud, S. (1940). *An outline of psychoanalysis*. New York: Norton.

Gekoski, M.J., Rovee-Collier, C.K., & Carulli-Rabinowitz, V. (1983). A longitudinal analysis of inhibition of infant distress: The origins of social expectations? *Infant Behavior and Development, 6*, 339–351.

Goldfarb, W. (1945a). Psychological privation in infancy and subsequent adjustment. *American Journal of Orthopsychiatry, 14*, 247–255.

Goldfarb, W. (1945b). Effects of psychological deprivation in infancy and subsequent stimulation. *American Journal of Psychiatry, 102*, 18–33.

Greenough, W.T., & Black, J.R. (1992). Induction of brain structure by experience: Substrates for cognitive development. In M.R. Gunnar & C.A. Nelson (Eds.), *Developmental behavioral neuroscience: Vol. 24. The Minnesota Symposia on Child Psychology* (pp. 155–200). Mahwah, NJ: Lawrence Erlbaum Associates.

Greenough, W.T., Black, J.R., & Wallace, C.S. (1987). Experience and brain development. *Child Development, 58*, 539–559.

Gunnar, M., Broderson, L., Nachmias, M., Buss, K., & Rigatuso, J. (1996). Stress reactivity and attachment security. *Developmental Psychobiology, 29*, 191–204.

Hodges, J., & Tizard, B. (1989a). IQ and behavioural adjustment of ex-institutional adolescents. *Journal of Child Psychology and Psychiatry, 30*, 53–75.

Hodges, J., & Tizard, B. (1989b). Social and family relationships of ex-institutional adolescents. *Journal of Child Psychology and Psychiatry, 30*, 77–97.

Immelmann, K., & Suomi, S.J. (1981). Sensitive phases in development. In K. Immelmann, G.W. Barlow, L. Petrinovich, & M. Main (Eds.), *Behavioral development: The Bielefeld Interdisciplinary Project* (pp. 395–431). Cambridge, UK: Cambridge University Press.

Isabella, R.A. (1995). The origins of infant-mother attachment: Maternal behavior and infant development. In R. Vasta (Ed.), *Annals of child development, 10*, 57–82. London: Jessica Kingsley.

Klaus, M.H., & Kennell, J.H. (1976). *Maternal-infant bonding: The impact of early separation or loss on family development*. St. Louis: Mosby.

Klaus, M.H., & Kennell, J.H. (1982). *Parent-infant bonding*. St. Louis: Mosby.

Knudsen, E.I. (1999). Early experience and critical periods. In M.J. Zigmond, F.E. Bloom, S.C. Landis, J.L. Roberts, & L.R. Squire (Eds.), *Fundamental neuroscience* (pp. 637–654). New York: Academic Press.

Kochanska, G., & Thompson, R.A. (1997). The emergence and development of conscience in toddlerhood and early childhood. In J.E. Grusec & L. Kuczynski (Eds.), *Parenting and children's internalization of values* (pp. 53–77). New York: John Wiley & Sons.

Laible, D.J., & Thompson, R.A. (2000). Attachment and self-organization. In M.D. Lewis & I. Granic (Eds.), *Emotion, development, and self-organization: Dynamic systems approaches to emotional development* (pp. 298–323). New York: Cambridge University Press.

Lamb, M.E., & Hwang, C.P. (1982). Maternal attachment and mother-neonate bonding: A critical review. In M.E. Lamb & A.L. Brown (Eds.), *Advances in developmental psychology, 2,* 1–39. Mahwah, NJ: Lawrence Erlbaum Associates.

Lamb, M.E., & Malkin, C.M. (1986). The development of social expectations in distress relief sequences: A longitudinal study. *International Journal of Behavioral Development, 9,* 235–249.

Lamb, M.E., Thompson, R.A., Gardner, W., & Charnov, E.L. (1985). *Infant-mother attachment.* Mahwah, NJ: Lawrence Erlbaum Associates.

Lieberman, A.F., & Zeanah, C.H. (1995). Disorders of attachment in infancy. *Child and Adolescent Psychiatric Clinics of North America, 4,* 571–587.

Maccoby, E.E. (1983). Let's not overattribute to the attribution process: Comments on social cognition and behavior. In E.T. Higgins, D.N. Ruble, & W.W. Hartup (Eds.), *Social cognition and social development* (pp. 356–370). New York: Cambridge University Press.

Maccoby, E.E. (1984). Socialization and developmental change. *Child Development, 55,* 317–328.

Main, M., & Cassidy, J. (1988). Categories of response to reunion with the parent at age 6: Predictable from infant attachment classifications and stable over a 1-month period. *Developmental Psychology, 24,* 415–426.

Marcovitch, S., Goldberg, S., Gold, A., Washington, J., Wasson, C., Krewich, K., & Handley Derry, M. (1997). Determinants of behavioural problems in Romanian children adopted in Ontario. *International Journal of Behavioral Development, 20,* 17–31.

Myers, B.J. (1984). Mother-infant bonding: The status of the critical period hypothesis. *Developmental Review, 4,* 240–274.

Rutter, M. (1981). *Maternal deprivation reassessed* (2nd ed.). Harmondsworth, England: Penguin.

Rutter, M. (1995). Maternal deprivation. In M.H. Bornstein (Ed.), *Handbook of parenting: Vol. 4. Applied and practical parenting* (pp. 3–31). Mahwah, NJ: Lawrence Erlbaum Associates.

Rutter, M., & the English and Romanian Adoptees (ERA) Study Team (1998). Developmental catch-up, and deficit, following adoption after severe global early privation. *Journal of Child Psychology and Psychiatry, 39,* 465–476.

Spitz, R.A. (1945). An inquiry into the genesis of psychiatric conditions in early childhood. I. Hospitalism. *Psychoanalytic Study of the Child, 1,* 53–74.

Sroufe, L.A., Carlson, E.A., Levy, A.K., & Egeland, B. (1999). Implications of attachment theory for developmental psychopathology. *Development and Psychopathology, 11,* 1–13.

Sroufe, L.A., Egeland, B., & Kreutzer, T. (1990). The fate of early experience following developmental change: Longitudinal approaches to individual adaptation in childhood. *Child Development, 61,* 1363–1373.

Sroufe, L.A., & Rutter, M. (1984). The domain of developmental psychopathology. *Child Development, 55,* 17–29.

Stern, D.N. (1985). *The interpersonal world of the infant.* New York: Basic Books.

Suomi, S.J. (1982). Abnormal behavior and primate models of psychopathology. In J.L. Fobe & J.E. King (Eds.), *Primate behavior* (pp. 171–215). New York: Academic Press.

Suomi, S.J. (1991). Early stress and adult emotional reactivity in rhesus monkeys. In G. Bock & J. Whelan (Eds.), *The childhood environment and adult disease* (Ciba Foundation Symposium 156) (pp. 171–188). Chichester, UK: John Wiley & Sons.

Suomi, S.J. (1999). Attachment in rhesus monkeys. In J. Cassidy & P.R. Shaver (Eds.), *Handbook of attachment: Theory, research, and clinical applications* (pp. 181–197). New York: The Guilford Press.

Teti, D.M., Sakin, J., Kucera, E., Corns, K.M., & Das Eiden, R. (1996). And baby makes four: Predictors of attachment security among preschool-aged firstborns during the transition to siblinghood. *Child Development, 67*, 579–596.

Thompson, R.A. (1998). Early sociopersonality development. In W. Damon (Ed.) & N. Eisenberg (Vol. Ed.), *Handbook of child psychology: Vol. 3. Social, emotional, and personality development* (5th ed., pp. 25–104). New York: John Wiley & Sons.

Thompson, R.A. (1999). Early attachment and later development. In J. Cassidy & P. Shaver (Eds.), *Handbook of attachment: Theory, research, and clinical applications* (pp. 265–286). New York: The Guilford Press.

Thompson, R.A. (2000). The legacy of early attachments. *Child Development, 71*, 145–152.

Thompson, R.A., & Limber, S. (1990). "Social anxiety" in infancy: Stranger wariness and separation distress. In H. Leitenberg (Ed.), *Handbook of social and evaluation anxiety* (pp. 85–137). New York: Kluwer Academic/Plenum Publishers.

Thompson, R.A., & Nelson, C.A. (in press). Developmental science and the media: Early brain development. *American Psychologist.*

Tizard, B., & Hodges, J. (1978). The effect of early institutional rearing on the development of eight-year-old children. *Journal of Child Psychology and Psychiatry, 19*, 99–118.

Tizard, B., & Rees, J. (1975). The effect of early institutional rearing on the behaviour problems and affectional relationships of four-year-old children. *Journal of Child Psychology and Psychiatry, 16*, 61–73.

Tizard, J., & Tizard, B. (1971). The social development of 2-year-old children in residential nurseries. In H.E. Schaffer (Ed.), *The origins of human social relations* (pp. 147–163). New York: Academic Press.

Tomasello, M., Kruger, A.C., & Ratner, H.H. (1993). Cultural learning. *Behavioral and Brain Sciences, 16*, 495–511.

Wartner, U.G., Grossmann, K., Fremmer-Bombik, E., & Suess, G. (1994). Attachment patterns at age six in South Germany: Predictability from infancy and implications for preschool behavior. *Child Development, 65*, 1014–1027.

Waters, E. (1978). The reliability and stability of individual differences in infant-mother attachment. *Child Development, 49*, 483–494.

Waters, E., Kondo-Ikemura, K., Posada, G., & Richters, J.E. (1991). Learning to love: Mechanisms and milestones. In M.R. Gunnar & L.A. Sroufe (Eds.), *Minnesota Symposia on Child Psychology: Vol. 23. Self-processes and development* (pp. 217–255). Mahwah, NJ: Lawrence Erlbaum Associates.

Yarrow, L.J., & Goodwin, M.S. (1973). The immediate impact of separation: Reactions of infants to a change in mother figure. In L.J. Stone, H.T. Smith, & L.B. Murphy (Eds.), *The competent infant* (pp. 1032–1040). New York: Basic Books.

Zeanah, C.H., Jr., Mammen, O.K., & Lieberman, A.F. (1993). Disorders of attachment. In C.H. Zeanah, Jr. (Ed.), *Handbook of infant mental health* (pp. 332–349). New York: The Guilford Press.

Zimmermann, P., Fremmer-Bombik, E., Spangler, G., & Grossmann, K.E. (1997). Attachment in adolescence: A longitudinal perspective. In W. Koops, J.B. Hoeksma, & D.C. van den Boom (Eds.), *Development of interaction and attachment: Traditional and non-traditional approaches* (pp. 281–292). Amsterdam: North-Holland.

6

Animal Models of Critical and Sensitive Periods in Social and Emotional Development

Maria L. Boccia
Cort Pedersen

CRITICAL PERIODS IN ANIMAL BEHAVIOR

Ethology, the study of animal behavior, is distinguished from comparative psychology by its roots in and emphasis on biology (Hinde, 1982). Konrad Lorenz, one of the founders of ethology, introduced the concept of a critical period into the study of behavior. He adapted the term from embryology to describe the phenomenon in which newborns of certain species of birds learn the characteristics of their species and develop a preference for an individual to whom they are exposed during a restricted period of time following hatching. Because subsequent research demonstrated greater flexibility in this type of learning than Lorenz originally proposed, many have switched to terms such as sensitive period, optimal phase, or window of opportunity.

In ethology, the study of bird song acquisition has been an intense focus of research for several decades. This research has helped define the application of critical periods to behavior development and has revealed interesting patterns of variability in the features of critical periods across species (Petrinovich, 1998). For example, some species can acquire new songs throughout their lives, while others are restricted to a more or less brief period in infancy. Some species must hear the song of an adult male of their own species during the critical period in order to acquire song, while others can develop species-typical song if they are exposed to a different species' adult song. Others need only to hear the sound of their own voice practicing to develop normal, species-typical song. These studies show that caution must be taken when discussing critical periods. Generalizations across species can be difficult and must be done after comparative research empirically documents the differences and similarities.

One area of human development that has received a great deal of comparative study is in the area of attachment and social and emotional development (see Chapter 5). Bowlby introduced ethological concepts and methods through his attachment theory. Comparative studies with non-primate and primate animals have provided information that has suggested features that are similar and dissimilar across human and nonhuman species. This chapter describes some of the most common animal models used to investigate critical periods in attachment and socioemotional development. Animal models may be particularly valuable in elucidating the neurobiological underpinnings of behavior and for studying how experience impacts these biological systems to produce long-term consequences. Following an introduction to the value and limitations of animal models, this chapter reviews the history of the study of critical periods in animal behavior. An overview of the significant findings in two animal models is provided, examining the role of early experience and possible critical periods in development, utilizing a rodent model and a nonhuman primate model. The chapter concludes with observations about the continuing value and limitations of using animal models in the study of critical periods.

INTRODUCTION TO THE CONCEPT OF ANIMAL MODELS

Animal models have been used with great effect in studying different phenomena in development (Sackett & Gould, 1991). Using animal models allows for greater experimental control, as well as control over and information about the early experiences and history of the organism being studied (Abramson & Seligman, 1977). Confounding variables typically observed in human research (e.g., health behaviors, drug abuse, smoking, prior experience, behavior outside the experimental setting) can be eliminated or studied systematically with animal models. Longitudinal studies can be conducted within feasible time scales and budgets because of the shorter life span of most species used as animal models. Furthermore, it is less problematic, depending on the species used as the model, to conduct certain types of research that would be ethically questionable or impossible with humans.

Criteria must be established, however, to evaluate the usefulness of any proposed animal model. Developmental psychopathologists have developed a set of four criteria that may be adapted to other domains of research

(McKinney, 1984; McKinney & Bunney, 1969; Suomi & Harlow, 1977). These criteria include symptoms, postulated etiology, neurobiological mechanisms, and treatment responses. Symptoms refer to the behavioral phenomena under study: Are the symptoms (behaviors) in the animal model the same as the symptoms in humans? The postulated etiology refers to the cause(s) of the behaviors. In the animal model, the causes of the phenomenon should be the same as in humans. Neurobiological mechanisms underlying the syndrome in the animal model should be the same as in humans. Finally, the treatment response should be the same. Of course, if all of these parameters about a particular phenomenon were known, then the animal model would not be necessary. However, this is typically not the case. Therefore, the model protocol is that one should match the animal model on what is known and utilize the animal model to explore unknown issues relevant to the human condition. For example, knockout mice (in which particular genes have been deleted or otherwise "knocked out") have been created that have a genetic defect known to cause certain human conditions. Researchers use these knockout mice to study how the genetic defect results in the phenotype of the disorder and to develop effective treatments.

There are several types of animal models (McGuire, Brammer, & Raleigh, 1983). *Homologous* models are those in which there is an assumed phylogenetic history that is shared. That is, there is a similarity of the system of interest because of the common ancestry between the species being utilized as an animal model and what you are interested in modeling in humans. This would suggest a common genetic and embryological/developmental background as well. Chimpanzees, for example, have been used in controversial experiments in vaccine development because they are the only species whose genetic background and immunological system is close enough to humans to become infected with certain human disease agents. A second type of animal model is an *analogous* model. In this case, there is no presumed genetic relatedness. Rather, there are environmental constraints or demands that are important in producing the outcome that you are interested in modeling. The model can be informative in terms of environmental process for which issues of phylogeny are irrelevant. For example, the relationship between experience and the development of learned helplessness as a cause of depression has been successfully explored using dogs and rats. The environmental contingencies and noncontingencies that produce this effect are independent of any common ancestry with these species. A *survey* model is one that involves a wide range of species that allows one to look at patterns of connections between different elements across the groups. This sort of cross-species study can be informative of principles one might miss by limiting one's research to just one species. In this chapter, such a survey of responses to maternal separation in several species of nonhuman primates is presented to examine patterns of response suggesting principles for understanding the consequences of attachment disruption. Finally, an *outcome* model is focused on examining relationships between independent and dependent variables, regardless of issues of phylogenetic relatedness, environmental constraints, or other factors. An example of this would include pharmaceutical studies, which look at the impacts of drugs on specific symptoms or physiological systems.

This chapter examines examples of the animal models of early sensitive or critical periods, focusing on attachment and social development. Not all models that have been developed in the past have been valid or generalizable to the human condition. In general, one may say that some of the models involving nonmammalian species and some models involving mammalian, nonprimate species have been problematic in terms of generalizing to the human condition. To some extent this has depended on how the model has been utilized to understand human development and is to some extent a question of definitions and criteria.

HISTORICAL BACKGROUND AND OVERVIEW

Imprinting was the earliest behavioral model used to study early social development (Salzen, 1998). Imprinting is the English translation of the term, *Prägung*, coined by Konrad Lorenz. He identified five important features of imprinting that made it a unique form of learning: 1) it is confined to a definite and brief critical period in development; 2) once established, learning is irreversible (or very stable); 3) it affects responses that appear later in development, such as choice of a sexual partner; 4) it is the learning of species characteristics (e.g., supra-individual); and 5) there is no apparent conventional reward or reinforcement.

Lorenz borrowed the term critical period from embryology. Contemporary researchers have suggested changing this to sensitive period or other variations, reflecting recognition of limitations of applying the embryological concept to behavior. Subsequent research on imprinting has called into question many of the classically defined features of imprinting. For example, sexual imprinting may be a distinct and separate process from filial imprinting, and although the initial imprinted preference is strong, it is not irreversible, with appropriate manipulations.

Recent research on imprinting has focused on examining the neural substrates (Salzen, 1998). These studies have identified particular brain centers associated with particular roles in the imprinting process. For example, one area of the chick forebrain (the intermediate medial hyperstriatum ventrale region) has been identified as involved in the initial process of imprinting but not in the expression of the imprinted preference after a consolidation period. The lateral neostriatal region, however, is involved in both of these components. Research on neural substrates also has identified component learning and memory processes that may help explain differences and similarities with traditional forms of learning.

Imprinting focuses on the infant's behavior toward the parent or the object of imprinting. Bonding in ruminants (e.g., goats, sheep, cattle, bison) focuses on the mother's attachment to the infant. Collias (1956) first identified this process and the critical role of contact during the first few hours after birth. Early studies demonstrated that, within a few hours of birth, a mother goat will bond to her infant, resulting in the female's accepting this infant for grooming and nursing and rejecting all others. This appears to be based on olfactory cues as she cleans the infant following birth (Kendrick et al., 1997). Although this process is limited to about 2 hours after birth, the critical period can be extended with appropriate manipulation (Hersher, Richmond, & Moore, 1963).

The concept of bonding was explored in human mothers and their infants by Klaus and Kennell (Klaus et al., 1972), who sought to determine whether there was a critical period for bonding in humans, which might explain aberrant maternal behavior in humans. The assumption was that a failure to have this early bonding experience would result in mothers and infants never developing strong attachments, with presumed negative consequences for the emotional development of the child. In that study, mothers were either provided early extended skin-to-skin contact or given standard maternity ward care. At the time, standard medical practice was to remove the infant immediately after birth, to separate mother and infant via the use of the nursery, and to permit minimal contact while in the hospital (30 minutes at 4-hour intervals for feeding). They found that 1 month later mothers in the extended care group exhibited more interest in and more contact with their infants. They concluded that there may be a "special attachment period in the human mother somewhat similar to that described in animals" (p. 463). The dissemination of this and additional studies changed the way the birthing process is treated. It is now standard practice to permit mothers to have extended contact with their infants at birth, to leave infants in their mother's room instead of putting them in the hospital nursery, and so forth. These changes may be seen as positive, in terms of how mothers and infants are treated at birth. However, problems with this original study led to questions about whether a brief critical period for bonding was a human phenomenon. Svejda, Campos, and Emde (1980) suggested that there were some methodological flaws in the Klaus and Kennell study, particularly with experimental control of attention. When they replicated this study with additional controls, no difference was found between the extended contact group and the control group. This suggests that the early skin-to-skin contact was not the critical parameter and that there is no early critical period for bonding phenomenon in humans comparable to that seen in ruminants.

Animal models of critical periods in human attachment described previously have been found to be inadequate in various ways. Human beings are primates, and there has been a considerable amount of research on attachment and social development in a number of nonhuman primate species, which have proved to be valuable animal models. The mother–infant relationship in monkeys is much more like human relationships than that seen in nonprimate species. The infants are very dependent on their mothers at birth and continue to be dependent for an extended period of time until they develop sufficient social and behavioral skills to become independent. Monkey mothers, in turn, provide a great deal of care for their infants, extending for a relatively long period of time (years in the case of apes).

Ross Thompson (see Chapter 5) provides definitions of attachments in humans that also describe well the relationship between a mother and infant monkey. An attachment between the mother and infant monkey develops during the first weeks of life and can endure for months or years. Female infants, in particular, will maintain relationships with their mothers throughout life, and it is not uncommon to find female monkeys who have strong relationships with their grandmother and great-grandmother. These enduring affectional ties in monkeys appear to be similar to those seen in humans.

The earliest use of monkey models of human infant attachment was to examine the nature of the attachment object and how manipulation of the object's characteristics affected the attachment. Prior to the 1960s, human attachment of an infant for the mother, regardless of what theoretical perspective one held, was assumed to be based on the role of the mother in feeding the infant. Whether one held to Freudian theories that focused on the breast as an object of gratification or Skinnerian theories that focused on the positive reinforcement qualities of milk, there was a common thread that the infant's attachment to the mother was the result of physical factors associated with feeding. All of these early theories assumed that the physical breast—the milk—was the foundation of the attachment. Harry Harlow and his colleagues, in a classic set of studies, demonstrated that this was not, in fact, the case (Harlow & Zimmermann, 1959). To test this feeding hypothesis, infant monkeys were given the choice of a terry cloth–covered surrogate and a wire surrogate. For half of the infants, the milk was provided by the cloth-covered surrogate, and for half of the infants the milk was provided by the wire surrogate. The infant monkeys spent almost all their time clinging to the cloth surrogate, regardless of which surrogate provided the milk. In addition, the cloth surrogate could be used by the infant as a secure base to explore a novel environment and to provide comfort in the face of fearful stimuli. The wire surrogates provided no such security. Of course, this all seems obvious now, but it was not at the time. Harlow coined the term *contact comfort* to describe this phenomenon. Understanding of attachments continues to include important functions in supporting social and emotional development (see Chapter 5).

Research with animal models of attachment has taken several new directions. As in other disciplines, there has been an explosion of neurobiological research in this area. Much of this research is inferential, based on peripheral measures such as peripheral blood components (Laudenslager et al., 1995), cardiovascular correlates (Boccia, Reite, & Laudenslager, 1989), or studies of neurotransmitter metabolites in cerebrospinal fluid (Clarke et al., 1996; Higley et al., 1993; Kraemer & Clarke, 1990). Some more direct studies of the central nervous system, however, are allowing new insights (Bachevalier, 1994; Beauregard & Bachevalier, 1996; Boccia, Reite, Kaemingk, Held, & Laudenslager, 1989; Siegel et al., 1993).

From this work, a convergence of research with rodents, nonhuman primates, and humans is emerging that is linking social affiliation, aggression, and stress reactivity to similar neurochemical systems in the brain (Nelson & Panksepp, 1998). A theoretical framework that is a valuable heuristic tool in this area is the notion of experience-expectant structures (Petrinovich, 1998). Experience-expectant structures are neurobiological structures designed to use environmental information that is so ubiquitous as to be universal. An example might be the mother as a stimulant for emotional development. Except in extraordinary circumstances, the mother of an infant is going to be present. The developmental process involved in experience-expectant structures takes a roughly shaped neurobiological system and refines it on the basis of experience. The developmental process of experience-expectant structures has been linked to overgeneration of the connections followed by pruning (see Chapter 11). It is presumed that the neurobiology of attachment will be found to involve experience-expectant structures as well (Schore, 1996). Two examples of this in early social experience include the long-term effects of altered maternal behavior in rats and attachment object separation and socialization in primates.

RAT MATERNAL BEHAVIOR AS AN ANIMAL MODEL OF THE IMPACT OF EARLY EXPERIENCE

Maternal care received in infancy affects adult stress responses and social behavior including maternal behavior. This conclusion has emerged from research in rodents on the consequences of daily maternal separations during the first 2–3 weeks of postnatal life. The initial, much-replicated observation was that brief daily separation (15–20 minutes or less per day, often referred to as "handling") during the postnatal period resulted in diminished hypothalamic-pituitary-adrenal (HPA) axis and anxious/fearful behavior responses to acute stress in adulthood (Ader, 1968; Levine, 1957). Specifically, corticosterone and ACTH levels increased less and returned to baseline more rapidly during and following stressors, such as immobilization while animals explored more freely when placed in a novel open field or elevated plus maze. These studies suggest a critical period for handling effects on stress, confined to a narrow window of time lasting about a week during the neonatal period. It is now well established that daily separation of rat pups from their mothers during the first few weeks after their birth permanently alters behavioral responses to stressors, including novelty. Adult rats who were handled this way in infancy do not have differing levels of corticosterone at baseline. When exposed to a stressor, however, they exhibit a smaller rise in this hormone and a quicker return to baseline levels than rats who were not handled as pups. Conversely, long periods of daily maternal separation (3–6 hours) during the first few postnatal weeks have opposite effects on adult acute stress responses (i.e., higher and more prolonged HPA axis responses as well as greater anxiety, fear, and avoidance) (Ladd, Owens, & Nemeroff, 1996; Ogawa, Mikuni, Kuroda, & Muneoka, 1994; Plotsky & Meaney, 1993).

It turns out that brief and long maternal separation (BMS and LMS) produce these contrasting lifelong consequences by exerting divergent effects on the amount of some components of maternal care received by pups. BMS increases and LMS decreases the amount dams orally groom pups and the amount they nurse in an arched-back posture over pups. Studies of rat dams that exhibit high versus low amounts of spontaneous pup-grooming and arched-back nursing (these animals were not subjected to maternal separation) have shown that the offspring they reared developed, respectively, low or high HPA axis and behavioral acute stress responses much like rats subjected as infants to BMS or LMS (Caldji et al., 1998; Liu et al., 1997). Contrasting developmental effects of early BMS and LMS experience on several neurochemical systems in the brain that regulate anxiety/fear and HPA axis activity are virtually identical to effects produced by receiving high versus low amounts of maternal grooming and arched-back nursing during infancy (Caldji et al., 1998; Caldji, Francis, Sharma, Plotsky, & Meaney, 2000). Cross-fostering studies have demonstrated that maternal behavior received, not genetic inheritance from the birth mother, dictates adult acute stress responses (Francis, Diorio, Liu, & Meaney, 1999).

The amount of pup-grooming and arched-back nursing exhibited by rat dams is related to their anxiety/fear levels and also determines the amount of these components of maternal behavior exhibited by adult females reared by these dams. Discovery of these connections has led to the hypothesis that the amount rat dams groom pups and nurse in an arched-back posture is a nongenomic mechanism whereby levels of acute stress responsivity and maternal care are transmitted from one generation to the next (Francis et al., 1999; Sharma et al., 1998). These effects are evident based on maternal behavior in the first week of life, suggesting a critical period for the effects of early experience on the development of these neurobehavioral systems.

There are important long-term behavioral and neurochemical correlates of early BMS and LMS experience. In addition to contrasting frequencies of maternal behavior, the decline in anxiety and increase in aggression during nursing differed significantly between rat dams subjected as infants to these contrasting early experiences (Boccia & Pedersen, 1999). Nursing dams subjected to BMS during infancy exhibited significantly less anxiety and significantly greater maternal aggression compared to dams subjected to LMS. Our observation on maternal aggression and the seminal report of Levine (1959) that early handling increased aggression between male mice suggest that maternal separation and associated alterations in maternal care received during this early critical period may exert effects on the development of a broader range of agonistic and other social behaviors than have been previously studied.

Research conducted by numerous investigators indicates that oxytocin, a small neuropeptide in the brain, is involved in activating social attachments. The onset of maternal behavior after birth in rats and sheep depend on oxytocin release within the brain (Kendrick et al., 1997; Pedersen, Caldwell, Walker, Ayers, & Mason, 1994; Van Leengoed, Kerker, & Swanson, 1987). The expression of maternal behavior in wild mice and perhaps monkeys (Holman & Goy, 1995; McCarthy, 1990) also is enhanced by central oxytocin administration. The activating effects of oxytocin on maternal behavior in rats is exerted within the brain in the medial preoptic area, ventral tegmental area, and olfactory bulbs (Pedersen et al., 1994; Yu, Kaba, Okutani, Takahashi, & Higuchi, 1996). Oxytocin receptors in the medial preoptic and ventral tegmental areas increase in number prior to parturition when maternal behavior is initiated (Pedersen et al., 1994; Pedersen, 1997). The establishment of monogamous pair-bonds brought about by sexual interaction in some species of rodents depends on oxytocin in the female brain and vasopressin (a molecule similar to oxytocin) in the male brain (Young, Wang, & Insel, 1998).

Interestingly, oxytocin also seems to be involved in stress responsivity by regulating other neurochemical systems in the brain that are involved in stress (Liberzon & Young, 1997; Neumann et al., 1998). This suggests a possible mechanism whereby affiliation plays a role in stress regulation, which is relevant to the suggestion of Thompson (see Chapter 5) regarding the importance of attachment in regulating the infant's fear response.

Research indicates that central oxytocin plays several key roles in the process whereby levels of maternal care, and perhaps even acute stress response levels, are transmitted intergenerationally. First, oxytocin in the rat mother's brain increases the amount of pup-grooming and arched-back nursing she exhibits. Intracerebroventricular administration of an oxytocin antagonist significantly and selectively diminishes (but does not eliminate) these components of maternal behavior (Pedersen & Boccia, 1999). Second, oxytocin receptor numbers are greater in the centromedial amygdala and the ventral tegmental area of females that were subjected as infants to BMS compared to females with early LMS experience (Boccia & Pedersen, 1999). This suggests that early maternal separation experience, and probably associated changes in the amount of maternal grooming and arched-back nursing received, influence the development of oxytocin receptors in brain areas involved in maternal behavior (ventral tegmental area) and in emotional and behavioral responses to stress (centromedial amygdala). Third, daily treatment with oxytocin or an oxytocin antagonist on postnatal days 2–10 resulted in rat dams exhibiting, respectively, significantly more or less pup-grooming toward offspring (Pedersen & Boccia, 2000). This finding implies that endogenous oxytocin activity in young female pups influences the development of their maternal behavior. If the amount of maternal grooming and arched-back nursing received influences oxytocin activity in infant rats, it may be a mechanism whereby early maternal care experience regulates maternal care exhibited as an adult.

These results, in combination with reports from others that oxytocin acts in the brain to diminish anxiety and HPA axis activation during stress (McCarthy, McDonald, Brooks, Goldman, 1996; Neumann, Torner, & Wigger, 2000; Uvnäs-Moberg, Ahlenius, Hillegaart, & Alster, 1994; Windle, Shanks, Lightman, & Ingram, 1997) and aggression (Lubin et al., 1999), suggest the following oxytocin-centered model whereby similar levels of maternal behavior and acute stress responses are transmitted from one generation to the next. Oxytocin activity in the rat mother's brain, which controls her levels of anxiety and aggression, determines how much she grooms pups and nurses in an arched-back posture, which regulates endogenous oxytocin activity in pups, which influences the development of oxytocin receptors and possibly other neurochemical systems in their brains and, thereby, their adult levels of maternal behavior, agonistic behavior, and acute stress responses. In other words, oxytocin activity in the pup brain transduces the amount of maternal care received into long-term effects on behavior and stress responses. There may be a critical or sensitive period during which mothering received influences the development of central oxytocin systems and, consequently, maternal and social behavior as well as stress-response systems.

PRIMATE MODELS OF EARLY EXPERIENCE AND SOCIAL DEVELOPMENT

Nonhuman primates offer unique advantages as animal model systems in terms of central nervous system structure, social behavior, and evidence of true social attachment. Another advantage of primate models is their variability. Humans demonstrate substantial individual variability in their responses to early deprivation or separation from an attachment object; nonhuman primates demonstrate similar variability. A systematic investigation into the sources of such variability in nonhuman primates may further enhance the utility of primate models in these areas and add to the understanding of the mechanisms underlying such variability in human behavior.

Research on early social development in primates can be seen within two different perspectives. One approach examines the characteristics of the attachment object, separating the different component stimuli that an attachment object provides, and examining the consequences for the emotional and social behavioral development of the infant. A second approach studies the consequences of separation once the attachment is formed and examines the short- and long-term consequences of this for socialization and emotional development. These two approaches have provided important information about critical periods and experience-expectant structures in the social and emotional development of primates.

Attachment Object Characteristic Manipulations

The first approach looks at the characteristics of the attachment object and how they influence infant development. Rhesus monkeys have been studied extensively in this regard. An adult rhesus monkey mother presents her infant with a complex array of stimuli. Of course, as noted previously, she provides contact comfort. She also is warm and provides thermal regulatory input. She provides vestibular stimulation through the effects of her typical movement patterns while the infant clings to her ventral surface. She provides experience with contingency as she varies her responses to the infant's behavior on a daily basis as well as over the course of development. Of course, she also provides exposure to mature species-typical behavior.

Adult female rhesus monkeys provide complex stimuli to their infants as attachment objects. Manipulations of the component characteristics of the attachment objects permit researchers to separate these features experimentally. Of course, the most extreme form is to remove the mother from the infant and give nothing in return, which is referred to as *social isolation* (Mason & Sponholz, 1963). The results are dramatic and devastating, with infants showing a range of social and emotional impairments. They exhibit many types of stereotypic behavior, are socially incompetent, are hyperfearful, and can exhibit inappropriate aggression. The first 6 months of life appear to be the critical period during which socializing input is required for normal development: If the monkeys are isolated for the first 3 months and then placed in social groups, they recover and develop normally. If the isolation occurs in the second half-year of life, following a period of mother rearing, they do not show these impairments. If the isolation occurs for the first 6 months, however, these effects occur. Although many, but not all, of the isolation effects can be reversed, the required intervention involves heroic efforts (Novak & Harlow, 1975; Suomi, Harlow, & Novak, 1974). This suggests that the first 6 months of life are a critical period for social development in rhesus monkeys.

Other types of attachment objects provide insights into the relationships between object stimuli and outcome for the infant. Infants provided with a cloth-covered surrogate cling to it and do not develop the self-clinging seen in isolate-reared monkeys. As noted previously, they are able to use the surrogate as a secure base for exploration so that they are not paralyzed with fear when placed in a novel environment. Furthermore, if the surrogate provides vestibular stimulation, by being hung from the top of the cage and allowed to swing, the infants do not develop rocking behavior stereotypies (Mason & Berkson, 1975). Mason and Capitanio (1988) conducted a study in which they cross-fostered rhesus monkeys to dogs and compared them with inanimate surrogates. This manipulation allows contingency to be separated from species-typical behavior. There is no experience of contingency with an inanimate surrogate. These animals, as one might expect, do better than the inanimate surrogate-reared ones, but not as well as ones raised with monkeys. They do show more appropriate behavior regulation. They are capable of forming a coherent social group with a dominance hierarchy, which animals raised with surrogates cannot do. Dog-reared monkeys do show limits in the complexity of the relationships formed, however, compared to normally reared monkeys.

Peer-rearing is a manipulation that has received increased attention as a model for examining neurobiological underpinnings of affiliation in monkeys (Champoux, Metz, & Suomi, 1991; Clarke, 1993; Clarke et al., 1996; Higley, Suomi, & Linnoila, 1991). This manipulation involves separating infants from their mothers at birth and raising them with other infants. This produces a variety of impairments in the monkeys. There is more typical behavioral development than seen with inanimate surrogates, but there are high rates of clinging, stereotypies, and alterations in the developmental trajectories of behaviors. Alterations in brain chemistry have been found that suggest there are neurobiological effects of this altered early experience that may relate to the behavioral deficits seen.

Although infants provide species-typical behavior, albeit in an immature form, they do not provide one important behavioral feature that adult females provide their infants: frustration. The frustration of goal attainment that the infant experiences developmentally (e.g., that experienced during weaning) probably plays an important role in the infant's development of independence and maturity.

These studies of altered attachment objects have provided a great deal of information about the relationship between different stimulus features of the attachment object and the consequences of these for the social and emotional development of the infant monkey. Research with situations of severe deprivation in human infants, such as the studies of Romanian orphans (Chisholm, 1998; Fisher, Ames, Chisholm, & Savoie, 1997; Kaler & Freeman, 1994; see Chapter 7), suggests that similar processes may be at work in human infant development, although recent long-term follow-up studies report significant, but not complete, recovery in these children once they are removed from the institutions (Groze & Ileana, 1996; Rutter, 1991). As Thompson notes in Chapter 5, the length of time spent in the orphanage prior to adoption affected how well the children were able to recover and form secure attachments to their adoptive parents. This parallels the finding with monkeys that the length and timing of the isolation are important in how the isolation affects the infants and what type of recovery is possible.

Attachment Object Separation

The second major approach in nonhuman primate model research employs the separation paradigm (Reite & Boccia, 1994). Rather than focusing on the formation of the attachment on the basis of the object's characteristics, this approach focuses on the disruption of the attachment relationship once it is formed. Typically, infants are raised in social groups for the first 3–6 months of life. At that time, the mother is removed from the social group and the response of the infant studied. Because the infant remains in the social group in which it was born and raised, social isolation and novel environments are eliminated as confounding factors. Harry Harlow and his colleagues first described the two-stage response to separation typically seen in rhesus monkeys, as well as some, but not all, other primate species (Seay & Harlow, 1965). Initial agitation, in which the infant gives distress vocalizations and exhibits high rates of locomotion, is followed by depression with characteristic slouched posture and sad facial expressions. In addition to the behavioral response, numerous physiological responses have been documented, ranging from cortisol and immune measures to neurotransmitter indices (Reite & Boccia, 1994). Table 6.1 presents the results of changes in neurotransmitter metabolites found in cerebrospinal fluid following separation in pigtail macaques (Reite, Boccia, & Laudenslager, unpublished data). Infants experiencing separations, but not the matched control animals, showed decreases in the serotonin metabolite (5HIAA) and dopamine metabolite (HVA) and an increase in the norepinephrine metabolite (MHPG).

These neurotransmitters, called biogenic amines, are involved in regulating behavioral systems that are important in modulating interactions with the environment (Rogenness & McClure, 1996). They participate in the regulation of motor activity, sleep, aggression, attachment, anxiety, and memory, to name a few behavioral systems. They have been implicated in several forms of psychopathology, such as affective disorders and schizo-

Table 6.1. Levels of neurotransmitter metabolites in cerebrospinal fluid during baseline and after 1 week of separation in separated pigtail monkey infants and unseparated control infants

Phase	5HIAA (serotonin metabolite)	MHPG (norepinephrine metabolite)	HVA (dopamine metabolite)
Baseline (N=15)	65.7± 4.0	18.8 ± 0.7	204.4 ± 13.7
Control infants after 1 week (N=2)	75.7 ± 15.1	15.8 ± 1.5	202.5 ± 29.8
Separated infants after 1 week (N=4)	54.9 ± 6.9	27.8 ± 6.9	180.3 ± 49.4

phrenia, and psychoactive drugs have their effects by operating on these neurotransmitter systems. These three neurotransmitter systems originate in a few central limbic areas of the brain and send projections to a wide range of other areas of the brain, including other limbic sites as well as cerebral cortex, cerebellum, and the spinal cord. Early experiences, then, can have broad-ranging consequences by affecting the development of the biogenic amine systems during critical periods in their development and maturation.

This 2-week separation experience, at approximately 6 months of age, produces long-term changes, both behavioral and physiological, that last into adulthood (Capitanio, Rasmussen, Snyder, Laudenslager, & Reite, 1986; Capitanio & Reite, 1984; Laudenslager, Capitanio, & Reite, 1985). Adults who are separated as infants play less, have smaller social networks, and have fewer significant positive social relationships. They also exhibit a variety of physiological differences, including altered cortisol and immune responses to challenge. Interestingly, as with the rats, maternal behavior is altered following the separation experience. A proximity index can be computed that reflects whether the infant or mother is more responsible for maintaining proximity in the relationship. If one examines this index at 15 months of age, following a separation experience at 6 months of age that lasted only 2 weeks, this index indicates that the mother is more responsible for maintaining proximity than in relationships in which no separation was experienced (Laudenslager, March, 2000, personal communication). As with the rats reported previously in this chapter, alterations in maternal behavior directed toward the infant are produced when the attachment bond is disrupted. This suggests that disruption of the relationship alters the mother's behavior toward the infant, which alters the neurobiological development of the infant that alters adult behavior. Furthermore, this may be a pattern that generalizes across a wide range of mammalian species including humans.

Animal models have been useful in studying possible critical periods in early development, although some problematic areas have produced some confusion. Comparative studies that include multiple species can be valuable in deriving general principles of development and learning about the nature and existence of critical periods. Such studies have led to the realization that behavior lies on a continuum, ranging from environmentally stable (e.g., unmodifiable by the environment) to environmentally labile (e.g., vary greatly with environmental variations) and that this lability may change over development (Hinde, 1982). Furthermore, because young individuals may be specialized for the task of growing and surviving to adulthood, these studies suggest it may be reasonable to expect that some aspects of their behavior will be irrelevant to their adult life. In fact, some of their behavioral characteristics may be seen as scaffolding whose importance is primarily related to the process of development and growth and may disappear as the adult functions emerge in the course of development.

Some generalizations from nonhuman primates to humans may not be valid. For example, if one studies only one species, the effect of separation experiences in that species may not generalize to the human condition. However, if we study a range of species, and examine the variety of factors that affect responses to separation, principles may be found that are applicable to humans. For example, it appears that one may generalize that the effects of separation are likely to be more severe, the more disturbed the mother–infant relationship. Another may be that the more disruptive the separation experience is in the immediate context, the more likely there will be long-term consequences of the separation.

In considering nonhuman primate research, several issues may be important for understanding human development. One is the apparent existence of a sensitive period for exposure to socializing influences, as described in the chapter. Another is the existence of clear and significant individual differences in the response to early experiences, such as altered attachment objects or temporary separations. These are in the area of generalizations rather than data, pointing to an important method of comparative research. The value of such research lies in the derivation of principles and generalizations rather than looking for one-to-one correspondences in the details of behavior.

In the context of discussions of attachment and early social and emotional development, the comparative data suggest that infants of a number of different species have periods of time in early development when they are particularly sensitive to the impact of varying social experiences. These experiences may influence later behavior by altering the development of the underlying neurobiological systems. Young individuals may be predisposed to receive certain kinds of socially relevant input, as in the notion of experience-expectant stimuli. If so, it would not be surprising to find behavioral and other mechanisms designed to keep the relevant environments more or less constant. For example, if the mother is an important developmental scaffolding stimulus, then proximity maintaining behaviors may be a critical behavioral component developmentally. Such mechanisms may lie more in the relationship the individual has with others than in the individual him- or herself. Furthermore, these requirements and the behavioral supports for maintaining these requirements will change over development.

The contemporary emphasis in animal models research in this area is on the neurobiological systems underlying these relationships and the timing and permanency of effects for critical periods. In addition, the role of neuronal pathways in the timing of critical periods is not completely understood and can be explored in these animal models. The concept of experience-expectant structures is a valuable heuristic and the types of research described in this chapter can help to expand the understanding of how processes function in the context of healthy social and emotional development, as well as the consequences when development goes awry. Animal model systems can help researchers evaluate both behavioral and neurobiological consequences of early traumatic events, and to develop and examine the efficacy of interventions designed to reverse the trauma effects.

REFERENCES

Abramson, L.Y., & Seligman, M.E.P. (1977). Modeling psychopathology in the laboratory: History and rationale. In J.D. Maser & M.E.P. Seligman (Eds.), *Psychopathology: Experimental models* (pp. 1–26). San Francisco: W.H. Freeman and Company.

Ader, R. (1968). Effects of early experiences on emotional and physiological reactivity in the rat. *Journal of Comparative and Physiological Psychology, 66*, 264–268.

Bachevalier, J. (1994). Medial temporal lobe structures and autism: A review of clinical and experimental findings. *Neuropsychologia, 32*, 627–648.

Beauregard, M., & Bachevalier, J. (1996). Neonatal insult to the hippocampal region and schizophrenia: A review and a putative animal model. *Canadian Journal of Psychiatry, 41*, 446–456.

Boccia, M.L., & Pedersen, C.A. (1999). Early maternal separation alters postpartum pup-licking and grooming, lactation-associated changes in aggression and anxiety, and central oxytocin binding in female offspring. *Proceedings of the Meeting of the Society for Neurosciences.* [Abstract No. 261.3].

Boccia, M.L., Reite, M., Kaemingk, K., Held, P., & Laudenslager, M. (1989). Behavioral and autonomic responses to peer separation in pigtail macaque monkey infants. *Developmental Psychobiology, 22*, 447–461.

Boccia, M.L., Reite, M., & Laudenslager, M. (1989). On the physiology of grooming in a pigtail macaque. *Physiology & Behavior, 45*, 667–670.

Caldji, C., Francis, D., Sharma, S., Plotsky, P.M., & Meaney, M.J. (2000). The effects of early rearing environment on the development of GABA and central benzodiazepine receptor levels and novelty-induced fearfulness in the rat. *Neuropsychopharmacology, 22*(3), 219–229.

Caldji, C., Tannenbaum, B., Sharma, S., Francis, D., Plotsky, P.M., & Meaney, M.J. (1998). Maternal care during infancy regulates the development of neural systems mediating the expression of fearfulness in the rat. *Proceedings of the National Academy of Sciences, USA, 95*, 5335–5340.

Capitanio, J.P., Rasmussen, K.L.R., Snyder, D.S., Laudenslager, M., & Reite, M. (1986). Long-term follow-up of previously separated pigtail macaques: Group and individual differences in response to novel situations. *Journal of Child Psychology and Psychiatry, 27*, 531–538.

Capitanio, J.P., & Reite, M. (1984). The roles of early separation experience and prior familiarity in the social relations of pigtail macaques: A descriptive multivariate study. *Primates, 25*, 475–484.

Carter, C.S., Lederhendler, I.I., & Pedersen, C.A. (1997). The integrative neurobiology of affiliation. *Annals of the New York Academy of Sciences, 807*, 614. New York: New York Academy of Sciences.

Champoux, M., Metz, B., & Suomi, S.J. (1991). Behavior of nursery/peer-reared and mother-reared rhesus monkeys from birth through 2 years of age. *Primates, 32*, 509–514.

Chisholm, K. (1998). A three-year follow-up of attachment and indiscriminate friendliness in children adopted from Romanian orphanages. *Child Development, 69*, 1092–1106.

Clarke, A.S. (1993). Social rearing effects on HPA axis activity over early development and in response to stress in rhesus monkeys. *Developmental Psychobiology, 26*, 433–446.

Clarke, A.S., Hedeker, D.R., Ebert, M.H., Schmidt, D.E., McKinney, W.T., & Kraemer, G.W. (1996). Rearing experience and biogenic amine activity in infant rhesus monkeys. *Biological Psychiatry, 40*, 338–352.

Collias, N.E. (1956). The analysis of socialization in sheep and goats. *Ecology, 37*, 228–239.

Fisher, L., Ames, E.W., Chisholm, K., & Savoie, L. (1997). Problems reported by parents of Romanian orphans adopted to British Columbia. *International Journal of Behavioral Development, 20*, 67–82.

Fleming, A.S., & Luebke, C. (1981). Timidity prevents the virgin female rat from being a good mother: Emotionality differences between nulliparous and parturient females. *Physiology & Behavior, 27*, 863–868.

Francis, D., Diorio, J., Liu, D., & Meaney, M.J. (1999). Nongenomic transmission across generations of maternal behavior and stress responses in the rat. *Science, 286*, 1155–1158.

Groze, V., & Ileana, D. (1996). A follow-up study of adopted children from Romania. *Child and Adolescent Social Work Journal, 13*, 541–565.

Harlow, H.F., & Zimmermann, R.B. (1959). Affectional responses in the infant monkey. *Science, 130*, 421–432.

Hersher, L., Richmond, J.B., & Moore, A.U. (1963). Modifiability of the critical period for the development of maternal behavior in sheep and goats. *Behaviour, 20*, 311–319.

Higley, J.D., Suomi, S.J., & Linnoila, M. (1991). CSF monoamine metabolite concentrations vary according to age, rearing, and sex, and are influenced by the stressor of social separation in rhesus monkeys. *Psychopharmacology, 103*, 551–556.

Higley, J.D., Thompson, W.W., Champoux, M., Goldman, D., Hasert, M.F., Kraemer, G.W., Scanlan, J.M., Suomi, S.J., & Linnoila, M. (1993). Paternal and maternal genetic and environmental contributions to cerebrospinal fluid monoamine metabolites in rhesus monkeys *(Macaca mulatta)*. *Archives of General Psychiatry, 50*, 615–623.

Hinde, R.A. (1982). *Ethology: Its nature and relations with other sciences*. New York: Oxford University Press.

Holman, S.D., & Goy, R.W. (1995). Experiential and hormonal correlates of care-giving in rhesus macaques. In C.R. Pryce, R.D. Martin, & D. Skuse (Eds.),

Third Schultz-Biegert Symposium. Motherhood in human and nonhuman primates (pp. 87–93). Kartause Ittingen, Switzerland.

Insel, T.R. (1997). A neurobiological basis of social attachment. *American Journal of Psychiatry, 154*, 726–735.

Kaler, S.R., & Freeman, B.J. (1994). Analysis of environmental deprivation: Cognitive and social development in Romanian orphans. *Journal of Child Psychology & Psychiatry, 35*, 769–781.

Kendrick, K.M., Da Costa, A.P., Broad, K.D., Ohkura, S., Guevara, R., Levy, F., & Keverne, E.B. (1997). Neural control of maternal behaviour and olfactory recognition of offspring. *Brain Research Bulletin, 44*, 383–395.

Klaus, M.H., Jerauld, R., Kreger, N.C., McAlpine, W., Steffa, M., & Kennell, J.H. (1972). Maternal attachment: Importance of the first post-partum days. *The New England Journal of Medicine, 286*, 460–463.

Kraemer, G.W., & Clarke, A.S. (1990). The behavioral neurobiology of self-injurious behavior in rhesus monkeys. *Progress in Neuro-Psychopharmacology & Biological Psychiatry, 14*, S141–S168.

Ladd, C.O., Owens, M.J., & Nemeroff, C.B. (1996). Persistent changes in corticotropin-releasing factor neuronal systems induced by maternal deprivation. *Endocrinology, 137*(4), 1212–1218.

Laudenslager, M.L., Boccia, M., Berger, C.L., Gennaro-Ruggles, M.M., McFerran, B., & Reite, M.L. (1995). Total cortisol, free cortisol, and growth hormone associated with brief social separation experiences in young macaques. *Developmental Psychobiology, 28*, 199–211.

Laudenslager, M.L., Capitanio, J.P., & Reite, M. (1985). Possible effects of early separation experiences on subsequent immune function in adult macaque monkeys. *American Journal of Psychiatry, 142*, 862–864.

Levine, S. (1957). Infantile experience and resistance to physiological stress. *Science, 135*, 795–796.

Levine, S. (1959). Emotionality and aggressive behavior in the mouse as a function of infantile experience. *The Journal of Genetic Psychology, 94*, 77–83.

Liberzon, I., & Young, E.A. (1997). Effects of stress and glucocorticoids on CNS oxytocin receptor binding. *Psychoneuroendocrinology, 22*, 411–422.

Liu, D., Diorio, J., Tannenbaum, B., Cladji, C., Francis, D., Freedman, A., Sharma, S., Pearson, D., Plotsky, P.M., & Meaney, M.J. (1997). Maternal care, hippocampal glucocorticoid receptors, and hypothalamic-pituitary-adrenal responses to stress. *Science, 277*, 1659–1662.

Lubin, D.A., Elliott, J.C., Fernandes, M.L., Johnson, A., Eustache, H., & Johns, J.M. (1999). An oxytocin antagonist infused into the amygdala parallels cocaine-induced increases of maternal aggression in rats. *Abstracts of the International Behavioral Neuroscience Society, 8*, 36.

Mason, W.A., & Berkson, G. (1975). Effects of maternal mobility on the development of rocking and other behaviors in rhesus monkeys: A study with artificial mothers. *Developmental Psychobiology, 8*, 197–211.

Mason, W.A., & Capitanio, J.P. (1988). Formation and expression of filial attachment in rhesus monkeys raised with living and inanimate mother substitutes. *Developmental Psychobiology, 21*, 401–420.

Mason, W.A., & Sponholz, R.R. (1963). Behavior of rhesus monkeys raised in isolation. *Journal of Psychiatric Research, 1*, 299–306.

McCarthy, M.M. (1990). Oxytocin inhibits infanticide in female house mice (*mus domesticus*). *Hormones and Behavior, 24*, 365–375.

McCarthy, M.M., & Altemus, M. (1997, June). Central nervous system actions of oxytocin and modulation of behavior in humans. *Molecular Medicine Today*, 269–275.

McCarthy, M.M., McDonald, C.H., Brooks, P.J., & Goldman, D. (1996). An anxiolytic action of oxytocin is enhanced by estrogen in the mouse. *Physiology and Behavior, 60*(5), 1209–1215.

McGuire, M.T., Brammer, G.L., & Raleigh, M.J. (1983). Animal models: Are they useful in the study of psychiatric disorders? *Ethopharmacology: Primate Models of Neuropsychiatric Disorders* (pp. 313–328). New York: Alan R. Liss, Inc.

McKinney, W.T. (1984). Animal models of depression: An overview. *Psychiatric Developments, 2,* 77–96.

McKinney, W.T., & Bunney, W.E. (1969). Animal model of depression. I. Review of evidence: Implications for research. *Archives of General Psychiatry, 21,* 240–248.

Meaney, M.J., Diorio, J., Francis, D., Widdowson, J., LaPlante, P., Caldji, C., Sharma, S., Seckl, J.R., & Plotsky, P.M. (1996). Early environmental regulation of forebrain glucocorticoid receptor gene expression: Implications for adrenocortical responses to stress. *Developmental Neuroscience, 18,* 49–72.

Meaney, M.J., Mitchell, J.B., Aitken, D.H., Bhatnagar, S., Bodnoff, S.R., Iny, L.J., & Sarrieau, A. (1991). The effects of neonatal handling on the development of the adrenocortical response to stress: Implications for neuropathology and cognitive deficits in later life. *Psychoneuroendocrinology, 16,* 85–103.

Nelson, E.E., & Panksepp, J. (1998). Brain substrates of infant-mother attachment: Contributions of opioids, oxytocin, and norepinephrine. *Neuroscience and Behavioral Reviews, 22,* 437–452.

Neumann, I.D., Johnstone, H.A., Hatzinger, M., Liebsch, G., Shipston, M., Russell, J.A., Landgraf, R., & Douglas, A.J. (1998). Attenuated neuroendocrine responses to emotional and physical stressors in pregnant rats involve adenohypophysial changes. *Journal of Physiology, 508,* 289–300.

Neumann, I.D., Torner, L., & Wigger, A. (2000). Brain oxytocin: Differential inhibition of neuroendocrine stress responses and anxiety-related behaviour in virgin, pregnant and lactating rats. *Neuroscience, 95*(2), 567–575.

Novak, M.A., & Harlow, H.F. (1975). Social recovery of monkeys isolated for the first year of life: 1. Rehabilitation and therapy. *Developmental Psychology, 11,* 453–465.

Ogawa, T., Mikuni, M., Kuroda, Y., Muneoka, K., Mori, K.J., & Takahashi, K. (1994). Periodic maternal deprivation alters stress response in adult offspring: Potentiates the negative feedback regulation of restraint stress-induced adrenocortical response and reduces the frequencies of open field-induced behaviors. *Pharmacology Biochemistry & Behavior, 49,* 961–967.

Pedersen, C.A. (1997). Oxytocin control of maternal behavior: Regulation by sex steroids and offspring stimuli. In C.S. Carter, I.I. Lederhendler, & B. Kirkpatrick (Eds.), The integrative neurobiology of affiliation. *Annals of the New York Academy of Sciences, 807,* 126–145.

Pedersen, C.A., & Boccia, M.L. (1999). Central oxytocin shifts maternal licking and grooming from self to pups: A mechanism for intergenerational transmission of stress responsivity. *Proceedings of the Meeting of the Society for Neurosciences.* [Abstract No. 247.6].

Pedersen, C.A., & Boccia, M.L. (2000). Oxytocin transcudes maternal care received in infancy into maternal care exhibited in adulthood. *Proceedings of the Meeting of the Society for Neurosciences.* In press.

Pedersen, C.A., Caldwell, J.D., Peterson, G., Walker, C.H., & Mason, G.A. (1992). Oxytocin activation of maternal behavior in the rat. In C.A. Pedersen, J.D. Caldwell, G.F. Jirikowski, & T.R. Insel (Eds.), Oxytocin in maternal, sexual, and social behaviors. *Annals of the New York Academy of Sciences, 652,* 58–69. New York: New York Academy of Sciences.

Pedersen, C.A., Caldwell, J.D., Walker, C., Ayers, G., & Mason, G.A. (1994). Oxytocin activates the postpartum onset of rat maternal behavior in the ventral tegmental and medial preoptic areas. *Behavioral Neuroscience, 108*, 1163–1171.

Pedersen, C.A., & Prange, A.J., Jr. (1979). Induction of maternal behavior in virgin rats after intracerebroventricular administration of oxytocin. *Proceedings of the National Academy of Sciences, USA*, 6661–6665.

Peterson, G., Mason, G.A., Barakat, A.S. & Pederson, C.A. (1991). Oxytocin selectively increases holding and licking of neonates in preweanling but not postweanling juvenile rats. *Behavioral Neuroscience, 109*, 470–477.

Petrinovich, L. (1998). Bird song development. In G. Greenberg & M.M. Haraway (Eds.), *Comparative psychology: A handbook* (pp. 566–575). New York: Garland Publishing.

Plotsky, P.M., & Meaney, M.J. (1993). Early, postnatal experience alters hypothalamic corticotropin-releasing factor (CRF) mRNA, median eminence CRF content and stress-induced release in adult rats. *Molecular Brain Research, 18*, 195–200.

Reite, M., & Boccia, M.L. (1994). Physiological aspects of adult attachment. In M.B. Sperling & W.H. Berman (Eds.), *Attachment in adults: Clinical and developmental perspectives* (pp. 98–127). New York: The Guilford Press.

Rogenness, G.A., & McClure, E.B. (1996). Development and neurotransmitter-environmental interactions. *Development and Psychopathology, 8*, 183–199.

Rutter, M. (1991). A fresh look at 'maternal deprivation.' In P. Bateson (Ed.), *The development and integration of behaviour: Essays in honour of Robert Hinde* (pp. 331–374). Cambridge, England: Cambridge University Press.

Sackett, G., & Gould, P. (1991). What can primate models of human developmental psychopathology model? In D. Cicchetti & S.L. Toth (Eds.), *Internalizing and externalizing expressions of dysfunction. Rochester Symposium on Developmental Psychopathology. Vol. 2* (pp. 265–292). Hillsdale, NJ: Lawrence Erlbaum Associates, Inc.

Salzen, E.A. (1998). Imprinting. In G. Greenberg & M.M. Haraway (Eds.), *Comparative psychology: A handbook* (pp. 566–575). New York: Garland Publishing, Inc.

Schore, A.N. (1996). The experience-dependent maturation of a regulatory system in the orbital prefrontal cortex and the origin of developmental psychopathology. *Development & Psychopathology, 8*, 59–87.

Seay, B., & Harlow, H.F. (1965). Maternal separation in the rhesus monkey. *Journal of Nervous and Mental Disorders, 140*, 434–441.

Sharma, S., Francis, D., Liu, D., Pearson, D., Plotsky, P.M., & Meaney, M.J. (1998). Variations in maternal care form the basis for a non-genomic mechanism of inter-generational transmission of individual differences in behavioral and endocrine responses to stress. *Abstracts of the Society for Neuroscience Annual Meeting, 176*, 12.

Siegel, S.J., Ginsberg, S.D., Hof, P.R., Foote, S.L., Young, W.G., Kraemer, G.W., McKinney, W.T., & Morrison, J.H. (1993). Effects of social deprivation in prepubescent rhesus monkeys: Immunohistochemical analysis of the neurofilament protein triplet in the hippocampal formation. *Brain Research, 619*, 299–305.

Suomi, S.J., & Harlow, H.F. (1977). Production and alleviation of depressive behaviors in monkeys. In J.D. Maser & M.E.P. Seligman (Eds.), *Psychopathology: Experimental models* (pp. 131–173). San Francisco: W. H. Freeman and Company.

Suomi, S.J., Harlow, H.F., & Novak, M.A. (1974). Reversal of social deficits produced by isolation rearing in monkeys. *Journal of Human Evolution, 3*, 527–534.

Svejda, M.J., Campos, J.J., & Emde, R.N. (1980). Mother-infant "bonding": Failure to generalize. *Child Development, 51*(3), 775–779.

Uvnäs-Moberg, K., Ahlenius, S., Hillegaart, V., & Alster, P. (1994). High doses of oxytocin cause sedation and low doses cause in anxiolytic-like effect in male rats. *Pharmacology Biochemistry and Behavior, 49*, 101–106.

Van Leengoed, E., Kerker, E., & Swanson, H.H. (1987). Inhibition of postpartum maternal behavior in the rat by injecting an oxytocin antagonist into the cerebral ventricles. *Journal of Endocrinology, 112*, 275–282.

Windle, R.J., Shanks, N., Lightman, S.L., & Ingram, C.D. (1997). Central oxytocin adminstration reduces stress-induced corticosterone release and anxiety behavior in rats. *Endocrinology, 138*, 2829–2834.

Young, L.J., Wang, Z., & Insel, T.R. (1998). Neuroendocrine bases of monogamy. *Trends in Neuroscience, 21*, 71–75.

Yu, G.Z., Kaba, H., Okutani, F., Takahashi, S., & Higuchi, T. (1996). The olfactory bulb: Critical site of action for oxytocin in the induction of maternal behaviour in the rat. *Neuroscience*, 72, 1083–1088.

7

Social and Emotional Development in Children Adopted from Institutions

Elinor W. Ames

Kim Chisholm

Because of the severe deprivation commonly found among children in institutions, studies of children reared in institutions during their early lives often have been regarded as real-life counterparts of experimental studies of deprivation. If it could be shown that the impact of early deprivation persists despite adoption into enriched family settings, then it might be claimed that infancy is a critical period.

There are limits to this analogy, however. Whereas variables in experiments are isolated and controlled, this is not the case in real-life situations. Being reared in an institution often means that children experience social, perceptual, nutritional, medical, and intellectual deprivation simultaneously. Because of these variables, it is difficult to discern which type of deprivation produces differences between institution-reared children and family-reared children.

A second problem is that institution studies depend on complex social factors, making it impossible to carry out the research design required to demonstrate a critical period. To prove the existence of a critical period, it is necessary to systematically vary not only the age at which deprivation begins, but also the duration of deprivation at each age. If, for example, it was found that children who spent their first 2 years in an orphanage still had attachment problems when they were adolescents, in spite of having been reared after age 2 in good homes, it would be tempting to say that the first 2 years represent a critical period for attachment. Actually, to conclude that deprivation at that particular age period mattered, one would have to demonstrate 1) a different duration (e.g., the first year alone, the first 15 months) was insufficient to produce the same problems in adolescence, and 2) the same duration would not have the same effect at another time. For example, 2 years spent in an orphanage at another time of life (e.g., from ages 1 to 3 or from ages 2 to 4) would not produce the same effects. In other words, to prove a critical period, one must be able to show both the exact ages that are important and the length of time the operative factor (in this case, institution life) must be in place for effects to occur.

The only published reports of socioemotional development of children adopted from orphanages or residential nurseries to private homes are those of Goldfarb (1943a, 1943b, 1944, 1945a, 1945b, 1947, 1955); Tizard (Hodges & Tizard, 1989a, 1989b; Tizard, 1977; Tizard, Cooperman, Joseph, & Tizard, 1972; Tizard & Hodges, 1978; Tizard & Joseph, 1970; Tizard & Rees, 1974, 1975; Tizard & Tizard, 1971); and three more recent studies of children adopted from Romania. In two of the studies, Romanian orphans were adopted to Canada (Ames, 1997; Chisholm, 1998; Chisholm, Carter, Ames, & Morison, 1995; Fisher, Ames, Chisholm, & Savoie, 1997; Marcovitch, Cesaroni, Roberts, & Swanson, 1995; Marcovitch et al., 1997). In the third study, they were adopted to the United Kingdom (O'Connor, Bredenkamp, Rutter, & the English and Romanian Adoptees [ERA] Study Team, 1999; O'Connor, Rutter, & the ERA Study Team, 2000; Rutter & the ERA Study Team, 1998). These sets of studies varied greatly in terms of the conditions in the institutions, the characteristics of the homes, the comparison groups employed, and the measures of socioemotional development used, so it is important to describe each of them before reviewing their results. Each of these studies is summarized briefly in Table 7.1. One disadvantage of these studies is that almost all of the children entered the institutions at a very young age and stayed there until they moved to their adoptive, original, or foster homes. Thus, there is a confound between the age of the children when they went to homes and the length of their institutionalization, and none of the studies allow us to tell which of two variables, age or duration, is the effective one.

This chapter looks at two areas of the socioemotional development of children who were adopted from institutions with reference to their behavior toward adults: 1) their attachment to their parents and 2) their behavior toward new adults (strangers). First, it reviews the theoretical background that suggests the possibility of a critical or sensitive period for the development of attachment. Then, the research results and the relation of the children's development to the time spent in institutions are discussed.

ATTACHMENT TO PARENTS

Attachment theory was partially derived from studies of children reared in institutions. John Bowlby (1953), widely recognized as the major theorist

Table 7.1. Socioemotional development of children adopted from orphanages or residential nurseries to private homes

Study	Design	Advantages	Disadvantages
Goldfarb's	Compared New York children who had been in institutions from infancy to age 3 and then transferred to foster homes with children who had been in foster homes from early infancy Poor conditions in institutions, including minimal interaction with caregivers (Goldfarb, 1943b)	Looked at long-term effects of children after removal from an institution Studied groups of children at different ages, from 43 months to adolescence (Goldfarb, 1943a, 1945a, 1945b, 1947)	Children experienced many types of institutional deprivation Children went to foster homes, where moves from home to home were common, rather than adoptive homes, where there was stability (Goldfarb, 1944) There is a possibility of halo effects from intellectual tests to social ratings Limited by the methodology of its time
Tizard's	Studied healthy children from residential nurseries in the United Kingdom Institution conditions were generally good Compared children who were adopted into middle-class homes with children who were restored to their birth families, which were usually of low socioeconomic status	Looked at long-term effects up to age 16 The only type of institutional deprivation was lack of close personal relationships with caregivers	Only healthy children were studied, so results are more positive than they might have been if all institution children had been studied Limited by the methodology of its time

(continued)

Table 7.1. *(continued)*

Study	Design	Advantages	Disadvantages
Romanian orphanage	Studied children adopted from Romanian orphanages to other countries Poor conditions in orphanages, including minimal interaction with caregivers Compared children from orphanages with nonadoptive children born in Canada (Chisholm, 1998; Marcovitch et al., 1997) or with children adopted domestically in the United Kingdom before age 6 months (O'Connor et al., 1999)	Used standard observational assessments of attachment Larger, more carefully selected samples of children than in earlier studies	Children experienced many types of deprivation in orphanages Measures were not designed to indicate the presence or absence of attachment but how secure an attachment was Measures of behavior toward new adults were not standard but were constructed by individual researchers (Chisholm, 1998; O'Connor et al., 1999)

in attachment, thought that the chief negative feature of group residential care for children was lack of opportunity for continuous personal caregiving so that a child was unable to attach to a particular caregiver.

The term *attachment* is used to indicate the loving bond that a child ordinarily develops with his or her parent(s). In popular literature, the term *bonding* often is used. There is a long history within the psychoanalytic tradition for the idea that the child's attachment to the parent is established within the first year of life and that its establishment has long-term consequences (Erikson, 1963; Freud, 1938). In his attachment theory, Bowlby (1969/1982) combined psychoanalysis with information from ethological studies of imprinting in animals, an area in which critical periods had been shown to exist. He noted, however, that boundaries of such periods in humans were not as abrupt as those found in animal imprinting studies. Bowlby, like most researchers studying human development, used the term *sensitive period* rather than *critical period* because he believed that development could occur later but would be harder to induce.

Clear-cut attachment is shown by children seeking to be physically closer to parents than to other people, being anxious with strangers or when separated from their parents, and using parents as a secure base from which to explore (i.e., exploring the environment with ease if the parent is present so that the child can return to him or her intermittently for emotional support). Because such signs do not appear until the second part of the first year, Bowlby (1953) concluded that it was only after the age of 6 months that separation of a child from his or her mother appeared to do harm. He reported that infants adopted between 6 and 9 months showed little or no socioemotional damage and proposed that the possibility of forming a first attachment might last through the end of the first year of life, perhaps even up to 18 months of age. If, however, good mothering was delayed until after the age of 2½ years, it was "almost useless" (Bowlby, 1953). Thus, a sensitive period was implied. A child was most ready to become attached quickly at least through the end of the first year (Bowlby, 1969/1982), but thereafter attachment would be increasingly more difficult (e.g., require a longer time or better parenting, take a less adaptive form), with the possibility that eventually even excellent parenting might not be able to remedy the child's problems.

As Bowlby's theory developed, the length he attributed to this sensitive period increased. By 1973, he stated that attachment behavior is most easily activated between 6 months and 5 years but that "sensitivity in this regard persists during the decade after the fifth birthday, albeit in steadily diminishing degree as the years of childhood pass" (Bowlby, 1973, pp. 202–203). Later, he viewed the end of the period as even more flexible, perhaps extending through adolescence (Bowlby, 1988).

Secure attachment in a child is related to the sensitive responsiveness of the mother or other important caregiver. *Sensitive responsiveness* refers to behavior that is not only responsive to an infant's signals and cues but also is appropriately or contingently responsive (Ainsworth, Blehar, Waters, & Wall, 1978; Belsky, 1999; Bowlby, 1969/1982). For example, a mother may respond often to her infant, but if her responses are not appropriate she may, through her insensitivity, distress rather than comfort the infant. Ainsworth et al. (1978) linked maternal sensitive responsiveness during the first year of life to the security of the infant's attachment. De Wolff and van IJzendoorn (1997), in a meta-analysis of 66 studies that examined the relationship between security and sensitive responsiveness, concluded that maternal sensitivity clearly contributes to the development of a secure attachment relationship. The work of van den Boom (1994) demonstrated that training sensitive responsiveness in mothers increased security in their infants. Belsky (1999) has acknowledged the evidence linking maternal sensitivity and security but has stated that one must also consider the social context within which the attachment relationship is developing. For example, stressors such as marital conflict, low socioeconomic status, lack of social support, and parents' poor psychological health will have a negative impact on parents' ability to respond sensitively to their infants (Belsky, 1999).

ATTACHMENT RESULTS

In order to use institution studies to study whether there is a sensitive period for first attachment, it is necessary to prove, or at least to assume, that children have not been able to make any significant attachments to their caregivers within the institution. There is little evidence on this point. It may be inferred from the very low caregiver-to-child ratio in Goldfarb's and the Romanian studies that caregivers would have little time to respond sensitively to any one child. In Tizard's studies, the limiting factors were high staff turnover and the institution's policy that caregivers were not to develop close personal relationships with specific children.

The only researcher who studied institutionalized children's behavior toward their caregivers was Tizard. Tizard and Tizard (1971) found that although it was possible to construct a small list of preferred persons (usually parents and grandparents) for family-reared 2-year-olds, a preference list could not be constructed for children in institutions because their lists included anyone the child knew well, including the nursery staff, cleaners, and gardeners. Their only favorites were adults who they saw very infrequently (e.g., a mother who visited), but significantly, these were the only adults who gave them the one-to-one attention that their regular nurses were forbidden to provide.

Children who were still in the institution at age 4½ followed their caregivers around, and some of them were described as very clingy (Tizard & Rees, 1975). Most of the children did show some preferences among nurses, but approximately half of them showed no distress when their group nurse left the institution permanently. In spite of the children's following and clinging, nurses reported that 70% of them did not care deeply about anyone. About half of the children constantly tried to make contact with any new adults and would follow after any staff member, but the other half seemed emotionally detached from all adults (Tizard & Rees, 1975). When the children were 8 years old, there were 7 institution children left to study. Only 3 of the 7 were reported by their institution housemother to be closely attached to her (Tizard & Hodges, 1978). Thus, children whose lives had been spent in institutions seemed to show generalized reactions to all adults, either showing interest in all familiar caregivers and strangers or becoming detached and showing little interest in any adults. In either case, they did not seem to have formed a deep attachment with a particular adult.

FOLLOWING REMOVAL FROM AN INSTITUTION

Chisholm et al. (1995) suggested several factors that might contribute to difficulties of children beyond age 1 or 2 developing a first attachment after moving from an institution to an adoptive home: 1) parents may not be as responsive to an older child's need for closeness as they would be to an infant's need; 2) some children adopted from poor institutions do not display behaviors such as smiling, making eye contact, or crying, thus making it more difficult for parents to determine the child's needs; and 3) because of their neglect in an institution, children may have developed expectations of others as untrustworthy, and this might promote difficult or passive interaction styles that would negatively affect their parents' responsiveness to them.

Goldfarb concluded that children who moved to foster homes after having been in orphanages for about 3 years were unable to attach to their new foster parents. This conclusion was based mainly on the results obtained from adolescents. Goldfarb (1943a) found that thirteen of fifteen 10- to 14-year-olds who had been moved from institutions to foster homes at about age 3, but none of the fifteen children who had been in foster homes since the first 6 months of life, were rated by their caseworkers as "removed" (e.g., emotionally withdrawn, cold, isolated), both with their families and with their caseworkers. They were not upset by a change in foster home or by threats of removal from foster homes in which they had been well accepted (Goldfarb, 1945b). By 1947, Goldfarb claimed that privation effects, including poor relationships to others, are permanent in institution children, being "analogous to the crippling physical loss of a limb that can never be stimulated to grow again" (1947, p. 449).

In contrast to Goldfarb, Tizard (1977) concluded that children could become attached to parents after leaving institutions. Twenty of twenty-five adopted children seemed to have formed a close mutually affectionate relationship with their new parents within a year of leaving residential nurseries (Tizard & Hodges, 1978). Eighty-three percent of mothers said that they felt their child was deeply attached to them at 4½ years of age (Tizard & Rees, 1975), 84% at 8 years old (Tizard & Hodges, 1978), and 81% at 16 years old (Hodges & Tizard, 1989b). At age 16, the adopted children were not significantly different from a middle-class comparison group in showing overt affection to their parents. Hodges and Tizard (1989b) concluded that lack of close attachments in the residential nurseries had not prevented them from making a close attachment to their parents.

There are several possible reasons for the difference between Goldfarb's and Tizard's conclusions. First, the institutions in which the children in Goldfarb's studies lived were deprived in other ways than lack of intense one-to-one interaction with adults. As a result, children had developmental delays when they left the institutions. Children from Tizard's institutions were chosen for good health and had average IQ scores when they left the institutions (Tizard et al., 1972). These factors may have made them more appealing to parents, who may then have been more responsive to them. Second, it is unclear whether the children from the institutions Tizard studied were totally deprived of the opportunity to form specific attachments in the institution. Tizard and Rees (1975) noted that the policy of discouraging staff from forming close relationships with specific children seemed not to have been completely successful, and there were some indications of children's preferences among their regular caregivers.

A third difference between the two studies was in the stability of placement after the children left the institution. Children in Tizard's studies went to stable adoptive homes. Hodges and Tizard (1989a) reported that only 14% of adoptive placements made after the age of 2 had broken down by age 16. Children in Goldfarb's studies went to foster homes that were not stable. By ages 10–14, about half of the children in both the institution and foster home groups had lived in three or more foster homes (Goldfarb, 1943a). It is probable that the making and breaking of attachments to a series of different parents was a factor that served to exacerbate the children's reported emotional coldness.

In the Canadian studies of children from Romanian orphanages, both Chisholm (1998) and Marcovitch (Marcovitch et al., 1997) used a more comprehensive method of evaluating children's patterns of attachment. This was a separation-reunion procedure in which preschool children first played with their mothers, then were separated from them for a short period of time and stayed in a room with a stranger, then were reunited with their mothers. The child's behavior during this procedure was videotaped and later coded by trained coders for the quality of the child's attachment to the mother. In the Chisholm (1998) research, children who each spent at least 8 months in a Romanian orphanage before being adopted to Canada between 1990 and 1991 were studied (Orphanage group). They were compared with two comparison groups: a group of never-institutionalized, nonadopted children living with their biological parents in British Columbia (Canadian-Born group), and a group of children adopted from Romania to British Columbia before the age of 4 months (Early-Adopted group). Children in each of these comparison groups were individually matched in sex and age to a child in the Orphanage group.

In the Marcovitch research (Marcovitch et al., 1995; Marcovitch et al., 1997), children who had been adopted from Romania between 1990 and 1991, and who lived within commuting distance of Toronto, were invited to come to a hospital laboratory for assessment. Children who had been in institutional care for more than 6 months comprised the Institution group. Children who had spent less than 6 months in institutions during the first

6 months of life were termed the Home group; these Home children were adopted at a variety of ages. In addition, a group of healthy Canadian 4-year-olds from another study in the same laboratory were used as a comparison for the Romanian adoptees' attachment patterns. Some basic characteristics of the institutionalized children and the procedure employed in the two Canadian studies are shown in Table 7.2. Attachment results for the United Kingdom study have not yet been published.

The classification of attachment styles obtained for the previously institutionalized children and their comparison groups in the two studies is shown in Table 7.3. Neither of the studies found any children who were judged by coders to be unattached (but it should be noted that both of the coding systems used were designed initially to measure types of secure and insecure attachment, rather than the presence or absence of attachment *per se*).

The first thing to note in Table 7.3 is that approximately one third of the previously institutionalized children in each study were classified as securely attached. This would certainly argue against Goldfarb's (1947) conclusion that early deprivation of the opportunity for a close contact with a specific caregiver necessarily produces permanent damage of the capacity to attach later.

At the same time, it is clear that the percentage of securely attached children in the formerly institutionalized groups was generally lower than in their respective comparison groups. One exception to this general finding is that no differences were found between the Institution and Home groups in the Marcovitch et al. study, a result the authors termed unexpected. This apparent failure to find a clear difference may be due to 1) the small number of children (N = 19) with more than 6 months of institutional

Table 7.2. Assessments of postadoption attachment in children adopted from Romanian orphanages

	Chisholm (1998)	Marcovitch et al. (1997)
Location	British Columbia, Canada	Ontario, Canada
Number of participants	43 (orphanage)	19 (institution) 37 (home)
Time in institution	Md (Median) = 17.5 months Range = 8–53 months	Mean = 27.3 months Range = 6–48 months
Age when tested	$4\frac{1}{2}$ years (n = 30) $5\frac{1}{2}$–9 years (n = 13)	3–5 years
Where tested	Home	Laboratory
Procedure	One separation (child with stranger)	Two separations (child with stranger and child alone)
Coding system	Developed by Crittenden (1992)	Developed by Cassidy and Marvin (1987, 1992)

Table 7.3. Attachment classifications obtained in two studies of children adopted from Romanian orphanages

	N	Secure	Typical insecure	Atypical insecure
Chisholm (1998)				
Orphanage	43	37%	30%	33%
Canadian-Born	43	58%	35%	7%
Early-Adopted	30	66%	30%	4%
Marcovitch et al. (1997)				
Institutionalized *and* "Home"	44	33%	25%	42% ("Controlling/ Other")[a]
Healthy 4-year-olds	38	50%	35%	15%

[a]Comparison of the patterns included in Chisholm's Atypical insecure and Marcovitch et al.'s Controlling/Other led to agreement among the researchers (S. Goldberg, personal communication, July 10, 1996) that they are approximately the same and are both similar to the Disorganized pattern described for infants by Main and Solomon (1990).

experience (Institution group) and 2) the mixed backgrounds of the Home children. Because the requirement for that group was only that the child had spent less than 6 months in hospitals and orphanages in the first 6 months of life, it is possible that there were some children in the group who spent almost 6 months in an institution so that the difference between the two groups in institutional experience may have been small. In addition, some of the Home children were adopted after 6 months of age, but nothing is known about the quality of their attachments to the biological parents who gave them up for adoption.

In both studies, a majority of the previously institutionalized children had attachments to their mother that were either secure or typical insecure (i.e., insecurely attached in a manner common in normative, nonclinical samples of North American children). In Chisholm's study, 67% of the children in the Orphanage group had either secure or typical insecure attachments; that is, they had the same types of attachments as approximately 95% of the Canadian-Born and Early-Adopted groups, which did not differ from each other. The corresponding percentages in Marcovitch et al.'s study were that 58% of Romanian adoptees had the same types of secure and typical insecure attachments that 85% of their comparison group had.

In spite of these positive results, it must be acknowledged that in each study a considerable percentage of the previously institutionalized children had made very unusual (atypical insecure) attachments to their adoptive parents, attachments that resemble those of only a small proportion of children in comparison groups. *Atypical insecure* indicates patterns of insecure attachment that are rare in normative samples of children and are often found in clinical samples of maltreated children (Cicchetti & Barnett, 1991; Crittenden, 1988a, 1988b). Such attachments have been suggested by some researchers to be risk factors in the development of psychopathology (Carlson & Sroufe, 1995; Crittenden, 1988b). It is clear, therefore, that although secure attachments are possible after institutionalization, they are not as easily accomplished as in comparison groups, and that in some cases the attachments are insecure in uncommon and maladaptive ways.

A SENSITIVE PERIOD FOR ATTACHMENT?

The Early-Adopted group (adopted before 4 months of age) in Chisholm's research showed a distribution of attachment classifications that was not different from that of Canadian-Born children. This finding fits with Bowlby's (1973) idea that any sensitive period for attachment does not begin in the first few months of life.

None of the attachment results give a precise answer concerning when a sensitive period might end. Tizard and Hodges (1978) found no relation between the age at which children had left the institution and whether the mother considered the child to be attached to her at age 8 years. Five of the nine children who left the institution after the age of 4½ were judged at age 8 to be closely attached to their parents.

Marcovitch et al. (1997) also reported that length of time in an institution (range birth to 48 months) was not related to attachment security. Chisholm et al. (1995) did not find a relationship between previously institutionalized children's age at adoption and their attachment security as scored by their parents' interview responses at approximately 1 year after adoption. Chisholm (1996) found that when attachment was measured by a separation-reunion procedure when children were 4½ or older, former orphanage children classified as insecure were no more likely than those classified as secure to have spent a longer time in an institution or to have been older when they were adopted.

Given that Chisholm (1996), Chisholm et al. (1995), Marcovitch et al. (1997), and Tizard and Hodges (1978) have all failed to find a relationship between length of time in an institution and the quality of the attachment relationships children later form with their adoptive parents, it appears that researchers have not discovered an age beyond which forming a first attachment *necessarily* becomes problematic, at least among children adopted up to age 7 or so. It should be noted, however, that the statistical analyses performed in most of these research studies are not ideal to investigate a sensitive period hypothesis, which is better explored by a careful inspection of data than by either correlations (that investigate how well data fit a straight line) or average differences between groups. In a reanalysis performed for this chapter, it was found that the medians and ranges of length of institutionalization in Chisholm's (1998) research were 16.5 (range of 9–39) months for securely attached children; 14 (range of 9–53) months for typical insecurely attached; and 21 (range of 8–53) months for atypical insecurely attached children. These differences were not statistically significant, but note that the oldest child who had formed a secure attachment had spent only 39 months in an orphanage. There were only five children who had spent longer than 39 months in an orphanage, all of whom had either typical insecure (n = 2) or atypical insecure (n = 3) attachments. Five children are not enough to conclude that there is an end of the sensitive period for secure attachment at 39 months. Insecure attachments of these children are more easily explained by other factors, which will now be explored.

Given the theoretical importance of sensitive responsiveness to the development of attachment, it should not be surprising that characteristics of both the child and the parent matter to security of attachment in institutionalized children. Children with lower IQ scores (Chisholm, 1998; Tizard & Hodges, 1978) and a larger number of behavior problems (Chisholm, 1998; Marcovitch et al., 1997) have more difficulty forming secure attachments to their parents, presumably because these problems may interfere with their parents responding sensitively to them. Reanalysis of Chisholm's (1998) data for this chapter also revealed another factor that may have interfered with parents being able to respond to an individual child: Although only 14% of securely attached and typical insecurely attached children were adopted by families that adopted another Romanian child at the same time, 57% of the atypically insecurely attached children had a sibling who had been adopted from Romania at the same time. Other family factors that were related to more insecure attachment were lower socioeconomic status of the family and a higher level of parenting stress (Chisholm, 1998). These stressors are among those believed by Belsky (1999) to have a negative impact on parents' ability to be sensitively responsive to their infants.

All five of the children in Chisholm's reanalysis who had more than 39 months in an orphanage had IQ scores lower than 85, some as low as 30 points below. In addition, three of the five had behavior problem scores indicating the need for professional help; each of these three children was one of two Romanian orphans adopted at the same time into a family, which necessarily limited the amount of specific responding to any one child. Four of the five had either family incomes or socioeconomic statuses that were lower than average for the Orphanage group as a whole, and three of the four for whom parenting stress scores were available had higher scores than average for the group. Thus, rather than assume that the insecure attachments of these five children were related to the length of time they spent in an orphanage, it seems more reasonable to suppose that the predominant explanation for their insecurity is that they went to families in which resources relative to children's problems were not enough to allow parents to provide them with the high level of sensitive responding that would have been necessary to promote secure attachment.

Chisholm's (1998) findings that family stressors are negative influences on the child's attachment are congruent with Tizard's finding that although children who went from residential nurseries to adoptive homes made close attachments to their parents, the picture was different for children restored to their biological mothers, whose mothers had usually been ambivalent or even reluctant to take them back (Tizard & Hodges, 1978). Restored children went home to families with larger numbers of children (Tizard & Hodges, 1978). Mothers in restored families were younger than adoptive mothers, and fathers had jobs indicating lower socioeconomic status than in adoptive families (Tizard & Rees, 1974). Restored parents spent less time playing with the children or engaging them in educational activities than did adoptive parents (Tizard & Hodges, 1978). This was not merely a class difference: Restored parents spent less time on these activities than their working class comparisons (Hodges & Tizard, 1989b).

In contrast, adoptive parents wanted the child; were affectionate; were willing and happy to devote a great deal of time to the child (even more than middle-class comparison parents); and seemed ready to accept and even enjoy dependent, young-for-age behavior (Tizard & Hodges, 1978). Tizard and Hodges concluded that a child's attachment did not depend as much on institutionalization as on the "willingness of the new parents to accept a dependent relationship and to put a lot of time and effort into developing it" (p. 115).

In summary, studies are fairly consistent in indicating that after children have been in institutions for many months with little or no opportunity to attach, they do show the capacity to attach to their adoptive parents. Such attachments may, however, be slow to develop, and a higher proportion of previously institutionalized children than family-reared children form insecure attachments, with some of those insecure attachments taking forms that are unusual in family-reared children. The length of institutionalization, or the child's age at first opportunity to attach, does not seem to be related to the security of the attachment that is established. Rather, the factors that are related to insecurity of attachment are those characteristics of children that make the parenting task more difficult (e.g., lower IQ scores, behavior problems, more than one child adopted at one time) and characteristics of their families (e.g., lower socioeconomic status, more parenting stress) that diminish their ability to deal with the children's problems. The overall message seems to be that it takes better-than-average parenting to promote secure attachment in children from institutions, especially when those children have several problems and family resources are not adequate for dealing with those problems.

BEHAVIOR TOWARD NEW ADULTS

Even when children in an institution have not had the prolonged interaction with a consistently present and responsive adult that would allow them to form an attachment relationship with him or her, at least they have encountered a number of different adults, including caregivers and visitors to the orphanage. As previously noted, children whose lives have been spent in institutions seem to show generalized reactions to all adults.

Children who have left institutions often display what Tizard (1977) termed *indiscriminate friendliness* (i.e., behavior that is friendly and affectionate toward all adults, including strangers, without the fear or caution characteristic of most children). Indiscriminate friendliness, often including attention-seeking and affection-seeking, has been reported by many researchers (Chisholm, 1998; Chisholm et al., 1995; Goldfarb, 1943b, 1945b; Marcovitch et al., 1995; Marcovitch et al., 1997; O'Connor et al., 1999; O'Connor et al., 2000; Tizard & Hodges, 1978).

In Chisholm's research (Chisholm, 1998; Chisholm et al., 1995), children were considered to be indiscriminately friendly to the extent that their parents reported that they 1) were very friendly with all new adults; 2) typically approached new adults, began talking, and asked questions of them; 3) had never been shy with new adults; 4) wandered away from parents in places in which new adults were present and did not show distress when they found themselves separated from parents; and 5) would be willing to go home with a stranger. At approximately 3 years after adoption, Orphanage children demonstrated more of these behaviors than did the Early-Adopted and Canadian-Born children, who did not differ from each other (Chisholm, 1998).

Using a measure similar to Chisholm's, O'Connor and his colleagues (O'Connor et al., 1999; O'Connor et al., 2000) studied what they termed *disinhibited attachment disorder behaviors*, measured with parent interview responses indicating children's 1) lack of differentiation between adults, 2) readiness to go off with a stranger, and 3) failure to check back with the parent in new (anxiety-provoking) situations. They found that scores on this measure were higher in 6-year-old children who had spent between 6 and 42 months in Romanian orphanages than in children of the same age who had been adopted from either Romania or the United Kingdom before the age of 6 months (O'Connor et al., 2000).

Both studies also found little or no change in indiscriminate friendliness over time. Chisholm (1998) found that the numbers of indiscriminately friendly behaviors shown by Orphanage children did not decline from its first measurement 11 months after adoption to the second measurement 3 years after adoption. O'Connor et al. (2000) found that scores remained stable from age 4 to age 6.

In short, indiscriminate friendliness seems to be characteristic of many children who have moved from institutions to home life. This characteristic seems resistant to change (Chisholm, 1998; O'Connor et al., 2000; Tizard & Hodges, 1978), sometimes persisting many years after the child leaves the institution (Goldfarb, 1943a).

RELATION OF INDISCRIMINATE FRIENDLINESS TO ATTACHMENT

Because infants who seek proximity with all adults were believed by Bowlby (1953) to be in the preattachment stage, it is legitimate to question whether the previously institutionalized child's indiscriminate friendliness with adults might be a sign of lack of attachment or of insecure attachment. Indiscriminately friendly behavior has been considered a symptom of attachment disorder. The *Diagnostic and Statistical Manual of Mental Disorders, Fourth Edition* (DSM-IV), from the American Psychiatric Association (1994) described the disinhibited/indiscriminate subtype of reactive attachment disorder of infancy and early childhood as indicated by the child's lack of selectivity among people from whom to seek support and nurturance and overfriendliness toward unfamiliar adults.

Tizard and Hodges (1978) found that while more than half of 8-year-old overfriendly children were said to be closely attached to their mothers, there was still a significant tendency for those who were not closely attached to their parents to be more overfriendly than children who were closely attached. Chisholm (1998) found that by 3 years after adoption, children who were more indiscriminately friendly were less secure as measured by parent interview. When attachment patterns measured in the separation-reunion procedure (Crittenden, 1992) were used as the measure of attachment, however, it was only the two most extreme measures of indiscriminate friendliness (wandering away and not showing distress when they found themselves separated from parents and being willing to go home with a stranger) that differentiated insecure from secure children. Both of those measures explicitly evaluate the child's use of the parent as a secure base, so it is reasonable that they would be related to attachment. The three measures that were more representative of simple friendliness (being friendly with new adults, eagerly approaching strangers, and never having been shy) were used equally by securely and insecurely attached children. Although data concerning the relation of attachment security and indiscriminate friendliness are not yet available from the United Kingdom study, O'Connor et al. (2000) have noted that of the three items they rated, only "would readily go off with a stranger" differentiated their Romanian sample from United Kingdom domestic adoptees, providing further evidence that perhaps not all of the items have the same origin or function in the same way.

Thus, although there is some evidence that insecurely attached children may be more likely to show indiscriminate friendliness than are securely attached children, the evidence is strong only for the more extreme forms of indiscriminate friendliness. Chisholm (1998), Marcovitch et al. (1997), and Tizard and Hodges (1978) have all found some securely attached children who are indiscriminately friendly in the sense of being generally friendly to new adults. For these reasons, it is unlikely that the indiscriminate friendliness of previously institutionalized children *necessarily* indicates an attachment disorder.

A SENSITIVE PERIOD FOR INDISCRIMINATE FRIENDLINESS?

There is some disagreement as to whether there is a relation between the length of time children spend in an orphanage (or their age at adoption) and the amount of indiscriminate friendliness they show. O'Connor and his colleagues (2000) have reported a modest correlation between the length of institutionalization and the number of *attachment disorder* symptoms Romanian adoptees showed at age 6. They also have expressed surprise at the wide variability among children, with a large proportion of children who stayed in an orphanage for more than 2 years not showing any symptoms, and a small number of children adopted within the first 6 months of life showing symptoms (O'Connor et al., 2000).

Neither Chisholm (Chisholm, 1998; Chisholm et al., 1995) nor Tizard (Tizard & Hodges, 1978; Tizard & Rees, 1975) was able to find a relation between the length of time children had spent in an orphanage (or their age at adoption) and the amount of indiscriminate friendliness they showed. Rather, indiscriminate friendliness seems to be a leftover from orphanage life or early postadoption days, whenever the child first learned that adults in general were interested in and attentive to him or her. Chisholm (1998) found that indiscriminate friendliness was positively related to the child's having been a favorite child in the orphanage, according to the parental report. Children perceived to be favorites of caregivers were those who had a small amount of increased interaction with them—an occasional hair tousle or a tickle to get them to laugh. Even this minimal increase over what most orphanage children received, however, was enough to show them that it was possible to get attention from adults. For other children, however, it was not until after adoption that they learned that adults generally cared about them.

There is only conflicting support for the assertion that indiscriminately friendly behavior is related to the length of time spent in an orphanage, but even if the relation were to be demonstrated more conclusively it would not provide evidence of a critical period for indiscriminate friendliness, because children in the studies of indiscriminate friendliness were not placed in the institutions at different ages, but all had been institutionalized from birth.

WHAT DO WE KNOW ABOUT ATTACHMENT OF CHILDREN FROM INSTITUTIONS?

According to present evidence, it appears that children removed from institutions to private homes before the age of 4 months do not experience problems in attaching to their new parents. Children removed at older ages, even after 4–7 years of institutionalization, seem able to become attached to new parents, but the process may be slower than normal. A higher proportion of them may have insecure attachments, with some having unusual insecure attachments that may portend psychological problems later. The major predictors of which children will have difficulty attaching, however, are not the length of institutionalization or the age of the child when adopted, but rather, how many problems (intellectual and behavioral) the child presents, how many children are adopted at one time, and how many resources (socioeconomic status and lack of stress) adoptive parents can bring to bear in dealing with the child's problems. Given children who have few problems when they leave the institution and parents who are able to respond sensitively, some children who move to adoptive homes when they are between 4½ and 7 years old are able to form attachment relationships (Tizard & Hodges, 1978). Previously institutionalized children's characteristic indiscriminate friendliness toward adults is not necessarily a sign of insecure attachment to their parents, except when it involves extreme behaviors like the willingness to go off with strangers. There is no evidence that there is a critical period for either attachment or indiscriminate friendliness.

WHAT DO WE NEED TO KNOW?

The results of institution studies on attachment reviewed here generally seem to fit Bowlby's theoretical predictions that 1) attachment to caregivers does not ordinarily occur until after the first few months of life; that 2) the formation of a first attachment may be made beyond 5 years of age; but that 3) the longer a child is prevented from making a first attachment, the more effort will be required from the child's parents to make that attachment a secure one.

Two factors that are important in determining a sensitive period for children from an institution who are placed into a home are the quality of the institution and the quality of the family into which the child is placed after institutionalization. The most positive report of how late the window for attachment may stay open has come from Tizard, who studied children from good institutions who went to attentive, devoted adoptive parents. The most negative report has come from Goldfarb, who studied children who left poor quality institutions with many problems and then went to a series of temporary foster homes. It is not known whether there are conditions in which the period of possible attachment might be extended through adolescence, as Bowlby (1988) suggested.

To map out all combinations of possible variables, it would be necessary to study more samples of children who entered and left institutions of different quality at different ages. Because most children are adopted from institutions before the age of 3, it would not be possible to study a large group of children adopted after that age without studying children from many different institutions with different criteria for admission and different standards of care. It is unlikely that this will be done any time soon, especially given that standard agreed-upon measures of attachment for older children and adolescents are not currently available.

Institution studies are not experiments with controlled variables. Because of this, trying to draw precise results from them is frustrating. Given the present state of knowledge, although prospective adoptive parents should be informed of the great effort and time that may be necessary to get a child from an institution to attach to them, there is no reason to tell them that there is any clear critical period after which it is impossible for a formerly institutionalized child to attach for the first time.

REFERENCES

Ainsworth, M.D.S., Blehar, M.C., Waters, E., & Wall, S. (1978). *Patterns of attachment: A psychological study of the strange situation*. Mahwah, NJ: Lawrence Erlbaum Associates.

American Psychiatric Association. (1994). *Diagnostic and statistical manual of mental disorders* (4th ed.). Washington, DC: Author.

Ames, E.W. (1997). *Development of Romanian orphanage children adopted to Canada*. Ottawa: Final Report to Human Resources Development Canada.

Belsky, J. (1999). Interactional and contextual determinants of attachment security. In J. Cassidy & P.R. Shaver (Eds.), *Handbook of attachment: Theory, research, and clinical applications* (pp. 249–264). New York: The Guilford Press.

Bowlby, J. (1953). *Child care and the growth of love*. Harmondsworth, England: Penguin Books.

Bowlby, J. (1973). *Attachment and loss: Vol. 2. Separation: Anxiety and anger*. New York: Basic Books.

Bowlby, J. (1982). *Attachment and loss: Vol. 1. Attachment*. New York: Basic Books. (Originally published in 1969)

Bowlby, J. (1988). Lecture 2: The origins of attachment theory. *A secure base* (pp. 20–38). New York: Basic Books.

Carlson, E.A., & Sroufe, A.L. (1995). Contributions of attachment theory to developmental psychopathology. In D. Cicchetti & D.J. Cohen (Eds.), *Developmental psychopathology: Vol. 1. Theory and methods* (pp. 581–617). New York: John Wiley & Sons.

Cassidy, J., Marvin, R.S., & Attachment Working Group of the MacArthur Network on the Transition from Infancy to Early Childhood. (1987, 1992). *Attachment organization in three- and four-year-olds: Coding guidelines*. Unpublished manual. University of Virginia, Charlottesville.

Chisholm, K. (1996). *Attachment security and indiscriminately friendly behavior in children adopted from Romanian orphanages*. Doctoral dissertation. Simon Fraser University, Burnaby, British Columbia.

Chisholm, K. (1998). A three year follow-up of attachment and indiscriminate friendliness in children adopted from Romanian orphanages. *Child Development, 69*, 1092–1106.

Chisholm, K., Carter, M., Ames, E.W., & Morison, S.J. (1995). Attachment security and indiscriminately friendly behavior in children adopted from Romanian orphanages. *Development and Psychopathology*, 7, 283–294.

Cicchetti, D., & Barnett, D. (1991). Attachment organization in maltreated preschoolers. *Development and Psychopathology, 3*, 397–411.

Crittenden, P. (1988a). Family and dyadic patterns of functioning in maltreating families. In K. Browne, C. Davies, & P. Stratton (Eds.), *Early prediction and prevention of child abuse* (pp. 161–189). Chichester, England: John Wiley & Sons.

Crittenden, P. (1988b). Relationships at risk. In J. Belsky & T. Networski (Eds.), *Clinical implications of attachment* (pp. 137–174). Mahwah, NJ: Lawrence Erlbaum Associates.

Crittenden, P. (1992). Quality of attachment in the preschool years. *Development and Psychopathology, 4*, 209–243.

De Wolff, M.S., & van IJzendoorn, M.H. (1997). Sensitivity and attachment: A meta-analysis on parental antecedents of infant attachment. *Child Development, 68*(4), 571–591.

Erikson, E.H. (1963). *Childhood and society*. New York: W.W. Norton & Company.

Fisher, L., Ames, E.W., Chisholm, K., & Savoie, L. (1997). Problems reported by parents of Romanian orphans adopted to British Columbia. *International Journal of Behavioral Development, 20*(1), 67–82.

Freud, S. (1938). Three contributions to the theory of sex. In A.A. Brill (Ed.), *The basic writings of Sigmund Freud* (pp. 553–629). New York: Modern Library.

Goldfarb, W. (1943a). The effects of early institutional care on adolescent personality. *Journal of Experimental Education, 12*(2), 106–129.

Goldfarb, W. (1943b). Infant rearing and problem behavior. *American Journal of Orthopsychiatry, 13*, 249–265.

Goldfarb, W. (1944). Infant rearing as a factor in foster home replacement. *American Journal of Orthopsychiatry, 14*, 162–166.

Goldfarb, W. (1945a). Effects of psychological deprivation in infancy and subsequent stimulation. *American Journal of Psychiatry, 102*, 18–33.

Goldfarb, W. (1945b). Psychological privation in infancy and subsequent adjustment. *American Journal of Orthopsychiatry, 14*, 247–255.

Goldfarb, W. (1947). Variations in adolescent adjustment of institutionally-reared children. *American Journal of Orthopsychiatry, 17*, 449–457.

Goldfarb, W. (1955). Emotional and intellectual consequences of psychologic deprivation in infancy: A reevaluation. In P. Hoch & J. Zubin (Eds.), *Psychopathology of childhood* (pp. 105–119). New York: Grune & Stratton.

Hodges, J., & Tizard, B. (1989a). IQ and behavioural adjustment of ex-institutional adolescents. *Journal of Child Psychology and Psychiatry, 30*(1), 53–75.

Hodges, J., & Tizard, B. (1989b). Social and family relationships of ex-institutional adolescents. *Journal of Child Psychology and Psychiatry, 30*(1), 77–97.

Main, M., & Solomon, J. (1990). Procedures for identifying infants as disorganized/disoriented during the Ainsworth Strange Situation. In M. Greenberg, D. Cicchetti, & M. Cummings (Eds.), *Attachment in the preschool years: Theory, research, and intervention* (pp. 121–160). Chicago: University of Chicago Press.

Marcovitch, S., Cesaroni, L., Roberts, W., & Swanson, C. (1995). Romanian adoption: Parents' dreams, nightmares, and realities. *Child Welfare, 74*, 993–1017.

Marcovitch, S., Goldberg, S., Gold, A., Washington, J., Wasson, C., Krekewich, K., & Handley-Derry, M. (1997). Determinants of behavioural problems in Romanian children adopted in Ontario. *International Journal of Behavioral Development, 20*(1), 17–31.

Morison, S.J., Ames, E.W., & Chisholm, K. (1995). The development of children adopted from Romanian orphanages. *Merrill-Palmer Quarterly, 41*(4), 411–430.

O'Connor, T.G., Bredenkamp, D., Rutter, M., & the English and Romanian Adoptees (ERA) Study Team. (1999). Attachment disturbances and disorders in children exposed to early severe deprivation. *Infant Mental Health Journal, 20*(1), 10–29.

O'Connor, T.G., Rutter, M., & the English and Romanian Adoptees (ERA) Study Team. (2000). Attachment disorder behavior following early severe deprivation: Extension and longitudinal follow-up. *Journal of the American Academy of Child and Adolescent Psychiatry, 39*(6), 703–712.

Rutter, M., & the English and Romanian Adoptees (ERA) Study Team. (1998). Developmental catch-up, and deficit, following adoption after severe global early privation. *Journal of Child Psychology and Psychiatry, 39*(4), 465–476.

Tizard, B. (1977). *Adoption: A second chance*. London: Open Books.

Tizard, B., Cooperman, O., Joseph, A., & Tizard, J. (1972). Environmental effects on language development: A study of young children in long-stay residential nurseries. *Child Development, 43*, 337–358.

Tizard, B., & Hodges, J. (1978). The effect of early institutional rearing on the development of eight year old children. *Journal of Child Psychology and Psychiatry, 19*, 99–118.

Tizard, B., & Joseph, A. (1970). Cognitive development of young children in residential care: A study of children aged 24 months. *Journal of Child Psychology and Psychiatry, 11*, 177–186.

Tizard, B., & Rees, J. (1974). A comparison of the effects of adoption, restoration to the natural mother, and continued institutionalization on the cognitive development of four-year-old children. *Child Development, 43*, 92–99.

Tizard, B., & Rees, J. (1975). The effect of early institutional rearing on the behaviour problems and affectional relationships of four-year-old children. *Journal of Child Psychology and Psychiatry, 16*, 61–73.

Tizard, J., & Tizard, B. (1971). The social development of two-year-old children in residential nurseries. In H.R. Schaffer (Ed.), *The origins of human social relations* (pp. 147–163). New York: Academic Press.

van den Boom, D.C. (1994). The influence of temperament and mothering on attachment and exploration: An experimental manipulation of sensitive responsiveness among lower-class mothers with irritable infants. *Child Development, 65*, 1449–1469.

IV

Critical Periods in Language Learning and Acquisition

8

Language Processing

How Experience Affects Brain Organization

Helen J. Neville

John T. Bruer

This book presents an opportunity to review what we know about critical periods and brain development in a range of areas, including vision, social-emotional development, and early literacy. One of the challenges confronting scientists is integrating research on these skills and their underlying brain systems to clarify what is and is not known. This chapter discusses research that is directed toward the underlying theme of taking a critical look at critical periods. This chapter focuses primarily on language processing but illustrates general principles of how experience influences brain organization by first summarizing some of the research on perceptual processing. Using this research as a basis, this chapter tries to offer answers to three questions: How do brain systems for perceptual and language processing arise during development? To what degree are these systems tightly constrained by biological factors? What is the role of experience in organizing these brain systems?

Philosophers, educators, and parents have debated issues of development, biological constraints, and the role of experience in development for millennia. These debates are often characterized, in a simple way, as the "nature versus nurture" argument. Systematic research on how and when experience might affect brain development began about 30 years ago with David Hubel and Torsten Wiesel's research on the development of the

The research discussed in this chapter has been supported by grants (nos. DC00128 and DC00481) from National Institutes of Health, National Institute on Deafness and Other Communication Disorders. The authors are grateful to their many collaborators on the several studies summarized here and to Linda and Julie Heidenreich for help in manuscript preparation.

visual system (Wiesel & Hubel, 1965; see Chapter 1). Thus, given this short history, it is not surprising that we do not yet know much about how and when experience influences brain development. Furthermore, until recently most of the research has been on rats, cats, and monkeys. Now, however, with the advent of noninvasive methods for imaging and recording from intact, functioning human brains, we can begin to answer questions more directly about how experience influences human brain development and organization.

Using these new technologies, we would like to answer the following questions: Do different brain systems possess intrinsic constraints that make them able to process certain kinds of information but not others? For example, can the brain's auditory systems only process auditory information, or are there circumstances under which it might come to process visual information? What is the role of environmental input, or experience, in the development and specialization of different brain systems? Is the influence of environmental input on brain systems limited to specific, critical periods in development, or can experience affect brain organization throughout the life span? Are some brain systems subject to critical period constraints, while others are not?

Before presenting the data that address these questions, let us briefly review what is known about the structural development of the brain. By every measure that neuroscientists have used, the human brain does not appear to be fully mature until 15–20 years of age. This holds true if one looks at the size and density of neurons, the extent of dendritic branching, the number and density of synapses, the pharmacological composition of the brain, and the electrophysiological responses of the brain (see Chapter 2). Fifteen to twenty years is a long developmental period during which environmental input could shape brain systems.

Figure 8.1 shows Peter Huttenlocher's oft-cited data on changes in synaptic density in the human brain over the life span (Huttenlocher & Dabholkar, 1997). Using electron-micrographic techniques, Huttenlocher and his colleagues counted the number of synapses in different brain areas in tissue samples taken at autopsy from individuals who died at different ages. These data illustrate that synaptic densities in the human brain change over the life span. Note that the curves depicting these changes do not asymptote, or settle at mature levels, until adolescence, showing the brain's long developmental time course. In every brain area that Huttenlocher studied, he found that there was an early period of rapid increase in synaptic density, followed by a gradual decrease. Maximal synaptic densities in the young brain are typically 50% greater than those found in adult brains. A working hypothesis of many scientists in this field is that this early overabundance of synapses provides the raw material for a mechanism whereby environmental input can shape brain systems. The hypothesis assumes that

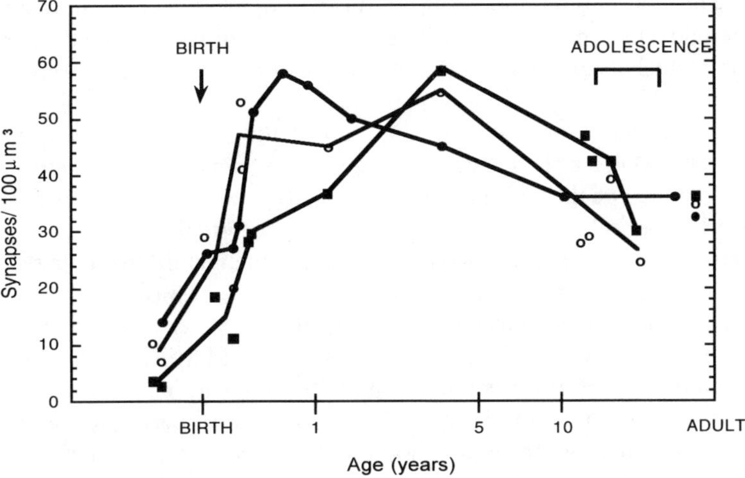

Figure 8.1. Mean synaptic density in synapses/100 μm³ in primary auditory (open circles), primary visual (filled circles), and prefrontal (squares) cortex at various ages. (From Huttenlocher, P.R., & Dabholkar, A.S. [1997]. Regional differences in synaptogenesis in human cerebral cortex. *Journal of Comparative Neurology, 387,* 170; reprinted by permission.)

environmental input contributes to determining which of the overabundant synapses are maintained or stabilized and which are lost.

An interesting feature of Huttenlocher's data is that the different brain regions he has studied show the same pattern of rapid increase followed by gradual decrease. However, the timing of that pattern follows different developmental time courses in different brain regions. For example, the visual cortex displays the increase and stabilization earlier than the prefrontal cortex, which shows a longer developmental time course. If these data are upheld, they imply that the time periods during which environmental input could shape developing brain systems differ, depending on the maturation of the brain region involved. Thus, we might expect that experience would have its effects on the developing visual system earlier than it would on the developing working memory and attentional systems that are mediated by neural circuitry in the frontal cortex.

The fact that there are different critical or sensitive periods for different brain systems, and even for subsystems within systems such as vision and language processing, is an important message that comes from the data scientists have collected (see Chapters 2 and 3). There appears to be extreme variability in how experience influences the development of different brain systems and their related functions. This is true even within the development of the visual system in which some aspects of development depend on input at one time while other aspects of this system's development depend on input at other times. For example, the development of ocular dominance preferences has a critical or sensitive period that is different from the period during which visual input can influence a neuron's orientation preference (Mitchell, 1981).

Furthermore, not only are there numerous critical periods within a system like vision or language, but some brain systems and their associated functions change throughout life. Not all systems and functions are subject to critical period constraints. Thus, some brain systems and their related functions are more constrained in their development and depend on receiving specific environmental input at specific times, whereas other brain systems do not. One important research goal is to determine which brain systems are subject to critical period constraints and which are not. These are complex questions. Keep in mind that it makes little sense to speak of *the* critical period for the visual system or *the* critical period for language acquisition. Given what we already know, this is too coarse a picture to guide research and its applications to policy and practice.

It is important to be aware that at the present time we know little about the neural mechanisms that underlie how experience influences brain development, or about the mechanisms responsible for the differences in modifiability by environmental input among brain systems. It is likely that when scientists do uncover these mechanisms they will involve factors such as the early and subsequent loss of excess synapses, changes in the balance of excitatory versus inhibitory connections within and among brain regions, and the degree of redundant connectivity within the brain. However, our current limited knowledge about the specific neural mechanisms involved in developmental brain plasticity does not prevent us from identifying different subsystems within the brain, drawing boundaries between them, and determining when, or if, these systems are subject to critical period constraints. We can identify which systems are changeable by experience and when they are most changeable. These findings will carry implications for the development and implementation of educational and rehabilitation programs.

There are at least two ways to study how experience affects brain organization during development. First, one can look at behavior and brain organization in adults who had different early experiences. For example, adults who have been deaf or blind from birth have had very different early sensory experience from that of hearing or sighted adults. In addition, many deaf people learn a sign language, a visual-spatial language, rather than a spoken, oral-aural language as their first language. Second, one can look directly at the behavior and brain organization in infants and children as they pass through different ages and specific milestones in perception and language.

In the work discussed here, scientists use two noninvasive techniques to study and observe brain organization. In the event-related potential (ERP) technique, scientists record the electrical events generated by neuronal activity in the brain from electrodes placed on individuals' scalps. As a technique, ERP has excellent temporal resolution. It allows them to track brain events rapidly at a millisecond-by-millisecond level. However, ERP's spatial resolution is not precise. Thus, to localize brain activity more precisely scientists use structural and functional magnetic resonance imaging (fMRI), which provides spatial resolution down to the millimeter level and in some cases even to the submillimeter level.

PRINCIPLES OF BRAIN SPECIALIZATION: PERCEPTUAL PROCESSING

With these research strategies and techniques, scientists have studied both language and perceptual processing. Although the focus of this chapter is on language processing, research on perceptual processing provides a useful model of how experience affects brain development. At the current time, it is reasonable to think, for reasons of scientific parsimony and in the absence of empirical evidence to the contrary, that similar principles govern the development of all highly specialized brain systems.

As mentioned previously, one of these general principles appears to be the variability, even within a perceptual system, in the extent and timing of a brain system's modifiability by experience. Research on visual processing in deaf subjects illustrates this principle. In studies such as these, it is important to have a homogeneous subject population in which we know the etiology of the perceptual problem. All of the deaf subjects who participated in the research discussed here were born to deaf parents and have been profoundly and bilaterally deaf since birth. Their condition is caused by a genetic abnormality that prevents the cochlea from developing normally. So, although they cannot hear because of this defect in the ear, their central nervous systems, including their brains, are not directly affected. The hearing siblings of the deaf subjects provide scientists with a control group. This control group is particularly important in studies of language acquisition, as will be evident in the next section.

Using a subject population like this allows us to ask the following questions: What impact does profound auditory deprivation have on the development of the remaining sensory systems? What happens to the auditory cortex in these subjects? What happens to the visual system when there is no auditory input early in development? We know there is a strong genetic bias for particular cortical structures to process acoustic information. Does this mean that these structures cannot process visual information? Is it possible to rewire the auditory system to process visual information? Are there limited temporal windows, or critical periods, during which rewiring in deaf subjects' brains can occur? Current research provides interesting answers to these questions.

In studies of visual processing in the deaf, scientists collected ERPs on congenitally deaf people and normal hearing controls as they processed visual stimuli (Neville, 1995). They found that the brain's electrical response to visual stimuli presented in the center of the visual field was the same in both populations. There were no major differences in brain organization after auditory deprivation for processing stimuli in the center of the visual field. However, in response to stimuli presented out in the visual periphery, deaf subjects showed much larger brain activation responses than did their hearing siblings. This finding suggests that auditory deprivation somehow affects the brain's representation of the visual periphery, but not the brain's representation of the center of visual space.

How might we explain this difference? The visual periphery is strongly represented along the brain's dorsal pathway that projects from V1, the primary visual area, up to the parietal cortex (see Figure 8.2). This dorsal visual pathway is important for processing motion and location in space. The center of the visual field is most strongly represented along the ventral visual pathway. This pathway is important for color and form perception. Comparing the brain activations of deaf subjects with those of their hearing siblings suggested the hypothesis that motion and spatial location processing are more plastic or more modifiable by experience during development than are color and form processing.

Scientists designed an experiment to directly test this hypothesis. They presented subjects with one set of stimuli designed to activate the motion sensitive dorsal system and another set of stimuli designed to activate the color sensitive ventral system. They found that deaf and hearing subjects had similar ERP brain response patterns to the stimuli that changed color and activated the ventral visual pathway. However, in response to the stimuli that displayed motion and activated the dorsal pathway, the deaf subjects showed a much larger brain response than did the hearing subjects (see Figure 8.3). From this experiment we can conclude that the ventral visual system was relatively unaffected, whereas the dorsal system was modified, by auditory deprivation. Thus, some parts of the visual system are radically changed after early auditory deprivation and others are not.

Functional MRI studies have allowed us to see more precisely where these changes are taking place in the brain (Neville & Bavelier, 1999). In normal hearing subjects, visual motion activates posterior visual areas and area MT, a motion center in the dorsal pathway of the brain. Deaf subjects have significantly larger activations in these visual areas as well as activations in areas extending up into parietal cortex, frontal cortex, and within

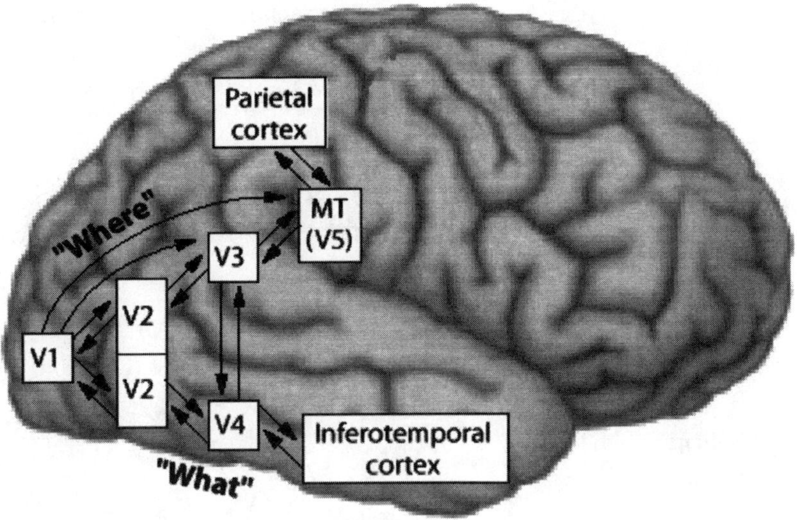

Figure 8.2. The dorsal ("where") and ventral ("what") pathway.

what would normally include the brain's auditory areas. If these results are upheld, they imply that strongly constrained sensory systems can change their functional properties when sensory experience is different.

There also may be a critical period after which rewiring of the sensory systems does not occur. Scientists have studied people who became deaf after the age of 4 due to the same genetic abnormality in cochlear development. In these cases the abnormal gene causes the cochlea to de-differentiate during development. When scientists examined brain recordings of these people who became deaf at a later age, they did not see the same enhanced visual responses to movement. Thus, there may be a limited time, within the first few years of life, when the auditory and visual sensory systems are being organized, during which incoming sensory stimulation plays a role in differentiating and defining these sensory systems.

If the dorsal visual pathway is more modifiable than the ventral visual pathway, then it also may be more vulnerable to abnormal experience. There is substantial evidence in the developmental literature that the dorsal visual pathway is vulnerable. Psychophysical studies (Lovegrove, Garzia, & Nicholson, 1990), physiological studies (Eden et al., 1996), and anatomical studies (Livingstone, Rosen, Drislane, & Galaburda, 1991) of dyslexic children suggest that dorsal pathway functions are deficient in these children, but their ventral visual pathways appear to be intact. Such children have not experienced sensory deprivation, but there is some abnormality in aspects of the visual system's development.

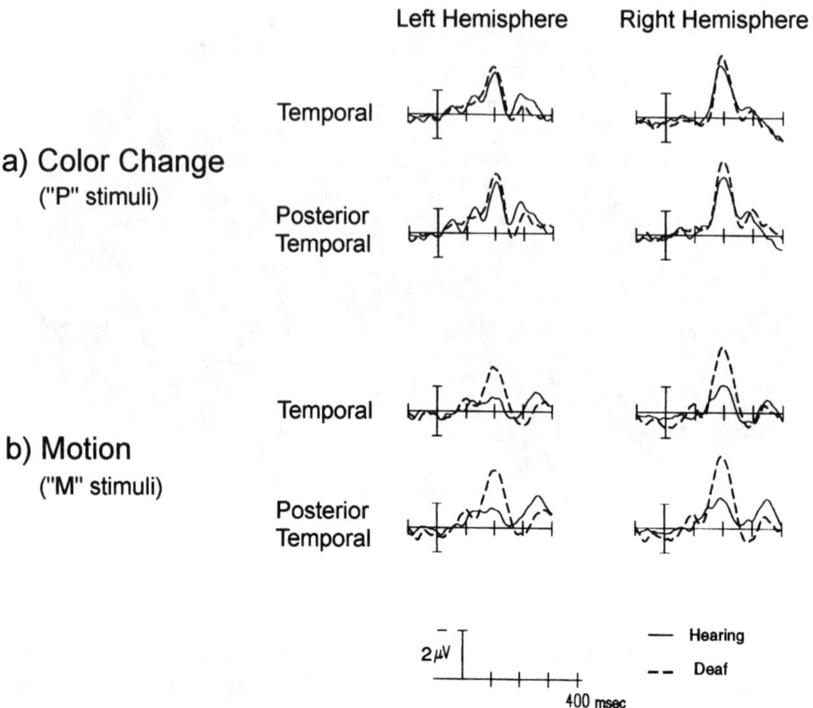

Figure 8.3. ERPs elicited by a) color change and b) motion in normally hearing and congenitally deaf adults. Recordings from temporal and posterior temporal regions of the left and right hemispheres. (From Neville, H.J., & Bavelier, D. [1999]. Specificity and plasticity in neurocognitive development in humans. In M.S. Gazzaniga [Ed.], *The new cognitive neurosciences* [2nd ed., p. 85]. Cambridge, MA: The MIT Press; reprinted by permission.)

Scientists are now using ERPs to study how developing infants and children respond to different sensory stimuli. These studies should reveal the time course of the differentiation and specialization of human sensory systems and provide insight into the neural substrate for sensory plasticity. So, for example, auditory stimuli in adults elicit large brain responses over the temporal cortex but little or no response over the visual cortex (see Figure 8.4). In a 6-month-old child, however, auditory stimuli elicit a large response over both the auditory and visual areas of the brain. This auditory response over the visual areas disappears during development over the period from 6 months to 36 months of age. Based on these studies, the first 3 years of life appear to be a time in development when the sensory systems are becoming organized and when sensory experience can play a role in the organization of these systems.

Studies that look at enhancements and vulnerabilities of systems during development can help us identify systems that are the most plastic and the most vulnerable to abnormal experience. Of course, visual and auditory processing are critical to many aspects of language processing.

THE DEVELOPMENT OF BRAIN SYSTEMS FOR LANGUAGE PROCESSING

In addition to auditory deprivation, deaf subjects also have had different early language experience. In these studies, the subjects, children of deaf

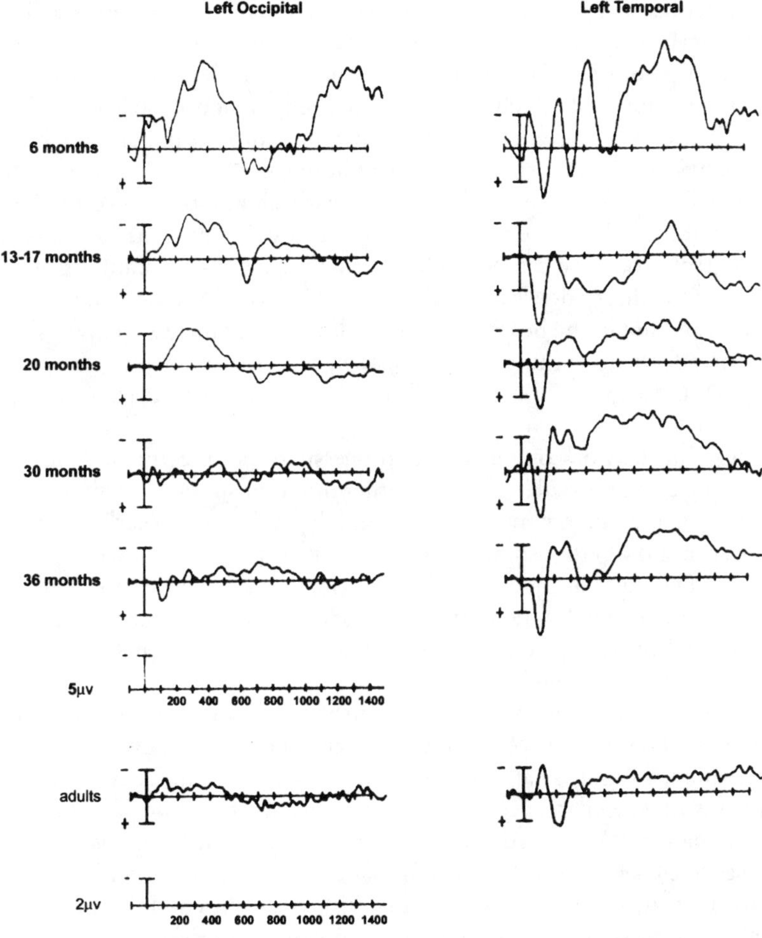

Figure 8.4. ERPs to auditory (speech) stimuli recorded over temporal and occipital regions in normal adults (bottom) and in children ages 6–36 months. (From Neville, H.J. [1995]. Developmental specificity in neurocognitive development in humans. In M.S. Gazzaniga [Ed.], *The cognitive neurosciences* [pp. 219–231]. Cambridge, MA: The MIT Press; reprinted by permission.)

parents, learned American Sign Language (ASL) rather than a spoken language as their first or native language, at the normal age for language acquisition in children. How might this experience affect the development of the brain's language systems? Would deaf subjects show the normal left-hemisphere specialization for language processing that is the ubiquitous pattern in normal hearing people?

There is a possible problem with using deaf subjects to study language processing. The deaf subjects sustained both early auditory deprivation *and* learned a signed, rather than a spoken, language. They have had both unusual early sensory experience and unusual early language experience. It is likely that the two kinds of experiences have different developmental effects on brain organization. How can one sort out which effects are due to auditory deprivation and which are due to learning a sign language? This is where that very important control group comes into the picture: the hearing siblings of the deaf subjects. These children also were born to deaf parents and learned ASL as a first language in early childhood. However, these hearing siblings did not experience any auditory deprivation. Thus, using this control group, we can be confident that the effects on brain organization due to auditory deprivation alone should be observed only in the deaf children and not in the hearing siblings, who are nonetheless "native" signers. Any effects of learning a visual-spatial, rather than an aural-oral, language should be seen in both the deaf subjects and their hearing siblings who used ASL.

As with the work on perceptual processing, the research on language processing attempts to determine whether different subsystems involved in language processing are modifiable by and dependent upon early language experience and whether some aspects of language processing are plastic and capable of change throughout life. Following the distinctions made about language processing by theoretical linguists and psycholinguists, scientists have looked in some detail at two subsystems—semantic processing and grammatical processing.

To study semantic processing, scientists have looked at subjects' brain responses when they process words that carry a lot of semantic and lexical information. Linguists call these words open-class words. They are nouns and verbs that refer to specific objects and events in the world (e.g., dog, banana, dance). We can contrast brain responses to these words with responses to closed class words; words that carry a lot of grammatical information (e.g., if, and, but). A person's inability to use closed-class words—no ifs, ands, or buts—is a clinical test for grammatical aphasia.

Open- and closed-class words are processed by different brain systems (Neville, Mills, & Lawson, 1992). In some ERP studies the subjects process sentences that are either semantically normal but contain grammatical errors (e.g., He gave it Joe to) or sentences that are grammatically correct but semantically anomalous (e.g., I like my coffee with sugar and cement). Scientists have found that semantic processing is associated with increased brain activity, specifically a negative electrical response over posterior brain regions of both brain hemispheres (see Figure 8.5). In contrast, grammatical processing is associated with increased brain activation over anterior regions of the left hemisphere (Neville, Nicol, Barss, Forster, & Garrett, 1991). Different brain systems mediate these different aspects of language processing.

Researchers have used the sentence processing tasks that place different demands on semantic versus grammatical processes to ask whether people who have learned a language late in life or who have had different early language experience show differences in how their brains process language. Does their different early language experience result in different brain organization for language processing? The answer is, just as with ventral and dorsal visual pathways, both no and yes.

In one study, scientists looked at Chinese-English bilinguals, native Chinese speakers who came to America at different ages (Weber-Fox & Neville, 1996). They found that the brain systems that mediate semantic processing were changed little by delays in exposure to the second language. Native Chinese speakers who learned English between 1 and 3 years of age showed the same normal bilateral brain activation for semantic processing as did native English speakers and as did the native Chinese speakers who learned English between 4 and 6 years and those who learned between 11 and 13 years. Researchers began to see slight differences in the brain responses only in subjects who learned English after age 16. Thus, semantic language processing appears to be invulnerable to delays in expo-

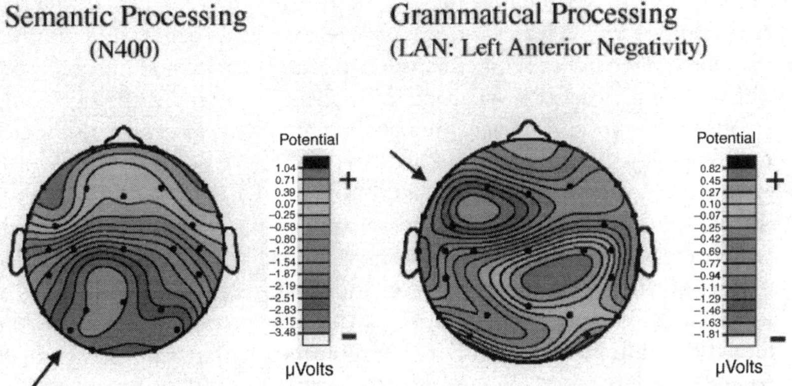

Figure 8.5. Processing semantic information in spoken sentences activates posterior areas of both hemispheres while processing grammatical information primarily activates anterior regions of the left hemisphere.

sure to a second language. In this way the semantic system is similar to the ventral visual pathway. Unusual early language experience does not have large effects on how semantic processing is organized in the brain.

However, grammatical processing appears to be more like the dorsal visual pathway. When scientists looked at brain responses during grammatical processing, they found that the Chinese subjects who learned English early, between 1 and 3 three years of age, developed the left-hemisphere activation pattern for grammatical processing just like native English speakers. However, delaying learning until 4–6 years of age resulted in a more bilateral pattern of brain activation. Among the Chinese immigrants who were first exposed to English between 11 and 13 years of age, scientists saw an aberrant activation pattern for English grammatical processing. These results are consistent with the finding in second language learning that later exposure to a second language results in marked deficits in grammatical processing and understanding (see Flege & Fletcher, 1992; see Chapter 10).

We can conclude that within the language processing system, the semantic and grammatical processing subsystems are affected differently by delays in language experience. The grammatical subsystem is more sensitive to early experience than the semantic system.

Researchers have just started to look at phonological processing, another important linguistic subsystem (see Chapter 10). They know that if they hear someone who pronounces English with a nonnative accent that the person most likely learned English after the age of 12. This aspect of phonological processing seems to be subject to a critical period effect. However, it also appears that not all aspects of phonological processing are time limited.

Scientists have looked at the ability to use stress to separate speech into distinct words (Sanders & Neville, in press). When we hear a language that we do not know, we cannot tell where one word begins and another ends. One cue we use to segment speech in languages we do know is stress, or the pattern of accent on syllables. In English, for example, the stress rule is strong, then weak: The accented syllable generally precedes the unaccented syllable—NA-tive, ENG-lish, SPEAK-er. We do have some words that show an atypical pattern—per-CENT, cor-RECT, re-CORD. As it turns out, linguists have shown that we can recognize the onset of words that follow the normal stress pattern more quickly than we can recognize the onset of words that follow the exceptional stress pattern.

Researchers have studied native Japanese speakers who came to the United States after the age of 12. These subjects were late English language learners. The Japanese language does not have any stress rules. Nonetheless, the Japanese subjects who learned English late picked up on the English stress rule quickly and showed no limitations in their ability to use stress to segment English speech. Again, we are reminded that there is a lot of variability in response to early experience, even within a language subsystem such as phonological processing. Some aspects of phonology can be learned with impunity at a later age, whereas other aspects are more constrained within a critical or sensitive period.

Scientists are now doing brain-imaging studies to investigate this phenomenon. For example, they also are looking at people who learned different stress rules—as in Spanish—to see if this rule would interfere with acquiring the English rule later in life.

Now let us return to the deaf subjects and how their unusual early language experience might have affected development of their language processing systems. Deaf subjects' experience with English is different from that of hearing people. For hearing people, English is an aural-oral, spoken-heard, language. For the deaf, English is a visual language, a language they read. Furthermore, when hearing people read they do a grapheme (written symbol) to phoneme (aural symbol) conversion. They convert written symbols into sounds. Obviously, deaf people do not perform this conversion when they read. Also, because most deaf people also learn English relatively late, they learn it imperfectly and often do not fully master English grammar.

How does this experience affect the organization of English semantic processing in deaf people's brains? The short answer is that it has no effect whatsoever. When engaged in semantic processing of English words, both deaf and hearing subjects showed exactly the same brain response pattern. The response has the same latency, amplitude, and scalp distribution in both hearing and deaf subjects. These results are consistent with those described previously in Chinese-English bilinguals' semantic processing. Again, this points to the conclusion that at least some aspects of semantic processing are robust in the face of altered early language experience.

However, when scientists looked at grammatical processing of English sentences in deaf subjects, they did not show the typical activity pattern over the left hemisphere as observed in hearing, native speakers of English. When processing English grammar, the deaf subjects responded like the late-learning Chinese-English bilinguals. This reinforces the conclusion that the grammatical processing system is more dependent upon early experience than is the semantic processing system (Neville et al., 1992).

By studying deaf subjects, we also can gain insight into another question: Why is it, as neuropsychologists have known for more than 100 years, that language processing systems are almost always localized to the brain's left hemisphere? What is the key factor or variable responsible for establishing language-processing systems in the left hemisphere? Is there something special about the left hemisphere with respect to language processing?

There has been a lot of discussion about these questions recently. One hypothesis is that the left hemisphere is the language hemisphere because it is well suited to process the high rates of auditory information that are typical of language use. In fact, the left hemisphere appears to be good at processing rapid auditory input of any kind, linguistic or not (Merzenich, Recanzone, Jenkins, Allard, & Nudo, 1988; Tallal, Saninberg, & Jernigan, 1991). A second hypothesis is that the left hemisphere is well suited for the grammatical encoding of information that is typical of all formal languages (Liberman, 1974). Thus, one hypothesis suggests that the left hemisphere is specialized for rapid auditory processing, the other that the left hemisphere is adept at grammatical encoding.

One way to test these hypotheses about left-hemisphere specialization for language is to look at how the brain is organized to process a sign language like ASL. ASL is not auditory and thus does not involve processing high rates of auditory stimulation, but it is highly grammatical (Klima & Bellugi, 1979). Sign language is made with the hands and perceived with the eyes. Both ASL's lexicon and grammar depend on the perception of location in space and movement. A sign language's grammar is temporally coincident with visual-spatial information. Researchers also know that in hearing people the right hemisphere plays an important role in visual-spatial processing. So, how does learning ASL reorganize the brain? Does processing ASL depend on the typical left-hemisphere language systems or, because it is visual-spatial, does it recruit right-hemisphere structures for language processing? Are the left-hemisphere language systems in the brain so constrained that they are used to process any language, regardless of its modality and structure?

To answer these questions, scientists have performed ERP, as well as fMRI, studies on deaf subjects and their hearing, ASL-using siblings (Neville et al., 1997, 1998). In these studies, deaf subjects and hearing subjects looked at written English sentences versus strings of English consonants. Thus, these two experimental conditions presented the same physical stimuli, but in one case the stimuli (sentences) carried linguistic information and in the other case (consonant strings) they did not. Scientists also presented these same subjects with signed ASL sentences versus nonsign gestures, again presenting physically equivalent stimuli, only some of which carried linguistic information.

In the fMRI images of these subjects, researchers looked for particular areas of the brain that were more active when the subjects were viewing linguistic input than when they were viewing the physically equivalent nonlinguistic input. Figure 8.6a shows the results for written English. There were three groups of subjects in the study—normal hearing native English speakers; deaf subjects, born to deaf parents, who were native ASL speakers and learned English later in life; and hearing siblings who learned ASL and English early in childhood (control subjects).

For the normal hearing subjects, there were no surprises in the pattern of brain activation that occurred when they processed English sentences. In these subjects, there was intense brain activity associated with the English sentences in the classical left hemisphere language areas, especially in Broca's area, Wernicke's area, and related posterior-temporal areas. They showed the classic left hemisphere pattern for language processing that many investigators reported in the late 1990s.

When deaf subjects read the English sentences they understood them perfectly well. However, in the fMRIs of the deaf subjects reading English sentences, scientists did not see activation in the classical, left hemisphere language areas. There was no significant activation of Broca's or Wernicke's area and little left-hemisphere activation.

However, they did see considerable posterior-temporal-parietal activation in the right hemisphere when the deaf subjects processed English sentences. Why might this be the case? Is it because deaf people learn a visual-spatial language as a first language, and this establishes a language system in the more visual-spatial right hemisphere? If this were the case, then we should also see this same right-hemisphere activation in response to English sentences in the hearing siblings who also learned ASL as a first language. However, the fMRIs of hearing native signers, in contrast to those of the deaf native signers, showed the typical left-lateralized activation pattern for processing English sentences, with little or no activity in the right hemisphere. So, learning a visual-spatial language as a first language does not account for the right-hemisphere activation and lack of left-hemisphere activation among the deaf subjects.

Maybe the deaf subjects show no left-hemisphere activation to English because for them English is a visual and not an auditory language. Maybe one has to learn an auditory language to organize the left-hemisphere language systems. However, the lack of left-hemisphere activation for English may be the result of having learned English later in life and thus not acquiring full mastery of English grammar. The deaf subjects might be showing the adverse effects of a missed critical period for grammar acquisition.

We can decide among these alternative explanations by comparing brain activation patterns for ASL versus nonsign gesture processing in these three groups of subjects (see Figure 8.6b). The fMRIs of the normal hearing subjects, who did not know ASL, showed no activation differences between ASL sentences and nonsign gestures. This is no surprise. However, when the deaf subjects looked at ASL sentences, scientists saw activation in the classical language centers of the brain's left hemisphere. When deaf subjects process ASL, their brains recruit classical Broca's, Wernicke's, and related areas that are associated with aural-oral language processing. This suggests that these left-hemisphere language centers are well designed and well suited to process formal language, independently of the language's modality or structure. It appears that these brain areas are biologically constrained or determined to process language. Thus, the feature that is special

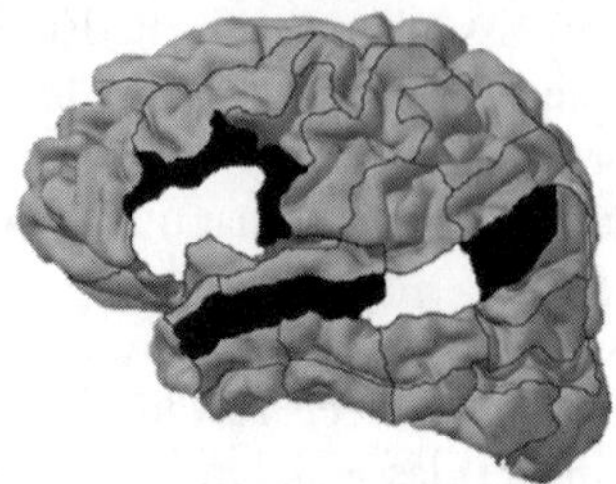
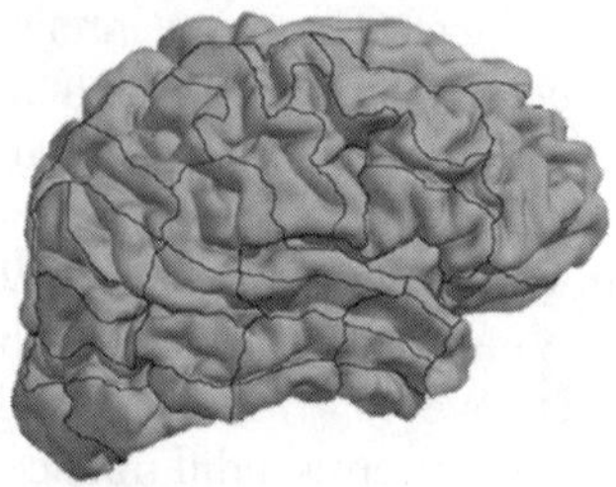

a. Hearing Subjects

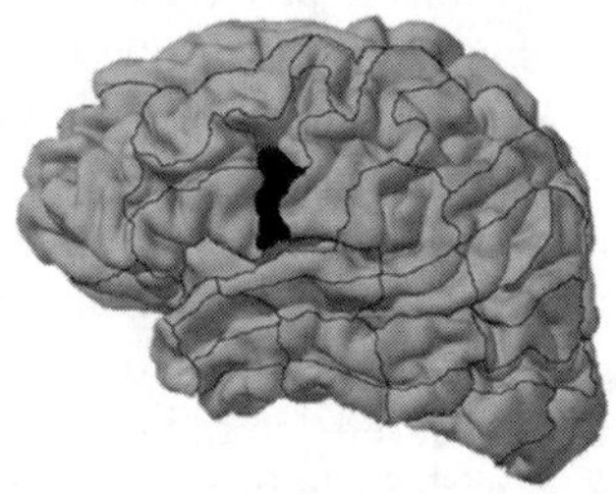
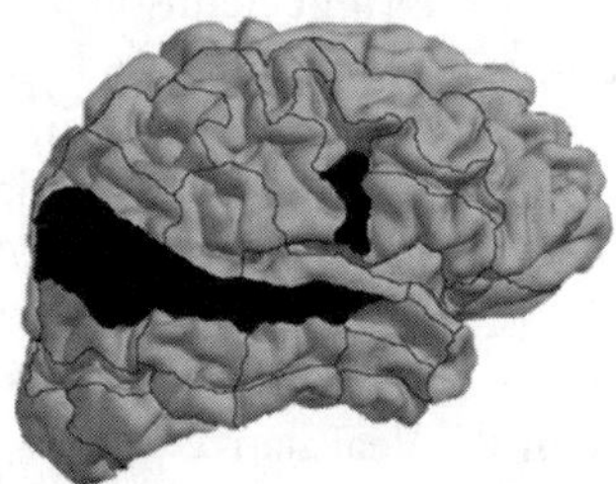

b. Deaf Subjects

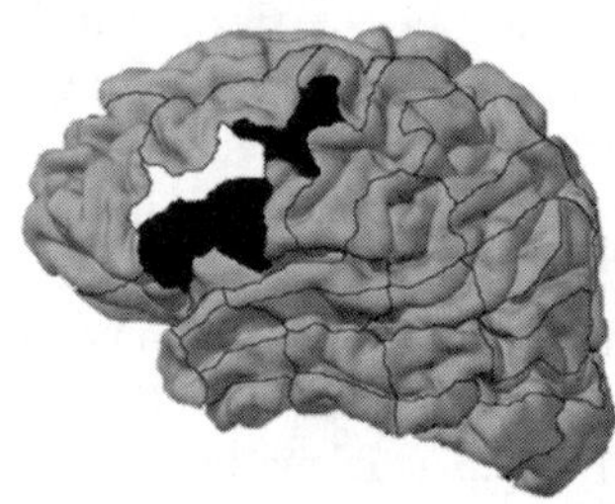
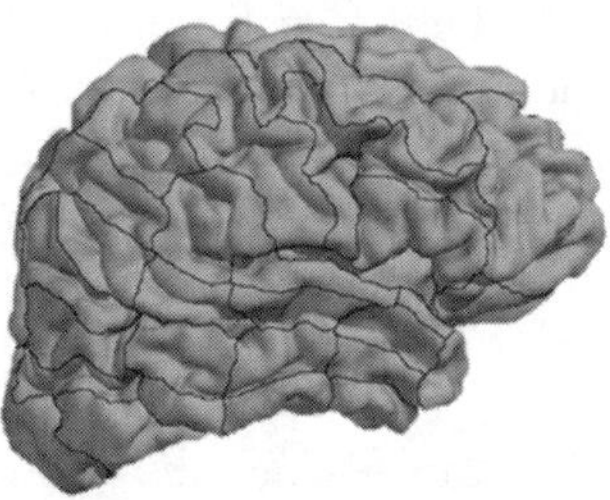

c. Hearing Native Signers

Figure 8.6a. Cortical areas displaying activation ($p < .005$) for English sentences (versus nonwords) for each subject group. (Key = ☐ $p<.0005$; ■ $p<.005$.) (From Neville, H.J., et al. [1998]. Cerebral organization for language in deaf and hearing subjects: Biological constraints and effects of experience. *Proceedings of the National Academy of Science, USA, 95*[3], 922–929; reprinted by permission.)

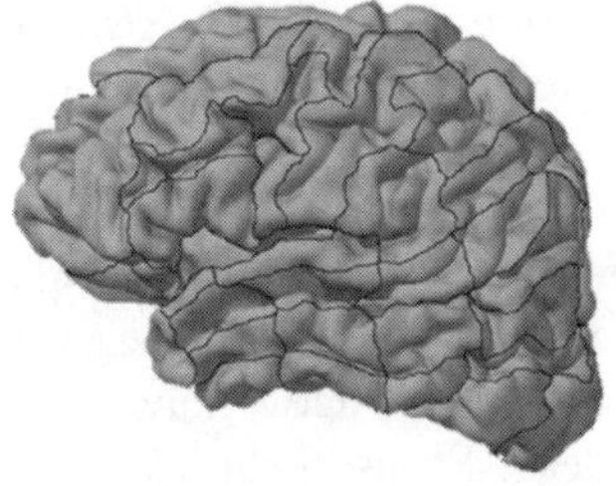

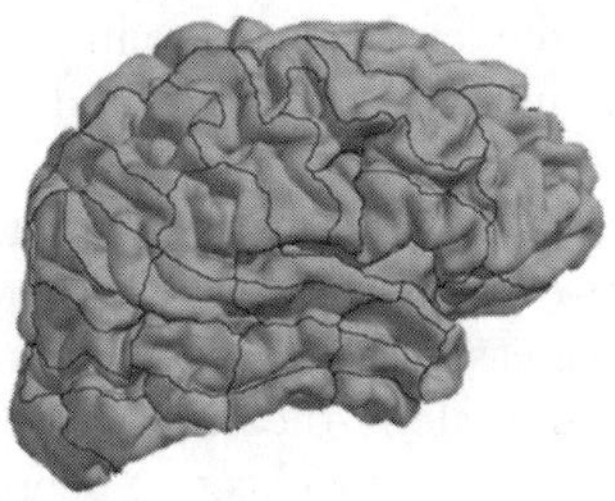

a. Hearing Subjects

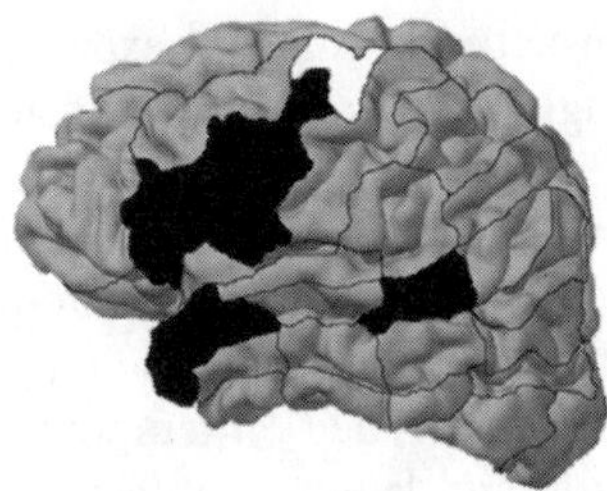

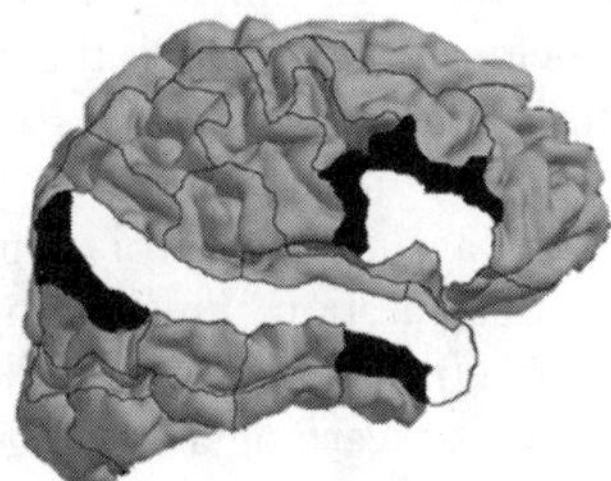

b. Deaf Subjects

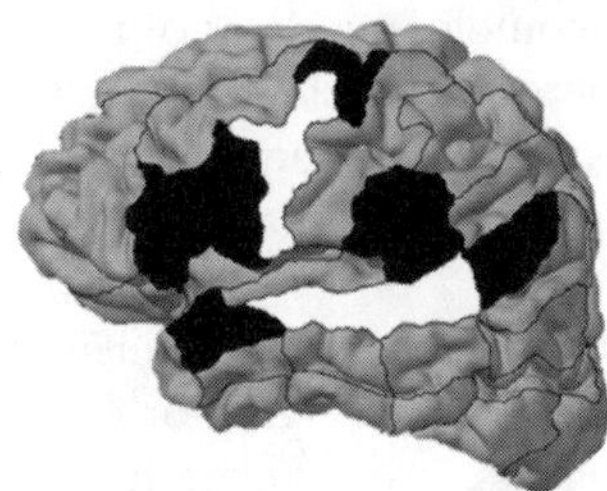

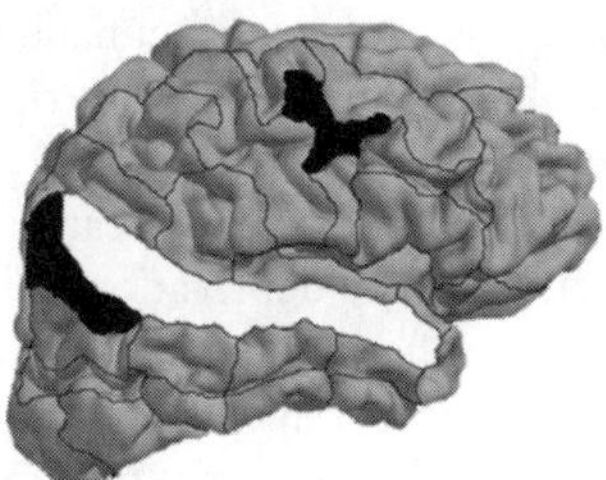

c. Hearing Native Signers

Figure 8.6b. Cortical areas displaying activation ($p < .005$) for ASL sentences (versus nonsigns) for each subject group. (Key = □ $p<.0005$; ■ $p<.005$.) (From Neville, H.J., et al. [1998]. Cerebral organization for language in deaf and hearing subjects: Biological constraints and effects of experience. *Proceedings of the National Academy of Science, USA, 95*[3], 922–929; reprinted by permission.)

about the left hemisphere in language processing appears to be its facility at grammatical encoding, and not a facility for processing rapid auditory input.

We see something else quite interesting when deaf subjects are processing ASL. Their fMRIs also show significant activation in right-hemisphere brain areas that are homologous to Broca's and Wernicke's areas, as well as activation along the entire superior temporal sulcus, activations that are not seen in normal hearing people. Do the deaf ASL users show this right-hemisphere activation because ASL is a visual-spatial language that recruits right-hemisphere structures for processing? Or, is this right-hemisphere activation the result of deaf people having hyperactive visual-spatial systems in their right hemisphere? That is, we would like to know whether this right-hemisphere activity is the result of unusual early language experience (learning visual-spatial ASL as a first language) or the result of early auditory deprivation.

Once again the control group of hearing, ASL-using siblings can help answer this question. The hearing siblings did not experience any auditory deprivation in infancy and childhood, but they did have the same unusual experience of learning a language whose grammar relied on temporal coincidences between visual-spatial information and language information. The fMRIs of the hearing siblings showed the same activation pattern as the deaf subjects as they process signed ASL sentences. When processing ASL sentences, the hearing native signers strongly recruit the classical language areas in the left hemisphere *and* the homologous areas of the right hemisphere. Therefore, the right-hemisphere activity seen when native signers (both deaf and hearing) process ASL sentences is an effect on brain organization due to early learning of a visual-spatial language and not due to early auditory deprivation.

In summary, what we learn from this is that when any individual processes sentences in his or her native language, whether English or ASL, the processing always recruits the classical language areas of the left hemisphere. This suggests that there is some biological constraint operating that makes these left-hemisphere structures well suited to process language, if the language is learned early in life. Yet, it also is clear that language experience plays a critical role in shaping the final form of the brain's language systems. We know this from the finding that an individual who learns a visual-spatial language, whether he or she is deaf or hearing, recruits the homologous right-hemisphere brain structures into language processing. There are biological constraints operating on how the brain is, or can be, organized to process language. The left hemisphere seems well suited and constrained to process grammatical information. However, language experience also is critical in determining the final organization of the brain's language processing systems. Clearly, when it comes to brain organization both nature and nurture play fundamental roles.

Given the interest in taking a critical look at critical periods, one might ask: Is there a critical period during development when learning a visual-spatial language recruits those right-hemisphere structures into the brain's language system? Scientists have begun to study this question by looking at people who learned ASL as a second language late in life. They are looking at hearing people who learned ASL after the age of 18 in order to become interpreters for the deaf. When these late learners process ASL, their fMRIs show that they do not recruit the right-hemisphere structures into their language processing systems to the same extent as native learners of ASL (Newman et al., 1998). When they process ASL, they use primarily the classic left hemisphere system. These people can function as interpreters, so they have acquired some fluency in ASL, but they are using different brain systems in processing ASL and are impaired on formal tests of ASL grammar. From these initial studies, it appears as if learning ASL before or after age 18 does make a difference. Scientists do not yet know exactly when this critical period ends, but they can find out by studying people who learned ASL at different ages prior to age 18.

They also have looked at how the language subsystems of the brain develop on-line, during infancy, and during childhood. For the semantic processing system, they study vocabulary development in children. Scientists find that there are shifts during development in how the brain's language systems are configured during the early years of life (Neville & Mills, 1997). These systems do not settle down into mature organization until children are 15 years old. For example, they looked at the children's ERPs when they processed words whose meanings they knew versus words they did not know. There are differences between these two classes of words in children's brain activation patterns. Thirteen-month-old children appear to use widely distributed brain regions within both hemispheres to make this distinction. There is activation of both the left and right hemispheres in frontal, temporal, and parietal regions (see Figure 8.7, top). If one looks at these same children at 20 months of age, quite a shift in the brain activation pattern can be seen. In these older infants, the only brain regions showing a difference for meaningful versus meaningless words is in the left hemisphere, and the difference is confined to the temporal and parietal regions (see Figure 8.7, bottom). This illustrates another general principle of brain development: As the brain develops, there is an increased focalization of the brain activity associated with a processing task. This focalization is an indicator of the increased specialization and fine tuning of functional brain systems.

Note, however, that the increased specialization of the brain systems is not predicted solely by the child's chronological age. We know this from comparing children of the same chronological age who differ in vocabulary size. The 20-month-old children already show this focusing and specialization of the left hemisphere. However, so do 13-month-old children with

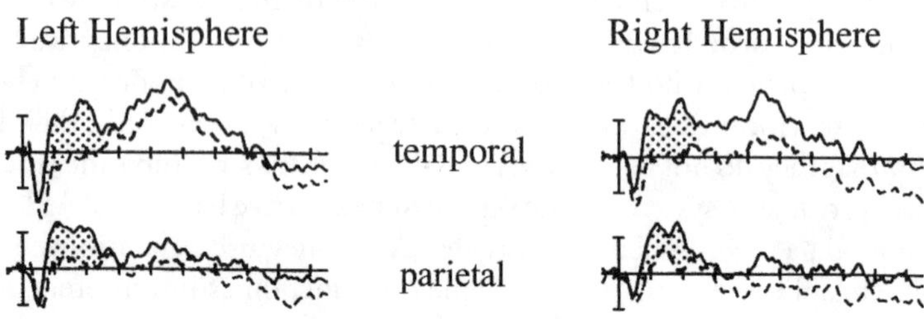

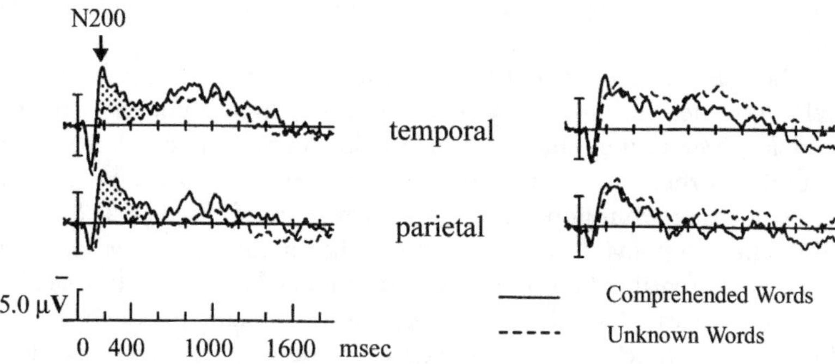

Figure 8.7. ERPs elicited by comprehended and unknown words in 13- to 17-month-old and 20-month-old children. At 13–17 months, ERPs to comprehended words are larger than to unknown words over several areas within both the left and right hemispheres. By 20 months, ERP differences to comprehended and unknown words are limited to temporal and parietal regions of the left hemisphere. (Neville, H.J., & Mills, D. [1997]. Epigenesis of language. *Mental Retardation and Developmental Disabilities Research Reviews, 3*[4], 282–292; reprinted by permission from Wiley-Liss, Inc., a subsidiary of John Wiley & Sons, Inc.)

comparably large vocabularies. The 13-month-old children who have small vocabularies, however, do not show this focalization specialization. So, while there are maturational changes in the brain that can be defined and that researchers have described, it is clear that language knowledge and experience also play a role in predicting the specialization and differentiation of these brain systems.

CONCLUSION

The story presented here seems complex and detailed. Nonetheless, the story represents what modern brain science does know about critical periods, early experience, and brain development. The short conclusion is that the effects of early experience on brain development are not as straightforward and transparent as the public has been led to believe, based on discussions of brain science in the policy and popular literature.

There are several principles to keep in mind when reading about critical periods in brain development or in language learning. First, research on how experience affects the brain is in its infancy. New noninvasive imaging techniques will facilitate studies of human brain development. Second, there is variability in how early experience affects brain organization. Some brain systems are subject to critical period constraints and others are not. This variability occurs both within systems such as vision and between systems. Third, within systems in which there are critical periods, these periods can differ for specific subsystems. Given this variability and complexity it makes little sense to speak of a critical period for brain development or even of a critical period for vision or language. Nor would it seem that these periods are limited to the first 3 years of life. Although this research does carry implications for rehabilitation, education, and child development, those implications, like the research itself, may not be straightforward or transparent. As scientists discuss the implications of this work for policy and practice, we must all remind ourselves that children's brains are not hard wired at birth, and that they are not always modifiable by experience either. Future research will identify and characterize the nature and extent of neuroplasticity within the several highly specialized brain systems important for human cognition.

REFERENCES

Eden, G.F., VanMeter, J.W., Rumsey, J.M., Maisog, J.M., Woods, R.P., & Zeffiro, T.A. (1996). Abnormal processing of visual motion in dyslexia revealed by functional brain imaging. *Nature, 382*, 66–69.

Flege, J., & Fletcher, K. (1992). Talker and listener effects on degree of perceived foreign accent. *Journal of the Acoustical Society of America, 91*, 370–389.

Huttenlocher, P.R., & Dabholkar, A.S. (1997). Regional differences in synaptogenesis in human cerebral cortex. *Journal of Comparative Neurology, 387*, 167–178.

Klima, E.S., & Bellugi, U. (1979). *The signs of language*. Cambridge, MA: Harvard University Press.

Liberman, A.M. (1974). The specialization of the language hemisphere. In F.O. Schmitt & F.G. Worden (Eds.), *The neurosciences third study program* (pp. 43–56). Cambridge, MA: The MIT Press.

Livingstone, M., Rosen, G., Drislane, F., & Galaburda, A. (1991). Physiological and anatomical evidence for a magnocellular defect in developmental dyslexia. *Proceedings of the National Academy of Science, USA, 88*, 7943–7947.

Lovegrove, W., Garzia, R., & Nicholson, S. (1990). Experimental evidence for a transient system deficit in specific reading disability. *Journal of the American Optometric Association, 61*, 137–146.

Merzenich, M., Recanzone, G., Jenkins, W., Allard, T., & Nudo, R. (1988). Cortical representational plasticity. In P. Rakic & W. Singer (Eds.), *Neurobiology of neocortex* (pp. 41–67). New York: John Wiley & Sons.

Mitchell, D. (1981). Sensitive periods in visual development. In R. Aslin, J. Alberts, & M. Petersen (Eds.), *Development of perception* (pp. 3–43). New York: Academic Press.

Neville, H.J. (1995). Developmental specificity in neurocognitive development in humans. In M.S. Gazzaniga (Ed.), *The cognitive neurosciences* (pp. 219–231). Cambridge, MA: The MIT Press.

Neville, H.J., & Bavelier, D. (1999). Specificity and plasticity in neurocognitive development in humans. In M.S. Gazzaniga (Ed.), *The new cognitive neurosciences* (2nd ed., pp. 83–98). Cambridge, MA: The MIT Press.

Neville, H.J., Bavelier, D., Corina, D., Rauschecker, J., Karni, A., Lalwani, A., Braun, A., Clark, V., Jezzard, P., & Turner, R. (1998). Cerebral organization for language in deaf and hearing subjects: Biological constraints and effects of experience. *Proceedings of the National Academy of Science, USA*, 95(3), 922–929.

Neville, H.J., Coffey, S.A., Lawson, D.S., Fischer, A., Emmorey, K., & Bellugi, U. (1997). Neural systems mediating American Sign Language: Effects of sensory experience and age of acquisition. *Brain and Language, 57*, 285–308.

Neville, H.J., & Mills, D. (1997). Epigenesis of language. *Mental Retardation and Developmental Disabilities Research Reviews, 3*(4), 282–292.

Neville, H.J., Mills, D., & Lawson, D. (1992). Fractionating language: Different neural subsystems with different sensitive periods. *Cerebral Cortex, 2*, 244–258.

Neville, H.J., Nicol, J., Barss, A., Forster, K., & Garrett, M. (1991). Syntactically based sentence processing classes: Evidence from event-related brain potentials. *Journal of Cognitive Neuroscience, 3*, 155–170.

Newman, A., Corina, D., Tomann, A., Bavelier, D., Braun, A., Clark, V., Jezzard, P., & Neville, H.J. (1998). Effects of age of acquisition on cortical organization for American Sign Language (ASL): A functional magnetic resonance imaging (fMRI) study. *NeuroImage*, 7(4), 5194.

Sanders, L., & Neville, H. (in press). Lexical syntactic and stress-pattern cues for speech segmentation. *Journal of Speech, Language, and Hearing Research.*

Tallal, P., Saninberg, R., & Jernigan, T. (1991). The neuropathology of developmental dysphasis: Behavioral, morphological, and physiological evidence for a pervasive temporal processing disorder. *Reading and Writing: An Interdisciplinary Journal, 3*, 363–377.

Weber-Fox, C., & Neville, H.J. (1996). Maturational constraints on functional specializations for language processing: ERP and behavioral evidence in bilingual speakers. *Journal of Cognitive Neuroscience, 8*(3), 231–256.

Wiesel, T., & Hubel, D. (1965). Comparison of the effects of unilateral and bilateral eye closure on cortical unit responses in kittens. *Journal of Neurophysiology, 28*, 1003–1017.

9

Sensitive Periods in First Language Acquisition

Heather Bortfeld
Grover J. Whitehurst

Research in developmental psychology has not actively addressed the topic of critical periods in development for many years. As evidence, neither the term *critical period* nor *sensitive period* appears in the index of any of the four volumes of the fifth edition of the *Handbook of Child Psychology* (Damon, 1998). The fourth edition of the *Handbook of Child Psychology* (Mussen, 1983), published 15 years earlier, has only one index reference to *critical period.* Therein about half of a page is devoted to explaining that the concept derived from Lorenz's work on imprinting (Lorenz, 1935) and has been replaced by the more popular term, *sensitive period*, which implies that "a given event produces a stronger effect on development or that a given effect can be produced more readily during a certain period than earlier or later" (Hinde, 1983, p. 41).

Among those who work in the field of language development, the concept of critical or sensitive periods also has not been a focus of attention. To the extent that it was considered at all, discussions of critical periods were blended inextricably with arguments for the nativist side of the nature versus nurture debate. Thus, it was assumed that if language acquisition were driven largely by biological mechanisms, there would be critical periods for its development. Lenneberg (1967) was a seminal figure in this tradition. He noted that language development has parallels in other domains, such as motor development, that are assumed to be driven largely by biological maturation. He pointed out that just as walking and grasping follow a relatively predictable maturational timetable, the same occurs for many aspects of language development.

A related argument, articulated most vividly by Chomsky (1959), was that many of the characteristics of language understood by mature speakers of all languages in the world are abstract and, in principle, could not be acquired through traditional social learning mechanisms. How is it, Chomsky wrote, that people can recognize nonsense sentences that they have never heard before as grammatical (e.g., colorless green ideas sleep furiously) unless humans are born with an innate language acquisition device that is prewired with the basic grammatical rules of language? Many researchers and theorists followed the nativistic lead of Lenneberg and Chomsky. Thus, Brown and Herrnstein stated, "One irresistibly has the impression of a biological process developing in just the same way in the entire human species" (1975, p. 479). Pinker maintained that language acquisition is such a robust process that "there is virtually no way to prevent it from happening short of raising a child in a barrel" (1994, p. 29).

Among recent research that has generated evidence for universality, and thus a probable biological basis for language development, is Goldin-Meadow and her colleagues' observations of deaf children (Butcher, Mylander, & Goldin-Meadow, 1991; Goldin-Meadow & Mylander, 1990, 1998). In these studies, profoundly deaf children with no exposure to sign language or oral language develop systems of manual sign communication that incorporate many of the formal features of spoken language. For example, Goldin-Meadow and Mylander (1998) observed deaf children of hearing parents in two cultures, American and Chinese, that differ in their child-rearing practices and in the way gesture is used in relation to speech. The spontaneous sign systems developed by children in these cultures shared a number of structural similarities: patterned production and deletion of semantic elements in the surface structure of a sentence, patterned ordering of those elements within the sentence, and linking of propositions within a sentence. The universality of these developments, which occur without linguistic input from parents, argues for a biological program for development of language structures.

A contrasting focus on the role of nurture has been present among many psychologists who study language development. Their work focuses on the role of the social and linguistic environment in shaping the course of language development. These empiricists have noted that the logical counterbalance to nativists' observation of universality in language development is the clear differences in language that are due to children's culture and environment. It may be obvious that French children grow up speaking French, while Japanese children grow up speaking Japanese, but it requires no less explanation than the commonalities in their abstract grammars.

Research on environmental determinants of language development examines such topics as motherese (the unique, simplified language that mothers speak to their young children that simplifies children's language learning task) (Snow, 1979), the role of conditions associated with economic poverty in the rate and form of children's language development (Whitehurst, 1997), the role of feedback in shaping the grammaticality of children's language (Bohannon, MacWhinney, & Snow, 1990), and the function of children's frequency of exposure to adult language in the rate of their language growth (Huttenlocher, Haight, Bryk, Seltzer, & Lyons, 1991).

One example of research on the latter topic is Hart and Risley's (1995) examination of the effects of frequency of parental talk to young children. Over a 2½-year period, vocal interactions in the children's homes were recorded for 1 hour each month for the 42 families in the study. Hart and Risley found a widening gap between the vocabulary growth of children from professional, working class, and welfare families across the first 3 years of the children's lives. This was strongly related to differences in the frequency of verbal interaction between parents and their children: The correlation between frequency of input and children's expressive language at 3 years of age was .84.

There was a difference of almost 300 words spoken per hour between parents with professional careers and those on welfare, which can be extrapolated to an estimate that the children in professional families heard approximately 11 million words annually, the children in working class families heard approximately 6 million words annually, and the children in welfare families heard approximately 3 million words annually. One observation from this study is that by age 3, the professional families' children had a larger recorded vocabulary than the welfare families' parents. In general, frequency and quality were aspects of parental speech that accounted for a large amount of the variance in the children's vocabulary growth, vocabulary use, and IQ scores at age 3 and were better predictors than race, gender, or birth order. These differences held up at age 9, when the children were tested again for vocabulary and language skills.

NATURE, NURTURE, AND CRITICAL PERIODS

The purpose of this brief introduction to the nativist and empiricist traditions in research and theory on language development is to frame the topic of sensitive periods.

One point is that equating sensitive periods with a strong maturational view of language development is unnecessary and unwarranted. Remember that a sensitive period refers to an effect of *environmental* stimulation that can be produced more readily during a certain period than earlier or later. To the extent that language develops in a lockstep maturational progression that requires little or no interaction with the environment, an inquiry into periods of special sensitivity to environmental stimulation is pointless.

A second point is that the methods of inquiry that have been characteristic of both the nativist and empiricist traditions are by themselves insufficient for determining the existence of sensitive periods. For instance, Lenneberg's (1967) catalog of the regular timetable for language milestones and related demonstrations that deaf children without exposure to sign language develop sign language with universal features (Goldin-Meadow & Mylander, 1998) does not answer the question of whether these progressions would be the same if somehow they could be prevented from starting until children were 5 years of age or whether the progression depends at all on interaction with environment. In other words, evidence that a developmental progression is driven primarily by biological events is neither necessary nor sufficient for the use of the construct of a critical period.

Likewise, evidence of the malleability of language development as a result of differences in children's social environments, seen in the work of Hart and Risley (1995), is not evidence against a critical or sensitive period. It is possible, for instance, that high frequency parent–child language interactions have their strongest effects during the preschool period, and that similarly rich verbal interactions at later points in a child's development might not make up for relative deprivation of these interactions during early childhood. In other words, Hart and Risley's results, or any other study demonstrating differences in language trajectories as a result of differences in experience within a common developmental epoch, are entirely consistent with the possibility that the epoch is a sensitive period for such development, without, of course, demonstrating the presence of a sensitive period.

Thus, demonstrations of regularity and universality, the meat of most arguments for biological models of language development, as well as demonstrations of malleability and individual differences, the heart of most environmental models of language development, do not argue for or against sensitive periods. This chapter addresses the methods that are suitable for answering questions about sensitive periods.

The third point is that critical periods may be determined exogenously (i.e., by external factors) as well as by an underlying biological process. For example, children in the United States who are failing in reading at the end of first grade are likely to be failing in reading at the end of third grade (Juel, 1988). Children who lag behind in their reading skills receive less practice in reading than other children (Allington, 1984), miss opportunities to develop reading comprehension strategies (Brown, Palincsar, & Purcell, 1986), encounter reading material that is too advanced for their skills (Allington, 1984), and acquire negative attitudes about reading itself (Oka & Paris, 1986). These children are caught in a downward spiral in which they are less prepared to accomplish their teacher's instructional goals than their more literate peers, more likely to experience failure and become discouraged, and likely to fall further behind at the next step in their academic journey.

Thus, one could argue that there is a critical period for learning to read: If children do not learn to read early in their elementary school careers, it is unlikely that they will learn to read well later. The stage for early reading success is set by experiences and resulting skills that are acquired during the preschool period (Whitehurst & Lonigan, 1998). However, this critical period is not determined by biological constraints—the worldwide success of adult literacy programs provides clear evidence that one can be taught to read at any age. In addition, there is little evidence that the underlying components of literacy are age graded. For example, Morais, Content, Bertelson, and Cary (1988) found that illiterate Portuguese adults could quickly learn to perform a pseudoword phoneme deletion task (this task measures phonemic awareness) when provided with corrective feedback and instructions. The reason that there is a critical period for acquisition of literacy skills is that schools provide an age-graded rather than skills-graded curriculum in which early delays are magnified at each additional step as the gap increases between what children bring to the curriculum and what the curriculum demands. Thus, the critical period for learning to read is cultural and exogenous, not biological and endogenous. It is in this context that the critical period question is addressed with regard to first language acquisition.

WHAT COUNTS AS EVIDENCE FOR CRITICAL PERIODS?

Evidence of critical periods in development ideally comes from controlled rearing studies. In such studies, organisms are reared in environments that differ only in the time during their life course in which they are exposed to a particular experience. If that experience has a stronger effect on behavior and the brain when presented during one developmental period than others, then that period can be said to be critical or sensitive with respect to that experience.

In the context of first language acquisition, a controlled rearing study would involve rearing children in environments that are normal and typical of the species in all respects except exposure to language. Children in an early exposure condition might be exposed to language from birth; children in a middle exposure condition might be reared without language input until they are 4 years of age, after which language interaction with adults would begin; and children in a late exposure condition might be first exposed to language as adolescents. Children in each condition would be followed for a fixed period after their first exposure to language, say 6 years, and their language development would be assessed. Evidence for a critical period would take the form of much greater competence in language at the end of the follow-up period for children exposed to language early compared with those exposed to it late.

Obviously, a controlled rearing study such as this cannot be conducted because ethics and human compassion would not permit it. Further, even if the experiment could be performed, difficulties of interpretation would remain. For example, given the central role of language in human interaction and development, how could one be sure that the children who were deprived of early language stimulation were not also deprived of opportunities for normal social or cognitive development. Effects on language learning at some later exposure to linguistic input might reflect the effects of abnormalities in socialization or thinking on the children's attention to language, rather than the closing of a biological window for language learning per se. This possibility would cloud the interpretation of the results, but not the demonstration of a sensitive period.

Given that even an ideally designed controlled rearing study would have interpretive difficulties, the actual evidence available on critical periods in the language development of humans is less than definitive. That evidence comes from four primary sources.

The first is from so-called "wild" children (i.e., rare cases of children who have been deprived of normal social and linguistic interaction during their first years of life). If such children are exposed to language later in life and do not develop normal language themselves, perhaps it is because they have passed a critical period for language acquisition. However, the possibility that these children had mental retardation to begin with cannot be discounted; neither can the likelihood that the effects of deprivation of language input during the first years are confounded with the effects of deprivation of other forms of experience.

The second source of evidence is from natural variation in the timing of exposure of deaf children to sign language. If deaf children have no exposure to a spoken language, and through differences in cultural or parental practice there are groups of children who are first exposed to sign language at earlier or later points in their life course, then researchers have a naturally occurring approximation of the ethically proscribed controlled rearing study. Of course, sign language may be acquired in different ways and have different features than vocal language. Also, deaf children who experience their first exposure to sign language later in life may have suffered the social or cognitive consequences of lack of early linguistic input that in turn affect their ability to acquire language.

A third method for examination of critical periods is loss of perceptual or learning capacities with age. If a young child can discriminate a speech sound or learn a linguistic skill that an older child or adult cannot learn as easily or as well, this suggests that a critical period for such learning occurs early in development. However, such a demonstration does not reveal whether the critical period is due to a biological window that closes with age, changes in motivation or opportunity (e.g., as in the case of learning to read described earlier in the chapter), or interference from subsequent learning. These questions speak to the reasons for a sensitive period, but not to the existence of the phenomenon itself.

A fourth methodology that permits inferences about critical periods involves examination of cerebral localization of language processing for individuals exposed to languages at different times in their life course. If individuals exposed to a language at a later time than usual utilize different areas of the brain or different neural pathways to process language, this is evidence that normal brain organization for language requires stimulation during critical periods. However, to the extent that individuals perform equivalently on language tasks, or at least perform within a normal range despite differences in brain organization, the critical period that has been demonstrated is neural, not behavioral.

FIRST LANGUAGE DEVELOPMENT: WHAT IS EXPECTED?

In order to discuss first language development, there needs to be clarification about language in general. First, language, like vision, is complex. Just as one cannot talk about vision without distinguishing among depth and color perception, binocular and monocular vision, and motion detection, language also is a system of components, each of which contributes to the whole. The base component of the language system is phonology—the patterning of sound combinations that are allowed in a particular language. Phonology generally embodies articulatory phonetics, which is the study of how sounds are produced in the world's languages. Syntax describes the grammatical rules specific to single languages and groups of languages. Morphology describes the rules of word formation. Semantics is the conventions for deriving the meanings of words and sentences. Finally, pragmatics is the rules for appropriate social use and interpretation of language in context.

Just as specific visual functions each have their own critical periods, a system as complex as language may be marked by different critical periods for different components. Furthermore, it is important to distinguish between a first or second language system because learning a first language is different from learning a language while having another language system already in place. Despite these differences, however, both types of learning are relevant to discussions about critical periods. This chapter focuses on first language development, though some references to second language research will be necessary and relevant to the discussion at hand.

Phonetics and Phonology: Normal Gains and Losses

An informative area of research regarding critical periods in first language development focuses on perception and production of speech sounds. Infants' perception of phonetic contrasts changes given specific linguistic input. Early work showed that infants have the capacity to discriminate phonetic contrasts that they have never heard before (Lasky, Syrdal-Lasky, & Klein, 1975; Streeter, 1976; Trehub, 1976). Subsequently, researchers demonstrated that adults are unable to perceive many nonnative phonetic contrasts (Flege, 1989; Logan, Lively, & Pisoni, 1989; Strange & Jenkins, 1978). The implications of these findings for the critical period debate should be apparent. That is, though much of the research on first language critical periods focuses on a cutoff point somewhere around adolescence, research on loss of perception of nonnative contrasts has made it clear that before puberty a lot happens to determine how fluent one is with the sounds of a particular language.

Werker and her colleagues set out to determine precisely when sensitivity to nonnative contrasts begins to decline. In an initial study, Werker (1981) tested Hindi-speaking adults, English-speaking adults, and English-exposed 7-month-olds on two Hindi contrasts (a voicing distinction and a place of articulation distinction). She found that whereas the Hindi-speaking adults and the English-exposed 7-month-olds could readily distinguish between each sound in the two sets of contrasts, English-speaking adults could not. In a subsequent study, Werker and Tees (1983) tested groups of English speakers between the ages of 4 years and adulthood on the same two contrasts. The researchers found that even the 4-year-old English speakers could not distinguish sounds in the two sets of contrasts.

Based on this work, it became clear that a lot happens to lay the groundwork for native-like fluency before puberty and even prior to the fourth year of life. In subsequent work, English-exposed 12-months-olds showed hardly any sign of discriminating non-English contrasts, while those same contrasts were easily distinguished by 12-month-olds exposed to the particular languages in which those contrasts occurred (Werker & Tees, 1984). Werker's studies were the first demonstrations of how early in a child's life exposure to the native language influences subsequent perception. The findings demonstrate a decline in sensitivity to nonnative speech contrasts when no exposure to them takes place. This decline in sensitivity was subsequently shown to take place systematically between the first 6–12 months of an infant's life, regardless of the infant's native language (Best & McRoberts, 1989; Werker & Lalonde, 1988).

Other work challenged just how clear cut this decline in sensitivity actually is. For example, Best and her colleagues (Best, 1991, 1995; Best, McRoberts, & Sithole, 1988) demonstrated that certain contrasts (e.g., between specific Zulu clicks [the Zulu language utilizes many tongue clicks]) continue to be distinguishable even to adult nonnative speakers. One can imagine (particularly if one has heard these clicks, which are decidedly non-speech sounding to a native English speaker) that this has to do with the lack of proximity of these sounds to any sounds in the native language of the listeners. Indeed, there is no sound in English that even approximates the Zulu click sounds. Other contrasts, like the Hindi voicing distinction tested by Werker and Tees, are similar enough to sounds that fall within some specific phonetic category in the listener's native language to be confused and, thus, not discriminated. Regardless, demonstrations of loss of sensitivity to nonnative contrasts in general are conceptually quite similar to the kinds of perceptual deficits described by Bruer (see Chapter 1) in other organisms when they are isolated from sufficient environmental stimulation. However, apparent from the work involving monkeys and kittens described by Bruer, it takes a lot to wipe out certain perceptual skills entirely. In fact, adult speakers can apparently regain the ability to distinguish certain nonnative contrasts when given enough appropriate training (Flege, 1989; Flege, Takagi, & Mann, 1995; McCandliss, Fiez, Conway, Protopapas, & McClelland, 1998; McClelland, 2001).

Some researchers have argued that such findings are indicative of the influence attentional factors can have on perceptual discrimination rather than of the actual loss of a biologically based sensory capacity (Jusczyk, 1985, 1992; Werker, 1981). This would mean that even if there were a period within which attention were fixed on features of one's native language phonology, this could be overridden given proper training even in adulthood. Regardless, the influence of this training is particularly noteworthy because the phonological system has traditionally been considered one of the most entrenched and sharply defined components of the language system.

EFFECTS OF LINGUISTIC ISOLATION ON FIRST LANGUAGE DEVELOPMENT

Numerous instantiations of linguistic input deprivation have been studied with the long-term goal of understanding whether critical periods for acquisition do, in fact, exist. Because such deprivation cannot be imposed in a laboratory setting, myriad situations in which deprivation has been imposed (most often naturally but, unfortunately, sometimes artificially) have been investigated by researchers interested in measuring developmental outcomes of such deprivation. Several of these deprivation studies and the principle language components affected by the deprivation will be reviewed.

Syntax and Semantics: Differential Outcomes of Deprivation

Genie In the late 1960s, social workers discovered a 14-year-old girl in California whose experience matched the criteria for the forbidden controlled rearing experiment. Genie had been tied to a chair for most of her life by her father. She was kept from the rest of the world, including the verbal input she would have received by being a part of that world. Whenever she tried to talk, Genie was severely reprimanded or beaten. Needless to say, she did not have much verbal ability at the time she was discovered. Years of work with Genie by psychologists and speech-language therapists produced little in the way of normal language development (Curtiss, 1977). Genie was unable to learn language—particularly syntactic constructions—to a normal, native-like level, even when given appropriate and abundant input and instruction. The common interpretation was that Genie was discovered past the critical period for developing a first language. Of course, Genie's experiences were abnormal in more areas than language alone, and one does not know whether she suffered some form of biological or congenital mental retardation. Thus, one cannot claim being past some critical period was the principal cause of Genie's stunted language capacity.

Deaf Studies

In all cases in which individuals such as Genie have been isolated specifically from linguistic input past adolescence, the circumstances under which such isolation occurred no doubt impacted their development in other, nonlinguistic ways. Given such abnormal upbringing, it is difficult to argue for the passing of some critical period as the sole source of the difficulties for subsequent language development. Deaf studies are an alternative to traditional case studies of deprivation.

Research by Bellugi and others (Bellugi, 1980, 1988; Klima & Belugi, 1979; Newport & Meier, 1986) shows that signed languages are characterized by the same complexities as spoken languages. In fact, there are notable similarities in specialization of brain functions between native users of signed and spoken languages (Poizner, Klima, & Bellugi, 1987). Moreover, there is evidence that hearing and nonhearing infants exposed to sign language engage in manual babbling (Pettito & Marentette, 1991). These similarities between signed and spoken languages have motivated researchers to look for, and find, what appears to be evidence for critical periods in the acquisition of sign (Mayberry & Fisher, 1989; Newport, 1991) and to argue that this evidence is relevant for spoken languages as well.

Some of the most compelling work in support of the hypothesis that acquisition of grammatical knowledge is constrained by a critical period is based on data collected from deaf speakers of American Sign Language

(ASL). Deaf and hearing children who learn sign language from their deaf parents follow the same learning course typical of spoken-language learning (Newport & Meier, 1985). The common reality, however, is that deaf children are born into hearing families in which parents do not know any sign language at all. In many cases, parents consciously decide not to allow their children access to sign language because they believe that their deaf children will come to learn a spoken language by lip-reading and then be able to make language-approximate pronunciations. The outcomes of such attempts vary because few completely deaf children ever learn to speak in a manner comprehensible to the rest of the speaking world. And because these children are not exposed to sign language, they are effectively deprived of linguistic stimulation. In this sense, children who have not been able to hear the language spoken around them (e.g., spoken English) and who are unable to learn a true alternative (e.g., ASL) because their parents have kept them from being exposed to it provide another opportunity for testing whether people can become fluent if their first opportunity to learn occurs after childhood.

Deaf children acquire most of their mature grammatical capacity within a very short period, just as hearing children do. They can do this even though they often lack access to either the kind of models or responses to poorly formed attempts at language that arguably help children rapidly learn such a complex system of behavior. Nonetheless, even though deaf children have the capacity to invent their own gestural forms for communicating meaning—and acquire words or signs at approximately the same time that children exposed to natural spoken or signed language would—Newport (1990) has shown that *when* one actually learns a formal signing language can influence ultimate attainment of fluency.

Newport compared the production and comprehension of ASL in three groups of people with congenital deafness. People in all three groups had been communicating in ASL for at least 30 years. The difference among the three groups was the age at which the individuals actually learned ASL. One group consisted of people who were born to deaf parents and learned ASL from birth. The second group consisted of early learners, defined as those who first came into contact with ASL between the ages of 4 and 6 years. The final group consisted of individuals who were first exposed to ASL after 12 years of age, which is commonly considered the cutoff point for a variety of proposed critical periods for language development. All of the individuals were older than 50 years of age at test time. Newport's results showed that only individuals in the first two groups, those who had been exposed to ASL prior to 6 years of age, demonstrated native-like fluency. The second group (those learning ASL between 4 and 6 years) showed subtle nonnative characteristics in their ASL. Those in the postcritical period group demonstrated significant deficits that are typically the mark of nonnative speakers. The majority of their problems had to do with ASL equivalents of function morphemes and complex syntactic structures within sentences. Individuals isolated from spoken language prior to adolescence (e.g., Genie) consistently have difficulties with these same things.

Neurobiological Perspective

Neville and her colleagues have approached questions about differences between grammatical and semantic processing from a neurobiological position (see Chapter 8). Their work relies in large part on the recording of event-related brain potentials (ERPs), which are the electrical currents generated through the scalp by neuronal firing. ERP recordings allow researchers to measure the timing and patterning of neuronal firing across developmental stages and behavioral tasks (Neville, 1995) and can be used in conjunction with more traditional behavioral measures to determine differences in cerebral processing associated with different forms of behavior. Ultimately, ERP recordings can provide information about the timing, sequence, and location of various forms of processing, including language. Neville has looked specifically at language processing and event-related brain potentials in normal adults, adults with congenital deafness, and typically developing children to determine whether cerebral subsystems specialized for either semantic or grammatical processing are differentially impacted by delays in language exposure.

In order to assess differences in the neural mechanisms used for processing different components of the language system, Neville and her colleagues (Holcomb & Neville, 1990; Neville, Mills, & Lawson, 1992) compared the timing and distribution of ERPs elicited from normal adults when they processed sentences containing anomalous open- or closed-class words. *Open-class* describes semantic content words, such as nouns, verbs, and adjectives that refer to specific objects and events. The term comes from the fact that in any language, this set openly admits new members. *Closed-class* describes grammatical function words, such as direct and indirect articles, conjunctions, and auxiliaries. The term comes from the fact that in any language, such function words belong to a closed set. Differences in semantic versus grammatical processing were assessed by comparing whether the differences between ERPs could be accounted for in terms of general processing differences (e.g., the frequency and length of the words) rather than in terms of the different functions the words perform (e.g., grammatical, semantic) when a person processes one or the other of the two classes of words. Results from this work indicate that notably different firing patterns occur when normal adults process grammatical and semantic information (Neville, 1995).

When processing grammatical information from their native language, people show localized firing in the anterior region of the left temporal lobe

(Neville, Nicol, Barss, Forster, & Garrett, 1991; Weber-Fox & Neville, 1996); this lateralized firing is not present when people process semantic information. Specifically relevant to the critical period question is the fact that the pattern for grammatical processing does not emerge until around age 11 and becomes solidly in place only around age 15 or 16. In contrast, native ASL users who learned English later in life do not manifest this lateralized firing pattern when processing English grammar (Neville, 1995). However, where the alteration in these deaf people's early language experience appears to have a pronounced effect on the development of systems relevant to grammatical processing, no such effect manifests for semantic processing. Taken together, these findings are consistent with behavioral evidence that adults continue acquiring lexical knowledge late into adulthood, while grammatical knowledge becomes markedly more difficult to acquire. Such findings provide some of the most compelling evidence to date in support of arguments for a critical period in grammatical development. They show differences in cerebral processing of grammatical information when that knowledge has been put in place before and after a particular point in developmental time, and no such differences in the processing of semantic information.

In another area of focus, Neville and her colleagues used typical developmental progression to determine whether there are differences in the time course for establishing grammatical versus semantic knowledge and whether the onset of one or the other form of processing varies from person to person. As mentioned, normal adults show highly lateralized firing during grammatical processing, such that ERPs reflect more electrical activity in the left cerebral hemisphere than in the right, while this lateralization does not hold for semantic processing (Neville, 1995). Furthermore, the grammatical asymmetry is correlated with levels of grammatical knowledge in 8- to 13-year-olds. Neville (1995) found that the higher a child's score on standard grammar tests, the more pronounced the left-sided asymmetry. In a group of 8- to 14-year-olds, ERP recordings that showed more left-sided asymmetry also were larger and correlated with lower volumes of cortical gray matter. On the other hand, there was no difference between patterns of electrical activation in 4-year-olds and adults processing semantic information.

This finding speaks directly to debates about the relevance of synaptic density across ages as well. Brain imaging studies have shown that the amount of gray matter in cerebral cortex (representing the density of synaptic connections) decreases starting around age 8 and continues decreasing until around age 30 (Jernigan, Trauner, Hesselink, & Tallal, 1991), a finding that is consistent with anatomical data (Huttenlocher, 1990; Rakic, Bourgeois, Eckenhoff, Zecevic, & Goldman-Rakic, 1986). It has been argued that this synaptic pruning is associated with functional consolidation, such that function becomes more streamlined and efficient even while brain plasticity decreases. Neville's (1995) work adds support to the view that the lower volume of gray matter associated with more pronounced left-side lateralization of grammatical processing is related to the so-called critical period for development of this kind of processing. It appears that native-like grammatical knowledge gets entrenched through the pruning of those synapses that are not being used for that processing.

Results from the studies reviewed here indicate different developmental time courses and sensitivities for grammatical and semantic processing. Processing of grammatical information appears to rely on different neural mechanisms than those relied on for processing semantic information. The semantic knowledge base continues to expand throughout life, and there apparently is no change in the neuronal firing pattern for processing semantic information from year to year as would be expected if there were a critical period for acquisition of semantic knowledge. Grammatical processing, however, shows gradually differentiated localized responses, reflecting a neural system where decreases in redundancy and increases in specificity manifest over developmental time. These data add support to the view long held by linguists and psycholinguists that language processing can be broken down into different subsystems. Furthermore, the findings reviewed here provide evidence for the biological basis of such distinctions and for component-specific critical period arguments.

INDIVIDUAL DIFFERENCES IN DEVELOPMENT

The concept of critical or sensitive periods focuses on age cutoffs or boundaries for effective stimulation. Much discussion of critical periods implicitly assumes an idealized, archetypal developing child, as if all children developed according to the same timetable. Examination of individual differences in language development divulges a more variable picture, suggesting that even if there are critical periods for language learning for the human species, they play out against a backdrop of individual differences in biological and environmental factors that must necessarily blur the effects of critical periods on individual children.

Evidence of just how flexible the brain is has led neuroscientists to suggest that a young brain can do its work with input that only needs to vaguely resemble a normal environment (Bruer, 1999). It takes pronounced genetic or environmental deprivation for normal firing patterns to go off track.

The phenomenon of expressive language delay is a prime example of such individual variability in the time course of language development. As reviewed by Whitehurst and Fischel (1994), children who will eventually achieve similar linguistic outcomes during the elementary school years may include those who will have hundreds of words in their vocabularies at 2 years of age and who are combining those words into multiword sentences, and those who will have virtually no expressive vocabulary at 2 years of age. Likewise, there are children who will have acquired mature expressive control over the phonology of their language by age 4, and others whose expressive phonology will be incomprehensible to others at this age, yet most of the children with articulation delays will catch up to their peers by elementary school. From an educational or policy perspective, it is particularly important not to confuse children at the slower end of the normal curve of language development with children who have missed some vaguely defined critical period for development.

Language development is multifaceted, as seen through the review of scientific literature on critical periods, with different patterns of development and different sensitivities to language input. Phonological sensitivity wanes to speech sounds not heard early in life (e.g., nonnative), but, given proper training, adults reacquire sensitivity to those contrasts. Grammar is the most difficult of all the components of the language system to develop past puberty. Nonetheless, people are able to learn second language grammars as if they were native speakers. In addition, semantic and pragmatic knowledge can be expanded as long as one is interested in doing so. The existing literature on sensitive periods in first language acquisition raises as many questions as it answers.

1. What kind of learning is occurring when individuals are able to acquire high levels of skill outside the normal sensitive period for grammatical or phonological development? An answer to this question would have clear implications for intervention and remediation in individuals who fail to acquire such competence either early or later in life.
2. How gradual (or sudden) is the drop-off in sensitivity to grammatical or phonological learning, and what are its age brackets? An answer to this question would have implications for the timing of educational and intervention programs.
3. What are the minimal levels of stimulation that are necessary to support learning during the sensitive periods of development, and what form must that stimulation take? Bruer (1999) argued that the development of the young brain is well buffered against an extremely wide range of environmental input. But how wide is that range? Consider this description by Heath (1989) of her research on the interactions between a mother and her preschool children. The mother is said to be prototypical of many poor urban African American mothers who live in small apartments or public housing, isolated from supportive family or community: "One mother agreed to tape record her interactions with her children over a 2-year period and to write notes about her

activities with them. Within approximately 500 hours of tape and over 1,000 lines of notes, she initiated talk to her three preschool children (other than to give them a brief directive or query their actions or intentions) in only 18 instances" (Heath, 1989, pp. 369–370). The rearing conditions in which three preschool children receive only 18 linguistically informative utterances over a 2-year period might fall outside the range of minimal stimulation needed to develop core linguistic competences. What then of the much higher frequencies of stimulation found among the welfare families in the research of Hart and Risley (1995)?

The existence of so many unanswered questions about the neuroscience of sensitive periods for first language acquisition places severe limits on inferences that can be drawn for educational policy. Clearly, deaf children should be exposed to sign language as early as possible in life if they are to acquire full sophistication in that language as adults. Clearly, hearing children should not be raised in a barrel or deprived of linguistic interactions with adults.

If researchers are willing to expand the concept of sensitive period to include exogenous and culturally framed windows of opportunity for learning, then the implications for early intervention and educational practice will expand tremendously. Decades of research have shown that children who start school behind are likely to fall further behind as they progress through their educational careers. Children who fail in school are likely to face economic difficulties in later life, and this relationship is strengthening as blue-collar jobs disappear in an economy that is increasingly knowledge based. Conditions associated with economic poverty are the single strongest predictors of children's success in school, and the differences produced by these conditions are present at the time children first walk through the school door. The preschool period is a critical window of opportunity for acquiring language and other skills, dispositions, and habits of learning that enable children to succeed in school. Knowledge is needed about how to enhance readiness for schooling in children whose families do not provide sufficient support. Future work in the neurosciences will enable researchers to better understand the neural substrates of early learning and development. The potential of that work for unifying the brain and behavioral sciences is exciting. However, the neurosciences are unlikely to reveal how to design preschool environments that provide optimal support for children in need. Researchers already know the critical importance of that task and have made some progress in solving it.

REFERENCES

Allington, R.L. (1984). Content, coverage, and contextual reading in reading groups. *Journal of Reading Behavior, 16*, 85–96.

Bellugi, U. (1980). The structuring of languages: Clues from the similarities between signed and spoken language. In U. Bellugi & M. Studdert-Kennedy (Eds.), *Signed and spoken language: Biological constraints on linguistic form*. Weiheim/Deerfield Beach, FL: Verlag Chemie.

Bellugi, U. (1988). The acquisition of a spatial language. In F. Kessell (Ed.), *The development of language and language researchers: Essays in honor of Roger Brown*. Mahwah, NJ: Lawrence Erlbaum Associates.

Best, C. (1991). *Phonetic influences on the perception of nonnative speech contrasts by 6-8 and 10-12 month olds*. Paper presented at the Biennial Meeting of the Society for Research in Child Development, Seattle.

Best, C. (1995). Learning to perceive the sound patterns of English. In C. Rovee-Collier & L. Lipsitt (Eds.), *Advances in infancy research*. Norwood, NJ: Ablex Publishing Company.

Best, C., & McRoberts, G. (1989). *Phonological influences on the perception of native and non-native contrasts*. Paper presented at the Biennial Meeting of the Society for Research in Child Development, Kansas City, MO.

Best, C., McRoberts, G., & Sithole, N. (1988). Examination of the perceptual reorganization for speech contrasts: Zulu click discrimination by English-speaking adults and infants. *Journal of Experimental Psychology: Human Perception and Performance, 14*, 345–360.

Bohannon, J.N., MacWhinney, B., & Snow, C. (1990). No negative evidence revisited—beyond learnability or who has to prove what to whom. *Developmental Psychology, 26*, 221–226.

Brown, A.L., Palincsar, A.S., & Purcell, L. (1986). Poor readers: Teach, don't label. In U. Neisser (Ed.), *The school achievement of minority children: New perspectives* (pp. 105–143). Mahwah, NJ: Lawrence Erlbaum Associates.

Brown, R., & Herrnstein, R. J. (1975). *Psychology*. Boston: Little, Brown and Company.

Bruer, J.T. (1999). *The myth of the first three years*. New York: Free Press.

Butcher, C., Mylander, C., & Goldin-Meadow, S. (1991). Displaced communication in a self-styled gesture system: Pointing at the non-present. *Cognitive Development, 6*, 315–342.

Chomsky, N. (1959). A review of B.F. Skinner's "Verbal Behavior." *Language, 35*, 26–58.

Curtiss, S. (1977). *Genie: A psycholinguistic study of a modern-day "wild child."* New York: Academic Press.

Damon, W. (1998). *Handbook of child psychology* (5th ed.). New York: John Wiley & Sons.

Flege, J. (1989). Chinese subjects' perception of the word-final English /t/-/d/ contrast: Before and after training. *Journal of the Acoustical Society of America, 86*, 1684–1697.

Flege, J., Takagi, N., & Mann, V. (1995). Japanese adults can learn to produce English /r/ and /l/ accurately. *Language and Speech, 38*, 25–56.

Goldin-Meadow, S., & Mylander, C. (1990). Gestural communication in deaf children: The non-effects of parental input on early language development. *Monographs of the Society for Research in Child Development, 49*, 3–4.

Goldin-Meadow, S., & Mylander, C. (1998). Spontaneous sign systems created by deaf children in two cultures. *Nature, 391*, 279–281.

Hart, B., & Risley, T. (1995). *Meaningful differences in the everyday experience of young American children*. Baltimore: Paul H. Brookes Publishing Co.

Heath, S.B. (1989). Oral and literate traditions among black Americans living in poverty. *American Psychologist, 44*, 367–373.

Hinde, R.A. (1983). Ethology and child development. In M.M. Haith & J.J. Campos (Eds.), *Handbook of child psychology. Fourth edition. Volume II. Infancy and developmental psychobiology*. New York: John Wiley & Sons.

Holcomb, P., & Neville, H. (1990). Auditory and visual semantic priming in lexical decision: A comparison using event-related brain potentials. *Language and Cognitive Processes, 5*, 281–312.

Huttenlocher, J., Haight, W., Bryk, A., Seltzer, M., & Lyons, T. (1991). Early vocabulary growth—relation to language input and gender. *Developmental Psychology, 27*, 236–248.

Huttenlocher, P. (1990). Morphometric study of human cerebral cortex development. *Neuropsychologia, 28*, 517–527.

Jernigan, T., Trauner, D., Hesselink, J., & Tallal, P. (1991). Maturation of human cerebrum observed in vivo during adolescence. *Brain, 114*, 2037–2049.

Juel, C. (1988). Learning to read and write: A longitudinal study of 54 children from first through fourth grades. *Journal of Educational Psychology, 80*, 437–447.

Jusczyk, P. (1985). On characterizing the development of speech perception. In J. Mehler & R. Fox (Eds.), *Neonate cognition: Beyond the blooming, buzzing, confusion*. Mahwah, NJ: Lawrence Erlbaum Associates.

Jusczyk, P. (1992). Developing phonological categories from the speech signal. In C. Ferguson, L. Menn, & C. Stoel-Gammon (Eds.), *Phonological development: Models, research, implications*. Timonium, MD: York Press.

Klima, E., & Belugi, U. (1979). *The signs of language*. Cambridge, MA: Harvard University Press.

Lasky, R., Syrdal-Lasky, A., & Klein, R. (1975). VOT discrimination by four to six and a half month old infants from Spanish environments. *Journal of Experimental Child Psychology, 20*, 215–225.

Lenneberg, E. (1967). *Biological foundations of language*. New York: John Wiley & Sons.

Logan, J., Lively, S., & Pisoni, D. (1989). Training Japanese listeners to identify /r/ and /l/. *Journal of the Acoustical Society of America, 85*, 137–138.

Lorenz, K. (1935). The companion in the bird's world. The fellow-member of the species as releasing factor of social behavior. *Journal fuer Ornithologie, 83*, 137–213.

Mayberry, R., & Fisher, S. (1989). Looking through phonological shape to lexical meaning: The bottleneck of non-native sign language processing. *Memory and Cognition, 17*, 740–754.

McCandliss, B., Fiez, J., Conway, M., Protopapas, A., & McClelland, J. (1998). Eliciting adult plasticity: Both adaptive and non-adaptive training improves Japanese adults' identification of English /r/ and /l/. *Society for Neuroscience Abstracts, 24*, 754.10.

McClelland, J. (2001). Failures to learn and their remediation: A competitive Hebbian account. In J. McClelland & R. Siegler (Eds.), *Mechanisms of cognitive development: Behavioral and neural approaches*. Mahwah, NJ: Lawrence Erlbaum Associates.

Morais, J., Content, A., Bertelson, P., & Cary, L. (1988). Is there a critical period for the acquisition of segmental analysis? *Cognitive Neuropsychology, 5*, 347–352.

Mussen, P.H. (1983). *Handbook of child psychology. Fourth edition*. New York: John Wiley & Sons.

Neville, H.J. (1995). Developmental specificity in neurocognitive development in humans. In M. Gazzaniga (Ed.), *The cognitive neurosciences* (pp. 219–231). Cambridge: The MIT Press.

Neville, H.J., Mills, D., & Lawson, D. (1992). Fractionating language: Different neural subsystems with different sensitive periods. *Cerebral Cortex, 2*, 244–258.

Neville, H.J., Nicol, J., Barss, A., Forster, K., & Garrett, M. (1991). Syntactically based sentence processing classes: Evidence from event-related brain potentials. *Journal of Cognitive Neuroscience, 3*, 155–170.

Newport, E. (1990). Maturational constraints on language learning. *Cognitive Science, 14*, 11–28.

Newport, E. (1991). Contrasting conceptions of the critical period for language. In S. Carey & R. Gelman (Eds.), *The epigenesis of mind: Essays on biology and cognition*. Mahwah, NJ: Lawrence Erlbaum Associates.

Newport, E., & Meier, R. (1985). The acquisition of American Sign Language. In D. Slobin (Ed.), *The cross-linguistic study of language acquisition*. Mahwah, NJ: Lawrence Erlbaum Associates.

Oka, E., & Paris, S. (1986). Patterns of motivation and reading skills in underachieving children. In S. Ceci (Ed.), *Handbook of cognitive, social, and neuropsychological aspects of learning disabilities* (Vol. 2). Mahwah, NJ: Lawrence Erlbaum Associates.

Pettito, L., & Marentette, P. (1991). Babbling in the manual mode: Evidence for the ontogeny of language. *Science, 251*, 1493–1496.

Pinker, S. (1994). *The language instinct*. New York: William Morrow & Company.

Poizner, H., Klima, E., & Bellugi, U. (1987). *What the hands reveal about the brain*. Cambridge: Bradford Books/MIT Press.

Rakic, P., Bourgeois, J., Eckenhoff, M., Zecevic, N., & Goldman-Rakic, P. (1986). Concurrent overprotection of synapses in diverse regions of the primate cerebral cortex. *Science, 232*, 232–235.

Snow, C. (1979). The role of social interaction in language acquisition. In W. Collins (Ed.), *Children's language and communication: Minnesota Symposia on Child Psychology*. Mahwah, NJ: Lawrence Erlbaum Associates.

Strange, W., & Jenkins, J. (1978). Role of linguistic experience in the perception of speech. In R. Walk & H. Pick (Eds.), *Perception and experience*. New York: Kluwer Academic/Plenum Publishers.

Streeter, L. (1976). Language perception of 2-month-old infants shows effects of both innate mechanisms and experience. *Nature, 259*, 39–41.

Trehub, S. (1976). The discrimination of foreign speech contrasts by infants and adults. *Child Development, 47*, 466–472.

Weber-Fox, C., & Neville, H. (1996). Maturational constraints on functional specializations for language processing: ERP and behavioral evidence in bilingual speakers. *Journal of Cognitive Neuroscience, 8*, 231–256.

Werker, J. (1981). The ontogeny of speech perception. In I. Mattingly & M. Studdert-Kennedy (Eds.), *Modularity and the motor theory of speech perception*. Mahwah, NJ: Lawrence Erlbaum Associates.

Werker, J., & Lalonde, C. (1988). Cross-language speech perception: Initial capabilities and developmental change. *Developmental Psychology, 24*, 672–683.

Werker, J., & Tees, R. (1983). Developmental changes across childhood in the perception of non-native speech sounds. *Canadian Journal of Psychology, 37*, 278–286.

Werker, J., & Tees, R. (1984). Cross-language speech perception: Evidence for perceptual reorganization during the first year of life. *Infant Behavior and Development, 7*, 49–63.

Whitehurst, G.J. (1997). Language processes in context: Language learning in children reared in poverty. In L.B. Adamson & M.A. Romski (Eds.), *Communication and language acquisition: Discoveries from atypical development* (pp. 233–266). Baltimore: Paul H. Brookes Publishing Co.

Whitehurst, G.J., & Fischel, J. (1994). Early developmental language delay: What, if anything, should the clinician do about it? *Journal of Child Psychology and Psychiatry, 35*, 613–648.

Whitehurst, G.J., & Lonigan, C.J. (1998). Child development and emergent literacy. *Child Development, 68*, 848–872.

10

A Critical Period for Second Language Acquisition?

Kenji Hakuta

The critical period hypothesis for second language (L2) learning has found resonance in a variety of policy positions regarding when an L2 should be introduced in the curriculum. For immigrant students, in a 1998 court declaration urging that such students be exposed to English as early as possible, an advocate wrote, "The optimal time to learn a second language is between age three and five or as soon thereafter as possible, and certainly before the onset of puberty" (Porter, 1998, p. 1). Porter is a leading advocate for English-only approaches to the education of language minority students and an opponent of bilingual education programs because they delay intensive instruction in English. She has found the critical period hypothesis to be in support of her position.

Advocates for the early introduction of foreign language in the elementary schools, dating back to the Foreign Languages in the Elementary Schools (FLES) programs of the 1960s, also have found an important ally in the critical period hypothesis. For example, the New Jersey State Department of Education's World Languages Curriculum Framework cited critical period research to make the following point: "With each year of growth, children are less able to filter out fine distinctions among the sounds of other languages. After early childhood, the language acquisition mechanism becomes highly structured creating an interference effect that may account for the difficulty in learning languages at a later time" (1999, p. 7).

Such statements draw on the critical period hypothesis for L2 acquisition, the origins of which are attributed to Penfield and Roberts (1959) and more prominently perhaps to Eric Lenneberg (1967), who amassed evidence in support of the view that first language (L1) acquisition is a biologically constrained process, with a specific timetable ending at puberty. In a single paragraph, Lenneberg speculated about the implications for L2 acquisition, noting that after puberty, second languages are acquired consciously and with great effort, and often not successfully (see Chapter 9). The purpose of this chapter is to make assumptions underlying this hypothesis and to highlight what is known and not known about its empirical status.

FIRST LANGUAGE (L1) ACQUISITION

A brief foray of the standard version of the critical period hypothesis for L1 acquisition is in order. The clearest account can be found in Pinker (1994). This view is based on Chomsky's account of linguistic competence—an abstract set of rules and representations that is highly specific to language (i.e., organized differently from other mental capacities, e.g., visual cognition) and an innate component of the human mind. The standard argument is that it is logically impossible for a child to acquire linguistic competence of this complexity through the types of exposure to language that children receive in their home environment. The argument states that a specialized biological program must exist for language acquisition, similar to the programmed course of development of physical systems such as vision, digestion, and respiration. As long as children are exposed to a threshold amount of linguistic exposure during the critical period, they will all uniformly acquire linguistic competence, much as children develop similar physical organs despite considerable variation in nutrition. And, if they are deprived of this exposure during the critical period, no amount of exposure after it can compensate for it.

Direct evidence in support of the critical period for L1 acquisition is thin and based on theoretical arguments and analogy to other well-explored developmental processes, such as visual development in the cat (Hubel, 1988). Most children are exposed to language early in life and acquire it successfully. Indeed, the first argument in favor of a critical period is its uniformity in spite of considerable environmental variation in the ways that parents talk to children. For ethical reasons, experiments in which infants are deprived of exposure to language during the putative critical period are not conducted. Other evidence in support of the hypothesis comes from unusual, tragic cases of language deprivation resulting from child abuse, and from studies of deaf children who are born to hearing parents, but who are exposed to American Sign Language (ASL) at a later age. Nevertheless, the hypothesis is commonly accepted. As Pinker stated, "Acquisition of a normal language is guaranteed for children up to the age of six, is steadily compromised from then until shortly after puberty, and is rare thereafter" (1994, p. 293).

ELEMENTS OF THE CRITICAL PERIOD HYPOTHESIS FOR SECOND LANGUAGE (L2) ACQUISITION

In theorizing about a putative critical period for L2 acquisition, a key framing question is whether L2 acquisition recapitulates the L1 acquisition process (a hypothesis known in literature as the L2=L1 hypothesis), or alternatively, whether L2 acquisition is a cumulative process that builds on the competence already developed in L1. If the L1=L2 hypothesis is correct, then the evidence for or against a critical period for L1 acquisition is relevant to L2 acquisition. However, if the cumulative model is correct, the evidence from L1 acquisition is irrelevant to answering the question about L2 acquisition.

The research evidence on the nature of L2 acquisition is clear on two points, but they are contradictory. First, with respect to rate of acquisition, there is evidence that linguistic similarity between the L1 and L2 matters (Odlin, 1989). A native speaker of Spanish will acquire English more rapidly than would a native speaker of Chinese, all other things being equal, because of the linguistic similarity between Spanish and English. This evidence would imply that the cumulative model is correct. Second, with respect to error patterns and the overall qualitative course of L2 acquisition, there is a similarity across speakers of different languages learning a given L2, indicating that more than a simple transfer from L1 to L2 is occurring (Bialystok & Hakuta, 1994). Indeed there is some sort of reenactment of the L1 acquisition process at work. As for Lenneberg, the originator of the critical period hypothesis for L2, it appears that he favored the cumulative model when he wrote that "we may assume that the cerebral organization for language learning as such has taken place during childhood, and because natural languages tend to resemble one another in many fundamental aspects, the matrix of language skills is present" (1967, p. 176). In any event, the jury is still out as to whether L2 is a recapitulation of L1 acquisition or an add-on process. What would be the key elements of a critical period in L2 acquisition?

1. *Clearly specified beginning and end points for the period:* Lenneberg suggested puberty, and others have followed suit. Johnson and Newport (1989) considered age 15 to be the end of the critical period. As noted previously, Pinker considered it to begin at age 6 and end at puberty. For present purposes, assume that the critical period hypothesis is set by puberty and ends at age 15. In any event, any claim to a critical period for L2 acquisition should be specific about an end point.

2. *Well-defined decline in L2 acquisition at the end of the period:* The ability to learn things declines with age, such as learning to ride a bicycle, yet it would not be stated that there is a critical period for cycling. *A general decline in learning is not strong evidence for a critical period for L2 acquisition.* The appeal of a critical period hypothesis lies in its specificity, that is, its ability to target specific learning mechanisms that get turned off at a given age (Birdsong, 1999). Thus, one important piece of evidence would be if a rapid decline could be found around the end of the critical period, rather than a general monotonic and continuous decline with age that continues throughout the life span.
3. *Evidence of qualitative differences in learning between acquisition within and outside the critical period:* A critical period is assumed to be caused by the shutting down of a specific language learning mechanism. Therefore, any learning that happens outside of the critical period must be the result of alternative learning mechanisms. If that were the case, then there should be clear qualitative differences in the patterns of acquisition between child and adult L2 learners. For example, if certain grammatical errors could be found among adult learners that are never found in child learners, or if child learners were able to learn specific aspects of the language that adults could not learn, then this would be strong evidence for a critical period.
4. *Robustness to environmental variation inside the critical period:* Another attraction of the critical period hypothesis is that there is a threshold level of exposure with uniformed outcomes, even with considerable environmental variation. The environment might play a larger role beyond that period and the outcomes would become more variable.

JOHNSON AND NEWPORT'S STUDY

A study by Johnson and Newport (1989) reported results consistent with the critical period hypothesis. The study's results are cited as authoritative evidence for a critical period in L2 acquisition. In their study of native speakers of Chinese and Korean who came to the United States at ages ranging from 3 to 39 years old, they asked individuals to identify grammatical and ungrammatical sentences that were presented auditorily. They reported that prior to age 15 there was a negative correlation with age, but after age 15 there was no correlation with age (satisfying conditions 1 and 2). In addition, the adult learners showed great variability in learning outcomes, whereas the child learners did not (condition 4).

A reanalysis of the data by Bialystok and Hakuta (1994), however, revealed some problems with the original interpretation. Bialystok and Hakuta argued that the data showed a discontinuity not at puberty but rather at age 20, and that there was statistically significant evidence for a continued decline in L2 acquisition well into adulthood. It is likely that the peculiarities of the sample (students and faculty from the University of Illinois at Urbana-Champaign) could have further complicated their results. A picture of the reanalysis is shown in Figure 10.1. The data show a continuous decline with age of arrival, which is not consistent with condition 2. Furthermore, the data patterns suggest two distinct groups of subjects, those before and after age 20, both of which show declining performance with age. The study should not be considered definitive in light of its sampling limitations.

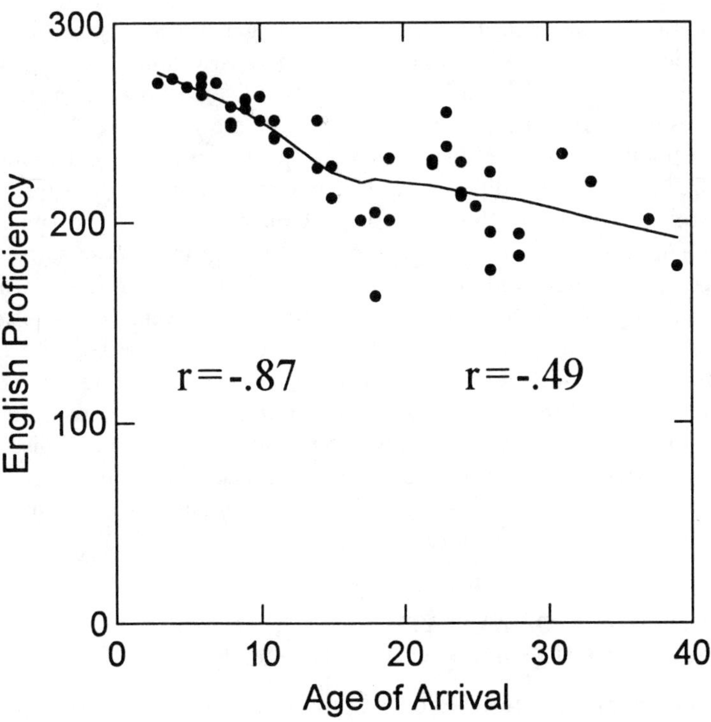

Figure 10.1. Reanalysis of Johnson and Newport (1989) study showing discontinuity at age 20, and continued decline in adult subjects. (From Bialystok, E., & Hakuta, K. [1994]. *In other words: The science and psychology of second-language acquisition.* New York: Basic Books; reprinted by permission.)

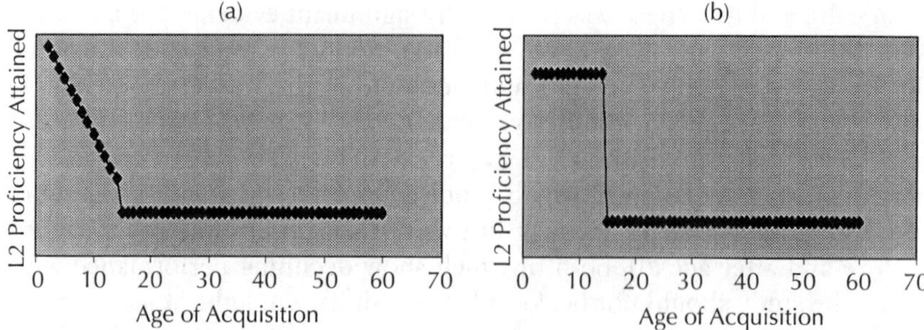

Figures 10.2a and 10.2b. Some theoretical predictions of the critical period hypothesis showing disruption at predicted end of the critical period.

CONDITIONS 1 AND 2: END POINT FOR THE CRITICAL PERIOD AND DISCONTINUITY AT THAT POINT

Theoretically, the critical period hypothesis generates a prediction that should look like Figure 10.2a or 10.2b, with a disruption occurring at the predicted age point. The difference may be in slope breaking at the age point, as in Figure 10.2a, or the slopes may be the same on either ends of the age point, but there could be a sharp drop-off at the age point, as in Figure 10.2b. A test of conditions 1 and 2 can be found in a study reported by Bialystok and Hakuta (1999) using the United States census data from 1990. The study looked at a large sample of immigrants whose native languages were Chinese and Spanish and who had immigrated to the United States at ages ranging from birth to 70 years old. The census bureau asked for a self-report of their English ability, which was converted to a four-point scale. The scale was validated by the census bureau against actual measures of English proficiency in a separate study. The data from this study showed continuous decline with age and no evidence of a discontinuity or sharp break at puberty as would be expected by conditions 1 and 2. The data are shown in Figure 10.3—it is essentially a straight line and there is no evidence for conditions 1 or 2.

CONDITION 3: QUALITATIVE DIFFERENCES BETWEEN CHILD AND ADULT LEARNERS

It is important for a critical period hypothesis to demonstrate that a specific learning mechanism is present during the period but not outside of the period, and one way to do so would be to show different patterns of acquisition in adults and children. Studies that compare the errors and performance patterns of child and adult L2 learners are informative in testing for the viability of condition 3.

One area of research is in the extent of native language influence L2 learning. The relevant question is whether children differ from adults in the extent to which native language influence can be found. The theoretical basis for this can be found in the late 1950s and 1960s when the predominant view of L2 acquisition was that of language transfer, based on the principles of behaviorist psychology (Hakuta & Cancino, 1977). In this view, the points of contrast between the native language and the target language determined the course of learning—positive transfer happened where the two languages were similar and negative transfer where they were different. For example, native speakers of Japanese have difficulty with the English determiner system (e.g., *a*, *the*, *some*) because there is no equivalent system in their native language. Native speakers of Spanish, however, do not have as much difficulty because a similar system exists in their native language. The question, then, is whether adult learners show more evidence of transfer errors than children because, according to the critical period hypothesis, children directly gain access to the target language whereas adults must go through their native language. This does not appear to be the case. Children who are learning a second language show evidence of transfer errors similar to adults and overall patterns of errors are not distinguishable between children and adults (Bialystok & Hakuta, 1994).

Another opportunity to look for differences between children and adults is in the pattern of development in the L2. In one study, Bailey, Madden, and Krashen (1974) compared the performance of adult and child

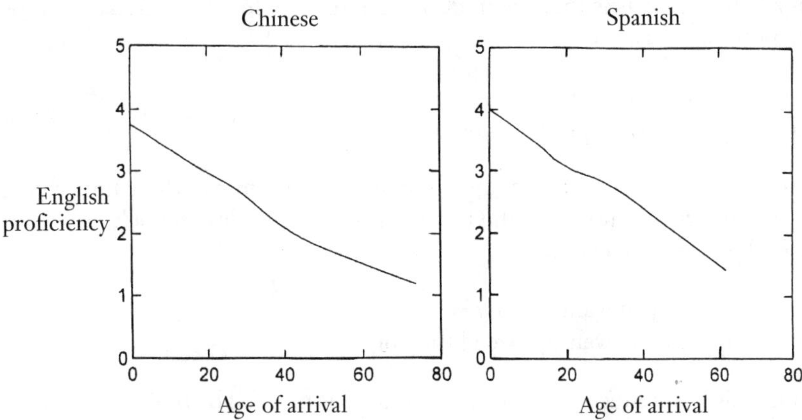

Figure 10.3. Self-reported English proficiency for U.S. immigrants as a function of age of arrival: Data from the 1990 U.S. census. (From Bialystok, E., & Hakuta, K. [1999]. Confounded age: Linguistic and cognitive factors in age differences in second language acquisition. In D. Birdsong [Ed.], *Second language acquisition and the critical period hypothesis* [pp. 161–181]. Mahwah, NJ: Lawrence Erlbaum Associates; reprinted by permission.)

learners of English as L2 on a test of English morphological structures. Specifically, they compared their ability to correctly use the present progressive *-ing*, forms of the verb *to be*, the plural *-s*, determiners (*a*, *the*), the past tense, the third person indicative (he run*s* every day), and the possessive *'s*. The results found a remarkable similarity in the rank ordered performance between children and adults, as can be seen in Figure 10.4. The native language background of students did not seem to affect the results. Overall, this study provides support for the fact that child and adult learners progress along similar paths of development.

A specific way to test the critical period hypothesis is by asking whether adult learners can demonstrate knowledge in the abstract aspects of language that are presumably accessible only through language-specific learning mechanisms (what linguists have come to call *universal grammar*). White and Genesee (1996) conducted such a test to see whether adult L2 learners of English had access to the following pattern of intuitions that all native speakers of English have:

1. Who do you want to see?
2. Who do you want to feed the dog?
3. Who do you wanna see?
4. *Who do you wanna feed the dog?

Number 4 (marked by *) is ungrammatical. Why, despite surface similarities, is 3 considered okay, but 4 is not okay? If grammatical intuitions were formed on the basis of analogy, 4 should be okay. The logical argument made by linguists is that the underlying structure for the sentences can be hypothesized as,

5. You want to see *who*?
6. You want *who* to feed the dog?

According to the theoretical model of universal grammar, these underlying forms of *who* are moved to the front of the sentence, leaving behind a trace *t* in the original location:

7. Who_i do you want to see t_i?
8. Who_i do you want t_i to feed the dog?

The rule that reduces *want to* to *wanna* for 8 is blocked by the trace between *want* and *to*. According to this analysis, this knowledge is needed in order to find 3 to be okay but 4 not to be okay. The abstractness of this rule makes it hard to learn without preexisting knowledge. The critical period hypothesis says that the learning mechanism that allows for this knowledge to be acquired is no longer present in adults.

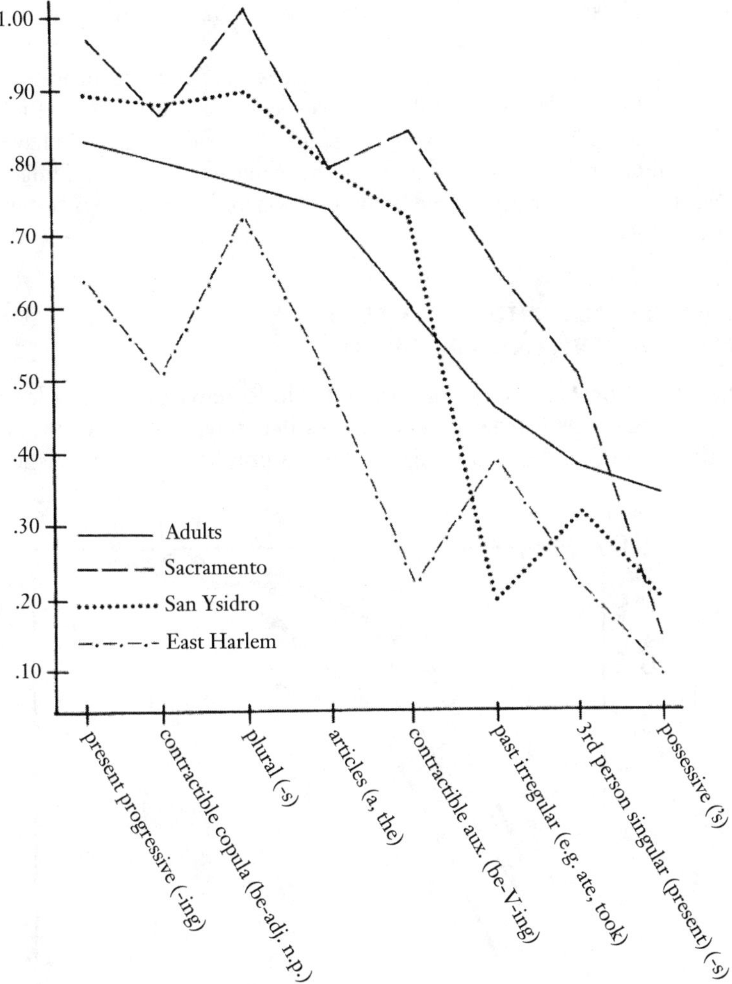

Figure 10.4. Comparison of performance on selected English grammatical structures in adult and child learners. (From Bailey, N., Madden, C., & Krashen, S. [1974]. Is there a "natural sequence" in adult second language learning? *Language Learning, 24,* 235–243; reprinted by permission.)

Using sentences like these, White and Genesee asked adults who had learned English at different ages to discriminate between grammatical and ungrammatical sentences based on abstract concepts. Although more adult learners had difficulty in distinguishing between these sentences than child learners, about one third of the adults who had acquired these rules showed equivalently high performance to child learners and native speakers of English. Thus, adults are capable of learning highly abstract rules that theory would say are accessible only with specialized language acquisition mechanisms.

There are no demonstrated differences between the process of L2 acquisition in children and adults, with respect to condition 3. As Bialystok and Hakuta concluded, "The adult learning a second language behaves just like a child learning a second language: he walks like a duck and talks like a duck, the only major difference being that, on average, he does not waddle as far" (1994, p. 86).

CONDITION 4: THE EFFECTS OF ENVIRONMENTAL VARIATION

The critical period assumes a minimal role for environment in learning, such that once the learner is exposed to a necessary and sufficient amount of stimulation, the learning is complete. An important variant in the envi-

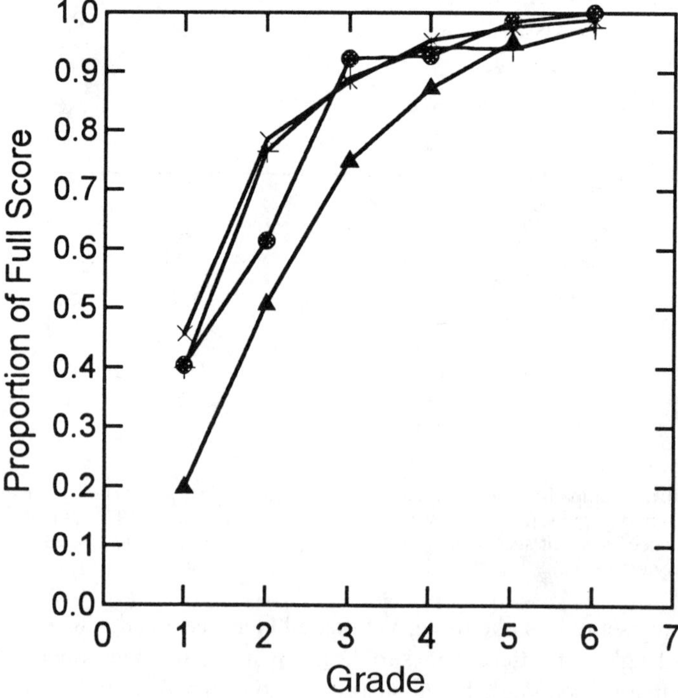

Figure 10.5. English oral proficiency development in immigrant students from a northern California school district, separated by poverty level in schools. This is a cross-sectional sample, but all subjects included in this analysis were enrolled in this school district since kindergarten. (Key: Poverty level: ▲ 70, + 50, × 25, ● 10.)

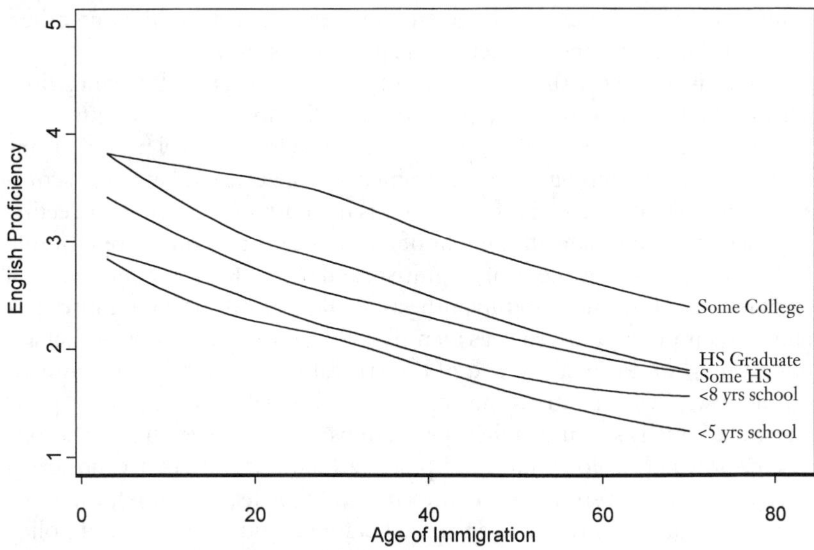

Figure 10.6. Self-reported English proficiency for native Chinese immigrants as a function of age of arrival, separated by educational attainment: Data from the 1990 U.S. census

ronment is socioeconomic status of the learner. Figure 10.5 shows oral proficiency data for immigrant students from a school district in northern California, varying by the socioeconomic environment of the school. This school district does not provide bilingual education and students are exposed only to English during the school day. The data show students who are from lower socioeconomic schools attain English proficiency a year slower than those students in higher socioeconomic schools.

Strong socioeconomic effects can be found in the census data as well. Figure 10.6 shows the same data as Figure 10.2, but they are separated by years of education attained as a proxy for socioeconomic status. There are effects for years of education—a regression analysis revealed that education accounts for the same amount of variance as the effects of age of immigration. In addition, the education effects are uniform across the life span and there is no indication, as might be suggested by the critical period hypothesis, that it works differently in child and adult learners.

CONCLUSION

The evidence for a critical period for L2 acquisition is scanty, especially when analyzed in terms of its key assumptions. There is no empirically definable end point, there are no qualitative differences between child and adult learners, and there are large environmental effects on the outcomes. None of the conditions are met by the present research.

This is not to say that there are not any age effects for L2 acquisition. All studies show that there is a monotonic decline in ultimate attainment in L2 with age. Failure to find supporting evidence for a critical period means that the view of a biologically constrained and specialized language acquisition device that is turned off at puberty is not correct. The gradual decline over age in the ultimate attainment of an L2 means that there are multiple factors at work—physiological, cognitive, and social. Researchers who wish to pursue the critical period hypothesis would need to become more specific in their predictions, such as identifying the linguistic processes that are putatively shut down at the end of the critical period. Yet, it is incumbent on those who wish to stress the cognitive and social factors in L2 acquisition to be equally specific in their predictions. Given the harsh implications of a critical period for policy and practice (i.e., not only that exposure is needed early, but also that exposure later in life is less valuable), the standards of evidence in this area must be held high and educators and policy makers who pay attention to this research should demand no less.

Beyond urging for the highest standards in research that bear on this theoretical question, policy makers and practitioners should also seek additional information related to age and L2 instruction, such as

1. What capabilities are there for staffing different program options at different grade levels?
2. Are students in different grade levels differentially responsive to technology-supported language learning environments?
3. In what ways does the relationship between language and content change as students progress through school?
4. What specific resources and needs exist in the community for L2s that can help motivate students at different ages?

Informed answers to such questions can help guide local communities and states in making decisions about optimal times for L2 instruction.

REFERENCES

Bailey, N., Madden, C., & Krashen, S. (1974). Is there a "natural sequence" in adult second language learning? *Language Learning, 24,* 235–243.

Bialystok, E., & Hakuta, K. (1994). *In other words: The science and psychology of second-language acquisition.* New York: Basic Books.

Bialystok, E., & Hakuta, K. (1999). Confounded age: Linguistic and cognitive factors in age differences in second language acquisition. In D. Birdsong (Ed.), *Second language acquisition and the critical period hypothesis* (pp. 161–181). Mahwah, NJ: Lawrence Erlbaum Associates.

Birdsong, D. (1999). Introduction: Whys and why nots of the critical period hypothesis for second language acquisition. In D. Birdsong (Ed.), *Second language acquisition and the critical period hypothesis* (pp. 1–22). Mahwah, NJ: Lawrence Erlbaum Associates.

Hakuta, K., & Cancino, H. (1977). Trends in second-language acquisition research. *Harvard Educational Review, 47*, 294–316.

Hubel, D. (1988). *Eye, brain, and vision*. New York: Scientific American Library.

Johnson, J., & Newport, E. (1989). Critical period effects in second language learning: The influence of maturational state on the acquisition of English as a second language. *Cognitive Psychology, 21*, 60–99.

Lenneberg, E.H. (1967). *Biological foundations of language*. New York: John Wiley & Sons.

New Jersey State Department of Education. (1999). New Jersey World Languages Curriculum Framework. Available: http://www.state.nj.us/njded/frameworks/worldlanguages/

Odlin, T. (1989). *Language transfer: Cross-linguistic influence in language learning*. Cambridge, England: Cambridge University Press.

Penfield, W., & Roberts, L. (1959). *Speech and brain mechanisms*. Princeton, NJ: Princeton University Press.

Pinker, S. (1994). *The language instinct*. New York: William Morrow & Company.

Porter, R. (1998). *Defendant declaration*. Valeria G. et al., v. Pete Wilson et al., No. C-98-2252-CAL, U.S. District Court, Northern District of California.

White, L., & Genesee, F. (1996). How native is near-native? The issue of ultimate attainment in adult second language acquisition. *Second Language Research, 12*, 233–265.

V

Early Intervention and the Relevance of Critical Periods

11

The Subtle Science of How Experience Affects the Brain

John T. Bruer

William T. Greenough

One of the most exciting advances in modern science is the progress neuroscientists have made in understanding the brain and its development. Given this exciting progress, it is no surprise that organizations and individuals interested in early childhood programs and polices have begun to consider what these neuroscience findings might imply for parenting, child care, and early childhood education.

Attempting to base policy and practice on research is desirable and commendable. However, it is seldom easy to determine the policy and practical implications of basic biological research. This is certainly the case in some recent attempts to use basic brain science to inform early childhood policies and programs.

One notion that has figured prominently in popular and policy discussions of early brain development is our emerging understanding of how and when experience influences brain development. When we read popular articles on brain science and child development, it is easy to become convinced that our neuroscientific understanding of how experience affects brain development leads straightforwardly to direct insights for improving

The work reported in this chapter was supported by Grant Nos. MH35321, AG10154, HD37175, awarded by the National Science Foundation, the FRAXA Research Foundation, the Illinois-Eastern Iowa District Kiwanis International Spastic Paralysis Research Foundation, and the Retirement Research Foundation. The authors thank Kathy Bates, Robert Galvez, Leslie Harms, and Marc Cohen for their assistance.

child care and parenting. Among other things, these articles suggest that early experience is important because it stimulates growth of neural connections in the brain. Or, we read that early experience, particularly early environmental enrichment, has a uniquely powerful and permanent influence on brain development, and that efficient learning is limited to the early years of life. We read that constant stimulation is important because when it comes to neural connections, we must either "use them or lose them." In popular discussions there also is a common belief that the more synapses a person has in his or her brain, the more intelligent he or she is.

In fact, although each of these statements is based on published neuroscience results, none of these insights are supported by what neuroscientists currently know about the effects of experience on brain development. Unfortunately, the popular press and many policy discussions tend to oversimplify the underlying brain science and overlook some fundamental distinctions that have guided research on how experience affects the brain.

Often, the problem is that when we think about the effects of experience, we tend to think simply about how the external, physical environment acts on an organism. We tend to think only about the interface between the body and its external surroundings. However, if we want to understand how experience affects brain development, we have to think more carefully about how experience acts on the nervous system. If we are to appreciate what neuroscience might be able to contribute to our thinking on brain development, early childhood, and critical periods, we must be more specific about the role experience plays in brain development.

Beneath the sensory interface between the organism and the external world there is a very complex set of interacting, internal environments. To tease out the practical implications of this research, we must first understand that different kinds of experience affect the brain in different ways and that for only some experiences are the effects on the brain limited to a critical or sensitive period during development. In thinking about experience and its effects on the brain, it is important to keep in mind that there are (at least) two different ways in which experience causes changes in the brain. One is called *experience-expectant* development and the other is called *experience-dependent* development. This distinction was introduced in one of the first interdisciplinary publications devoted to brain science and child development (Greenough, Black, & Wallace, 1987) but often has been overlooked in subsequent popular and policy discussions, much to the detriment of those discussions.

There are aspects of brain development that require or, better, *expect* certain kinds of experiences to occur at specific times during development, if normal development is to occur. *Experience-expectant* development is the aspect of brain development that has typically been thought about in the tradition of "critical periods" for experience in development. Experience-expectant development is limited to developing skills and neural systems that are characteristic of a species. Typically, sensory and motor systems (e.g., vision, audition, first language learning in humans) develop in part via experience-expectant processes. In the overwhelming number of cases these systems develop normally because the expected, required experiences are reliably present in any typical human environment and readily available to all typical members of a species in their typical environments. Claims about critical or sensitive periods are claims about experience-expectant development. Research shows that experience-expectant development involves losing preexisting synapses (see Figure 11.1).

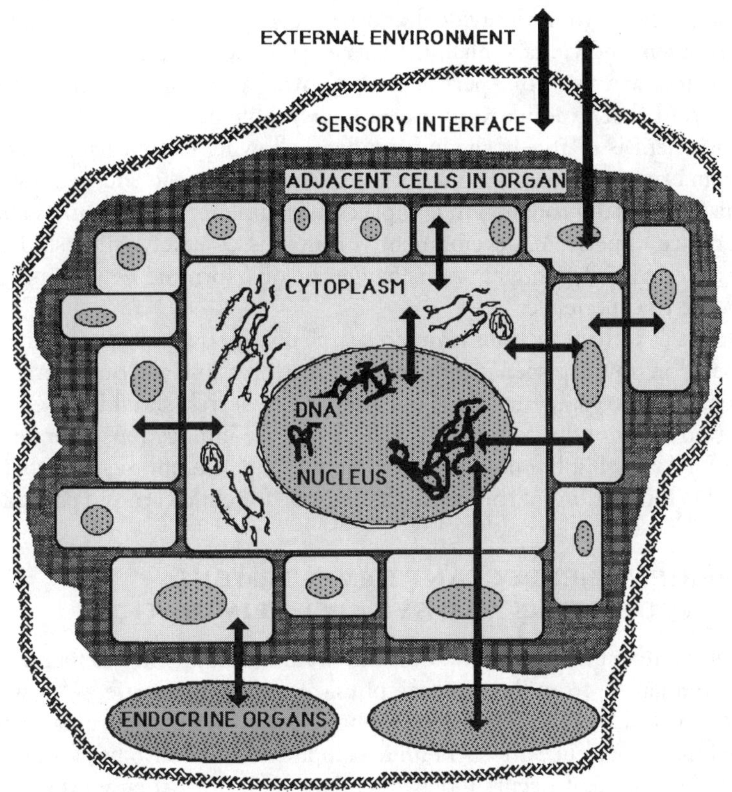

Figure 11.1. The chromosomes of a cell that contain its genes exist in a hierarchy of interacting environments extending from their immediate environment in the cell nucleus to the environment surrounding the organism. Each of those environments can influence the expression of genes. The environment acts on the organism largely by regulating gene expression directly or via intermediary processes. (From Greenough, W.T. [1991]. Experience as a component of normal development: Evolutionary considerations. *Developmental Psychology, 27*[1], 14–17; reprinted by permission.)

Ultimately, however, experience affects the brain by causing chemical changes within cells that influence cell function and structure. Experience brings about these effects by regulating the expression of genes, which govern protein synthesis. *Protein* is not just something we eat; rather, it is the chemical substance that gives character to living cells. One case of experience-expectant change appears to involve a defect in a gene that encodes a protein that may be necessary for the normal developmental process of synapse elimination, discussed later in this chapter. This example involves the role of the fragile X mental retardation protein in brain development, which helps to illustrate that, in some cases, losing synapses is crucial for normal brain development.

In contrast, *experience-dependent* development is driven by experiences that are unique to an individual and to the physical, social, and cultural environment individuals inhabit. Experience-dependent brain changes allow us to learn from our personal experiences and store information derived from that experience to use in later problem solving. This type of development is relatively age independent, allowing us to learn and benefit from experience throughout our lives. Research on the effects of raising animals (normally rodents) in complex environments tells scientists about experience-dependent development. From this research scientists know that experience-dependent brain changes involve forming new synapses in response to experience.

The next three sections review research on experience-expectant development, on how experience influences gene expression, and on experience-dependent development; point out how this research should cause us to question many of the popular ideas regarding the implications of brain science for early childhood policy and practice; and attempt to state what, in fact, the implications of this research might be for child care and parenting.

EXPERIENCE-EXPECTANT DEVELOPMENT: SYNAPTOGENESIS AND SYNAPSE ELIMINATION

Popular interest in early childhood and brain development has focused on how stimulation from the external, physical environment affects "how the brain is wired," as the popular metaphor puts it. Brain science has established that experience affects brain development, but it also has found that much development occurs independently of and prior to any experience. Neuroscientists have confirmed that much of the brain's basic circuitry is formed under genetic control and does not depend on experience, stimulation, or neural activity of any kind. Neuroscientists also have found that even some specific neural connections develop independently of sensory stimulation from the external environment. Early in development neural cells begin to fire spontaneously, without receiving any external stimulation. Based on the principle that "cells that fire together, wire together," this spontaneous activity results in the formation of some neural circuitry. For example, in some animal species this spontaneous firing of nerve cells contributes to the development of the visual system even before the animal's eyes are open. In monkeys, researchers have found that spontaneous neural activity forms primitive ocular dominance columns—brain structures that support binocular vision—before monkeys are born (Horton & Hocking, 1996). In kittens, when researchers applied drugs to block spontaneous neural activity within their visual systems, primitive ocular dominance columns failed to form (Stryker & Harris, 1986). Of course, these structures also are influenced by later experience, as noted in the following paragraphs.

Early in development, genetic factors and spontaneous neural activity contribute to the neural substrate that experience modifies later in development. Genes are responsible for another aspect of this neural substrate. We have all read that in the early months and years of life there is a rapid increase in the number of neural connections or synapses in the brain. Neuroscientists call this phenomenon *developmental synaptogenesis*. This rapid increase in brain connectivity also occurs largely independently of experience.

Developmental synaptogenesis results in a substantial overproduction of synapses in the young brain. *Overproduction* means that in this early phase of development there are more synapses in the brain than when the animal reaches maturity. The early excess of synapses provides the raw material for experience-expectant development. As development proceeds, a selection process occurs that determines which of these synapses survive and which die. Diagrams such as the one in Figure 11.2 illustrate how the number of synapses in the brain changes across development.

Reading recent issues of *Newsweek* or *Time*, it would appear that neuroscientists had just discovered developmental overproduction and subsequent elimination of synapses. In fact, scientists have known about this phenomenon for more than 25 years. In 1975, Brian Cragg measured the number of synapses per neuron in the developing cat visual cortex. He found that there was an overproduction of synapses in that brain area and noted that this synaptic excess lasted until the time that critical or sensitive periods for visual ocular dominance column organization ended in the cat. A few years later, Boothe, Greenough, Lund, and Wrege (1979) showed a similar pattern of synaptic overproduction and loss in the monkey brain. In that same year, Peter Huttenlocher (1979) published the first study that described a pattern of synaptic overproduction and elimination in the human brain. This study, and subsequent work by Huttenlocher and his colleagues,

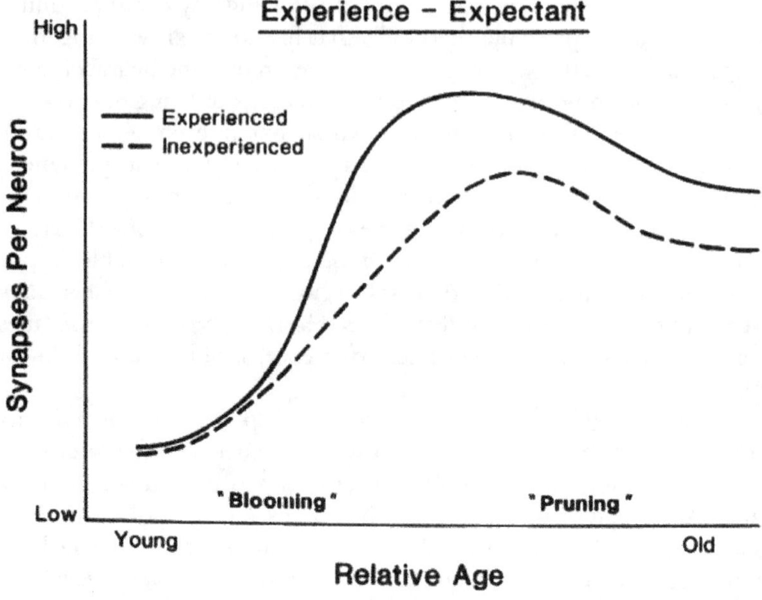

Figure 11.2. Schematic illustrating overproduction and loss of synapses in experience-expectant developmental processes. Synapses are produced prior to some normally occurring developmental event such as exposure to patterned visual experience. The event causes synapses that are appropriately activated by the experience to become stable and survive while synapses that have not been appropriately activated are eliminated. (From Greenough, W.T., Black, J.E., & Wallace, C.S. [1987]. Experience and brain development. *Child Development, 58*[3], 539–559; reprinted by permission. ©1986 by Lawrence Erlbaum Associates.)

is mentioned throughout this book (Huttenlocher, 1990; Huttenlocher & Dabholkar, 1997; Huttenlocher & de Courten, 1987; Huttenlocher, de Courten, Garey, & van der Loos, 1982).

When we see studies of how synaptic densities or numbers change over the life span (such as the one previously mentioned), however, we must always remember that the methods scientists used to measure synapse formation have varied with the knowledge available at the time the studies were conducted. Many studies of synaptic change have used measures based on the number of synapses per unit volume of brain tissue, which provide only measures of the distance between synapses. Such relative measures are unreliable because the brain's volume changes during development, and these changes in volume are due to changes not only in synapses, but also to changes in blood vessels and glial, or support cells, in the brain. These different types of tissue grow at different rates during development and thus vary in how much they contribute to brain tissue volume at different times. Therefore, synaptic density does not accurately reflect synaptic numbers.

Scientists can avoid this methodological problem by using more rigorous and more accurate measures of how synaptic connectivity in the brain changes over time. If they count both the number of nerve cells per unit volume of brain tissue and the number of synapses per same unit volume, then divide the number of synapses by the number of neurons per unit volume, scientists can compute the number of synapses per neuron. This is an absolute rather than a relative measure of connectivity, because when scientists do the division the unit volumes of brain tissue cancel out. This eliminates the problem created by different kinds of brain tissue growing at different rates. (The studies of synaptic change due to rearing in complex environments discussed next use this absolute measure. Note that if the number of neurons were changing in the neocortex then the synapse per neuron measure would not reflect the total picture. However, it appears unlikely that the number of neurons changes to any great extent in the neocortex.)

Thus, from a neuroscientific perspective, we should keep three things in mind about developmental synaptogenesis. First, a significant amount of synapse formation is under intrinsic, not environmental, control. Second, the finding of synapse overproduction and loss cannot be called *new neuroscience* (2 decades is a long time in a rapidly advancing field such as neuroscience). Third, many studies of synapse formation and loss over the life span are plagued by methodological problems.

Scientists also know, at least from isolated examples, how experience-expectant development affects which synapses live and which die. The most common example they cite is how visual deprivation affects brain connections in the formation of ocular dominance columns (LeVay, Wiesel, & Hubel, 1980; see Chapter 3). In this case, the eye-to-brain connections are diffuse and overlapping in early development and the overlapping connections are eliminated with visual experience.

Scientists have shown that visual experience is essential to the organization of these connections because, if during the period of excess synaptic connections, visual experience is biased or unbalanced in some way, there is a relative loss of neural connections into the deprived part of the visual system and a relative survival of connections in the experienced part of the visual system. Depriving one eye of visual experience causes the eye that remains open to dominate the connections the eyes make to the appropriate visual information processing areas in the brain.

Another example of experience-expectant change is how experience affects dendrites in "whisker barrels" in rodent brains. If you have ever looked closely at a mouse, you have seen that mice have a number of long whiskers protruding from their faces as depicted schematically in Figure 11.3a. These whiskers are not merely cosmetic but are, in fact, highly sensitive organs that the mouse uses, for example, to find its way about in the

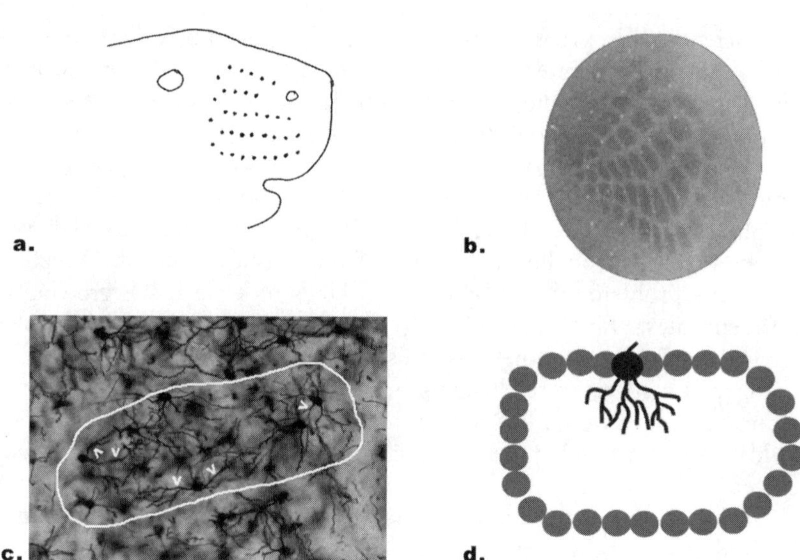

Figure 11.3. a) Schematic pattern of whiskers on the snout of a mouse; b) "Barrel"-like pattern of cellular organization is revealed by cytochrome oxidase staining of mitochondria, which are more concentrated in synaptic terminals and dendrites; c) Neuronal cell bodies make up the walls of the barrels. In this Golgi impregnated barrel, dendrites (some marked by arrows) of neurons are oriented largely toward the center or "hollow" of the barrel in an adult mouse; d) Schematic depiction of neuronal cell bodies making up the barrel wall and dendrites extending into the hollow of the barrel.

darkness of its burrow. The whiskers grow in rows on the mouse's face and are connected to rows of nerve cell groups organized in cylinders (like the walls of a barrel) in the somatosensory area of the mouse's brain, the part of the brain that processes sensations of touch (see Figure 11.3b). Each barrel is responsible for processing sensory information coming to the brain from a particular whisker. Under a microscope, scientists can see that the barrels of a mature mouse consist of a relatively dense wall of nerve cell bodies that surround a hollow in which there are relatively few cell bodies, but which one finds most of the dendrites of these cells (see Figure 11.3c).

Moreover, the cell bodies in the barrel walls specifically tend to project their dendrites into the barrel hollows. These dendrites receive connections from the axons of other nerve cells that carry information from the whiskers. Thus, in the mature mouse the cells in the barrel walls tend to send their dendrites in only one direction, toward the hollows (see Figure 11.3d). Presumably, these cells could send their dendrites in any direction, but they choose (so to speak) to send them in a specific, single direction. Thus, we might ask: Do these cells send their dendrites in a single direction throughout their existence? Or, early in development do these cells send their dendrites in all directions and then "choose" the directions that most fruitfully interact with the proper axonal inputs? To address how dendrites develop, Greenough and Chang (1988) measured how much dendritic material from barrel wall neurons projected toward the barrel hollow during development versus maturity.

Figure 11.4 shows that the pattern of the dendrites did change with age. As the animals grew from 10 days old to 30 days old, the number of dendrites increased in the hollow and decreased in the direction oriented away from the hollow. Also, during this same developmental period, there was a reduction in the number of dendrites originating from the cell bodies, and the reduction was considerably greater on the side of the cell body away from the whisker barrel hollow. So, dendrites growing in the wrong direction were eliminated at the same time that dendrites growing in the right direction increased in size. This suggests that the amount of synapse overproduction and loss might be underestimated in studies that just count synapses because some synapses could be lost at the same time that others were being added, and only the net change at any point in time would be

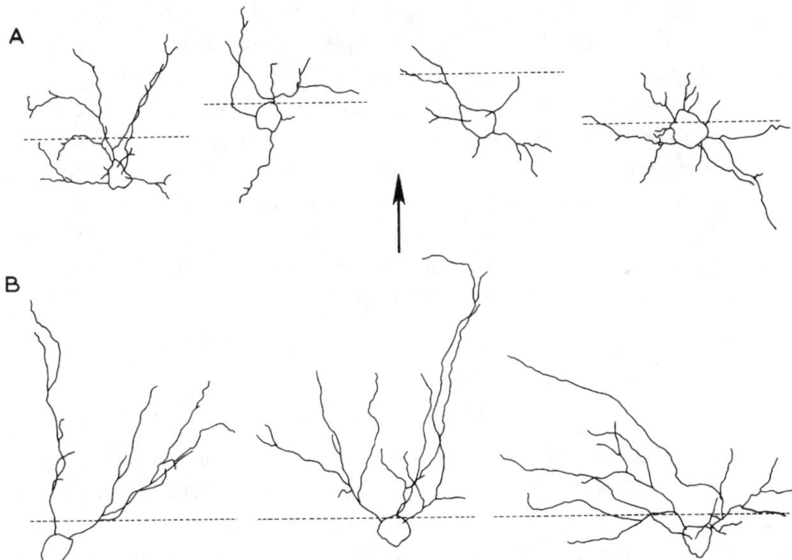

Figure 11.4. Tracings of dendritic fields of representative neurons from whisker barrels of mice at two ages—10 days old in A and 30 days old in B. The dashed line is a tangent to the inner edge of the wall of cell bodies surrounding the barrel hollow. At 10 days of age, dendrites are nonsystematically oriented in all directions around the cell body. By 30 days of age, dendrites are largely oriented toward the cell hollow indicated by arrow. (From Greenough, W.T., & Chang, F.L.F. [1988]. Dendritic pattern formation involves both oriented regression and oriented growth in the barrels of mouse somatosensory cortex. *Developmental Brain Research, 43,* 148–152; reprinted by permission from Elsevier Science.)

seen in mere counts of synapses. Only because we could see the orientation of dendrites with respect to the barrel was the full extent of dendritic loss evident in this study.

Thus, what happens to the whisker barrels during development provides an example of experience-expectant development. Early in development, dendrites, where synapses form, are produced in overabundance in expectation that experiences will occur that select the dendrites and synapses that should survive. During development, sensory stimulation results in the loss of dendrites, and their associated synapses that project away from the hollow of the whisker barrel, whereas there is selective preservation and embellishment of dendrites that are oriented toward the hollow of the barrel. In this way, the early overabundance of synapses that results from developmental synaptogenesis provides the raw material that "expected" experience shapes and refines to fine tune this rodent sensory system. It seems unlikely that this sort of mechanism would have evolved unless developing animals almost always received sufficient stimulation for typical development in their natural environment, and most evidence in mammalian sensory systems supports this.

One lesson we should draw from the examples of ocular dominance columns and whisker barrels is that experience-expectant development involves the *loss* of preexisting synapses. Other critical or sensitive period experience-expectant phenomena also have been shown to involve loss of preexisting synapses (e.g., Horn, Bradley, & McCabe, 1985). Another lesson to be drawn is that synapse loss is often underestimated in studies in which they are merely counted, even if the procedure is correctly and meticulously performed. The reason is that some dendrites and their associated synapses are being lost even as others are growing; and only the number of synapses present at any point would be counted.

EXPERIENCE, GENES, AND PROTEIN SYNTHESIS: LESS IS MORE

As mentioned previously, when thinking about the effects of experience on brain development, we should keep in mind that ultimately experience affects the brain by influencing gene expression, most of which results in the synthesis of protein. As previously noted, the proteins that a cell makes give that cell its particular characteristics. Under some conditions, both during development and in adulthood, protein synthesis occurs in the spines of the dendrites, the location where many synaptic inputs connect. Using a special preparation of concentrated, purified synapses, it is possible to see that synapses respond to stimulation by rapidly increasing the amount of proteins that they produce. In one case, we can see how stimulation causes protein synthesis that may contribute to experience-expectant brain development (Comery et al., 1997; Weiler et al., 1997; see Figure 11.5).

One of the proteins (not the only one) synthesized at synapses is the fragile X mental retardation protein. Individuals who, because of a mutation, are unable to produce the protein have fragile X syndrome and experience mild to severe mental retardation. (It is called fragile X because the gene responsible for synthesizing the protein is carried on the X chromosome, and, in people with fragile X syndrome, this region is "fragile," or subject to impaired replication [under some conditions] during cell division.) Fragile X syndrome is the most common cause of inherited mental retardation.

Using a molecular biological technique called a Western blot, shown in Figure 11.6, we can measure the amount of a particular protein that is

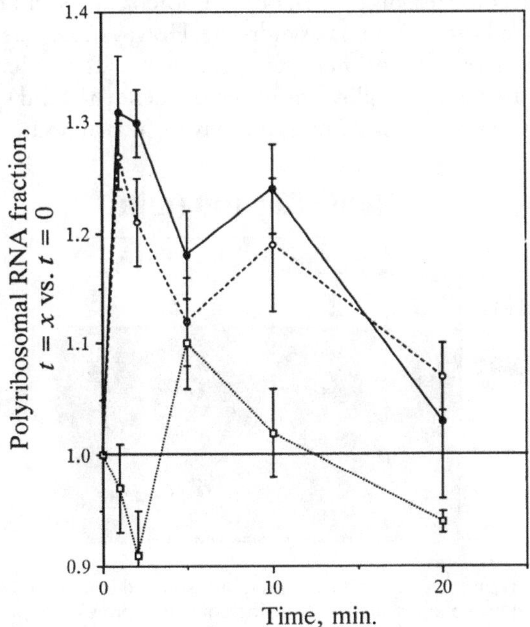

Figure 11.5. In a preparation of purified synapses, stimulation that mimics or causes release of the chemical neurotransmitter activates the synthesis of protein (in this case measured as increased RNA being translated into protein) in the postsynaptic cell. Potassium (filled circles, solid lines) releases the neurotransmitter glutamate. Glutamate (open circles, dashed lines) likewise increases synthesis. NMDA (squares, dotted lines), which affects a different glutamate pathway, initially depresses protein synthesis. (From Weiler, I.J., & Greenough, W.T. [1993]. Metabotropic glutamate receptors trigger postsynaptic protein synthesis. *Proceedings of the National Academy of Sciences [U.S.], 90,* 7168–7171; reprinted by permission.)

produced at the synapse under various conditions. If the preparation of purified synapses is not stimulated, the amount of fragile X mental retardation protein present at the synapse remains stable. If the preparation of purified synapses is stimulated, however, the amount of protein increases relative to the control condition. Thus, the fragile X mental retardation protein is synthesized at synapses in response to synaptic activity.

To determine what the function of a protein might be in brain development, scientists study *knockout mice*—mice in which one or more genes, in this particular case the gene for the fragile X mental retardation protein, have been knocked out of the animals' chromosomes. Fragile X knockout mice cannot synthesize the protein and thus can serve as an animal model for studying human fragile X syndrome (Consortium, 1994).

Fragile X knockout mice have no detectable gross abnormalities in brain structure. They survive at birth and have a typical life span. They show impairments on some learning tasks, but not others, and seem to be mildly affected compared with the human syndrome. However, aspects of the morphology, or fine structure, of their nervous systems are particularly interesting. We used a stain that allows us to see the dendrites and spines of the neurons in the brains of these mice and have similarly examined human

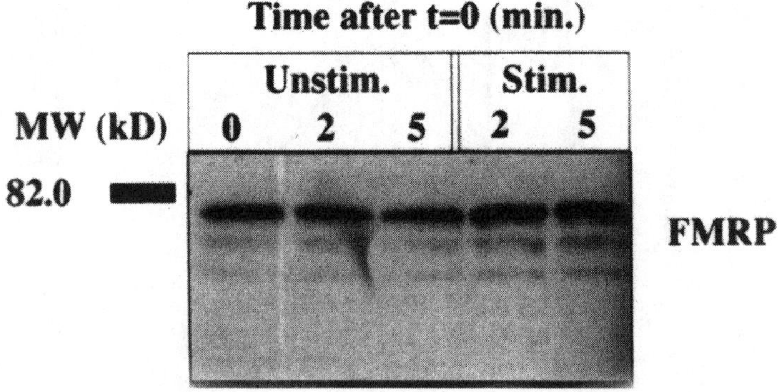

Figure 11.6. A "Western blot" uses antibodies to measure the amount of protein present. Each of the five vertical columns labeled at the top contains a protein sample from purified synapses that has been separated into its constituent proteins based on their size. The dark horizontal bands in each column, three clearly identifiable bands and a fourth somewhat obscured by the top band, represent slightly different molecular forms of the fragile X protein (labeled FMRP). The right three columns are unstimulated samples taken at 0, 2, and 5 minutes after the point at which the left two columns were stimulated with an artificial neurotransmitter. The left two columns show darker bands 2 and 5 minutes after stimulation, indicating that the amount of the fragile X protein was increased by neurotransmitter stimulation. (From Weiler, I.J., Irwin, S.A., Klintsova, A.Y., Spencer, C.M., Brazelton, A.D., Miyashiro, K., Comery, T.A., Patel, B., Eberwine, J., & Greenough, W.T. [1997]. Fragile-X mental retardation protein is translated near synapses in response to neurotransmitter activation. *Proceedings of the National Academy of Sciences [U.S.], 94,* 5395–5400; reprinted by permission.)

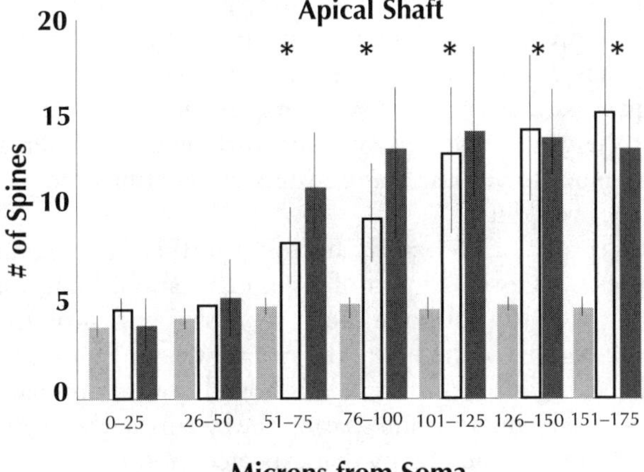

Figure 11.7. The density of spines along pyramidal cell apical dendrites, at different distances from the cell body in human fragile X autopsy samples from temporal (white bars) and visual (dark gray bars) cortex compared with control temporal cortex (light gray bars). Spine density, and presumably spine synapse number, is greater in the fragile X patients. This condition, in which mentally deficient individuals have more synapses than controls, appears to be unique to fragile X syndrome but definitely dispels the notion that more synapses is invariably an indication of better brain function. (From Irwin, S.A., Patel, B., Idupulapati, M., Harris, J.B., Cristostomo, R., Kooy, F., Willems, P.J., Cras, P., Kozlowski, P.B., Swain, R.A., Weiler, I.J., & Greenough, W.T. [in press]. Abnormal dendritic spine characteristics in the temporal and visual cortex of patients with Fragile-X Syndrome: A quantitative examination; reprinted by permission from Wiley-Liss, Inc., a subsidiary of John Wiley & Sons, Inc. Modified draft version of a contribution to be published in the forthcoming *American Journal of Medical Genetics, 98,* 2.)

fragile X autopsy brain samples. Two characteristics stand out. First, in individuals with fragile X syndrome and in the knockout mice, the dendritic spines tend to maintain a developmentally immature appearance; that is, the dendritic spines are thin and elongated relative to the spines seen in their genetically normal counterparts. Second, and perhaps most important, in humans the density of the spines, the number of spines per unit length of dendrite, is higher in those with fragile X syndrome than in those who are genetically intact, as shown in Figure 11.7. (In the knockout mouse there is no consistent, statistically reliable spine density difference.) What we have in the human fragile X syndrome, then, are individuals who have *more* spines, and presumably more spine synapses per neuron, than typical individuals, but who have mental retardation.

We can infer from these studies that the production of the fragile X mental retardation protein at synapses probably occurs in response to synaptic activity. We hypothesize that this protein contributes in some way to the maturation of some synapses and to the elimination of others. In the absence of the protein, synapses appear immature and there are more of them. Thus, in individuals with fragile X syndrome there is a failure to create mature synapses, and a failure of either normal synapse elimination or some other process that regulates synapse number. One interpretation is that, without the gene, experience cannot work its developmental magic, causing some spines to become mature while eliminating others, as it does when the gene is working.

If this interpretation is correct, this result further indicates that eliminating synapses is an essential part of brain maturation. In normal development, during the early period of excess synapses per neuron that occurs in at least some regions of the brain, the neural wiring diagram in animals and in people, as far as scientists know, is honed toward optimal function by eliminating noisy synapses, and sparing the synapses whose importance has been determined by the activity that expected experience causes within the nervous system. Fragile X syndrome appears to prevent this process from occurring. Although other interpretations of the data also are possible, if our interpretation is correct, synapses that should be eliminated are not because fragile X syndrome results in mental retardation. An individual with fragile X usually has excess synapses and is incapable of normal functioning. Results such as this argue against popular claims that more synapses inevitably translate into higher intelligence, and that children should be stimulated to preserve synapses that might otherwise be lost.

EXPERIENCE-DEPENDENT DEVELOPMENT AND COMPLEX ENVIRONMENTS

At one time or another, most people have heard about the experimental evidence that supports the existence of *experience-dependent* brain development. That evidence originally came from studies of rats that had been raised in different kinds of environments. In these studies, rats raised in *complex* environments—that is, rats raised in groups and in large cages filled with toys or obstacles—are compared with rats raised either in groups (socially) or individually in standard laboratory cages. The basic result, shown in Figure 11.8, was that these different rearing conditions have clear effects on the number of synapses per neuron in brains of young rats. Rearing conditions cause experience-dependent changes in the brains of these animals. In particular, animals raised in complex environments add dendrites to neurons and have more synapses per neuron than do animals raised socially or in isolation (e.g., Turner & Greenough, 1985; Volkmar & Greenough, 1972). Thus, we can conclude that the experience available to the rats in the complex environment causes additional synapses to form.

Using a different measure of synaptic change, we also have determined what happens to *adult* rats exposed to complex environments. In this case

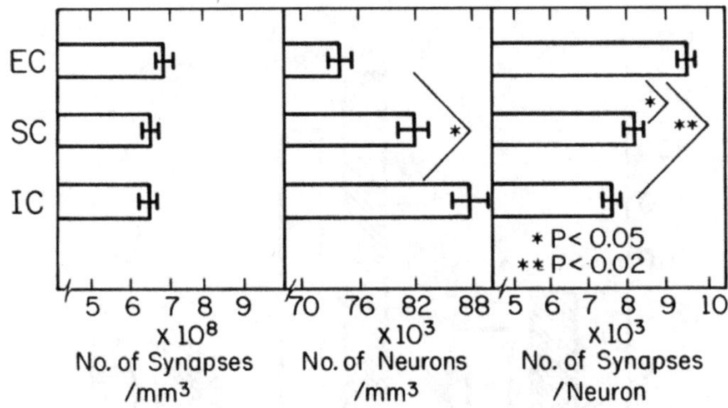

Figure 11.8. Effects of rearing in environmental complexity (EC), a social cage (SC), or an individual cage (IC) on the number of synapses per neuron (right panel) in the rat visual cortex. Neuron density is lower in the EC rats because there are more blood vessels, glia, as well as synapses axons and dendrites, separating the neurons. Because the overall thickness, length, and width of the cortex increases, space for these new additions is available and there is no discernible difference in the number of neurons in the visual cortex across these three groups. (From Greenough, W.T. [1985]. The possible role of experience-dependent synaptogenesis, or synapses on demand, in the memory process. In N.M. Weinberger, J.L. McGaugh, & G. Lynch [Eds.], *Memory systems of the brain: Animal and human cognitive processes* [pp. 77–103]. New York: The Guilford Press; reprinted by permission.)

we measured the amount of dendrite per neuron, assuming that total dendritic length per neuron reflects the total number of synapses per neuron. What we found, even in the adult rat, was that for a variety of cell types, exposure to complex environments as compared with laboratory cage environments causes total dendritic length to increase (Green, Greenough, & Schlumpf, 1983; Juraska, Greenough, Elliott, Mack, & Berkowitz, 1980). Hence, we can conclude that exposure to complex environments also causes an increase in the total number of synapses in adult rats (see Figure 11.9). (Soon to be published data support this with direct measurement of synapses per neuron.)

With experience-dependent change, as evidenced by these complex rearing studies, synapses are not generated in advance of experience or in expectation of experience but rather are generated in response to experience. Most important, the finding of new synapse formation in adult rats demonstrates that experience-dependent brain changes, unlike experience-expectant changes, are not age-dependent and are not subject to critical or sensitive period constraints. Moreover, similar results occur in middle-age rats (Green et al., 1983). Experience-dependent brain development can occur essentially throughout the life of an animal.

Experience-dependent brain changes are not limited to neurons but also occur in other types of cells found in the brain. These are the changes

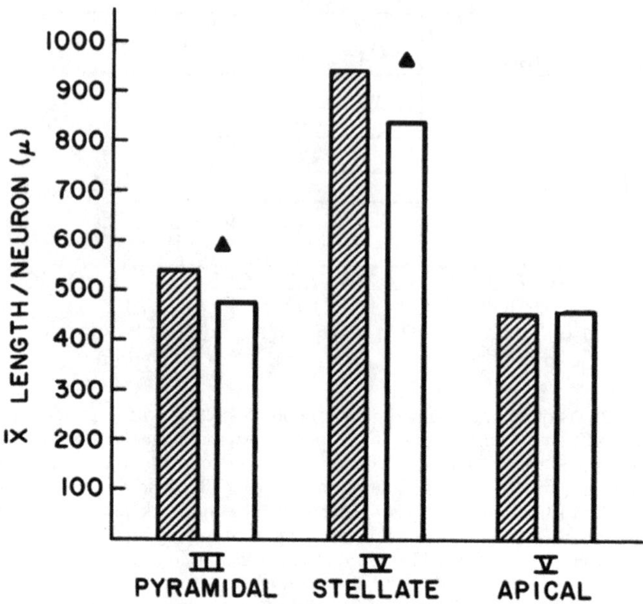

Figure 11.9. Total dendritic length of layer V pyramidal neurons and layer IV stellate neurons in visual cortex of rats placed in the complex environment for 30 days beginning in young adulthood. Effects of a complex environment are not limited to development. (Key: ▲ P<.01; ▨ EC; ☐ IC.) (From Juraska, J.M., Greenough, W.T., Elliott, C., Mack, K.J., & Berkowitz, R. [1980]. Plasticity in adult rat visual cortex: An examination of several cell populations after differential rearing. *Behavioral and Neural Biology, 29,* 157–167; reprinted by permission.)

that push neurons apart in the environmental complexity (EC) rats. If scientists look at the brain's vascular system, they can measure the amount of brain tissue that is devoted to carrying blood. When we measured the amount of capillary volume per neuron, we found that the rats exposed to complex environments have substantially more capillary volume per neuron than the socially or individually housed animals (Black, Sirevaag, & Greenough, 1987; see Figure 11.10). The mean distance to the nearest capillary from a random point in tissue—a measure of how far away cells are from this nutrient source—was lower (closer) in the EC rats and capillaries were slightly larger on average (see Figure 11.10). Hence, oxygen, blood sugar, and other nutrients are more readily available to the cells of the brain in the EC rats. This is an aspect of the brain's readiness to function that is not often discussed. Maybe neurons and synapses seem closer to the action in the brain's vascular, but there is every reason to believe, given how responsive the system is to experience, that it is also important to brain function. This capillary effect is largest in young animals, and is progressively reduced in size as animals grow older, but never disappears entirely (Black, Polinsky, & Greenough, 1989).

Similarly, we examined how experience affects glia, the cells in the brain that support the neurons. Astrocytes are one type of glial cell, and are responsible both for nutrient exchange between capillaries and neurons and for maintaining the "microenvironment" of the neuron to optimize function. We measured the amount of astrocyte surface per neuron in brains of animals raised in complex, social, or isolated environments, using an antibody to an astrocyte-specific protein to visualize them. Animals raised in a complex environment had a greater amount of astrocyte per neuron than did animals raised socially or individually (Sirevaag & Greenough, 1991; see Figure 11.11).

Experiments such as these tell us that the entire cellular makeup of the brain, not just the neurons, is responsive to experience, and that this responsiveness is something that the brain retains postdevelopmentally and well into maturity. The brain's capacity to be plastic, or to adjust to experience, is not something that goes away early in development, when critical periods for basic sensory development end. The brain is a dynamic organ and all, or at least most, of its cellular constituents seem to be experience-sensitive throughout life.

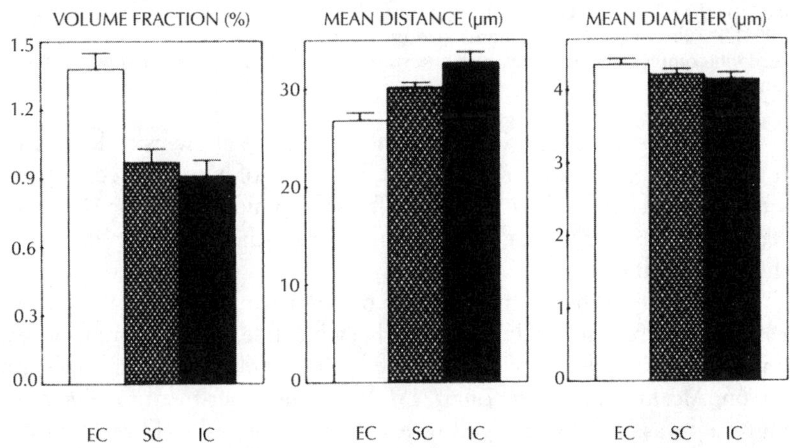

Figure 11.10. Effect of experience on capillaries, the blood carrying vessels that supply nutrients to cells in visual cortex. Volume fraction indicates the amount of blood available under conditions of peak demand (EC>SC, IC, statistically). Mean distance to the nearest capillary indicates how readily available blood-borne nutrients are to brain cells (EC<SC<IC). Diameter and number of capillaries together comprise volume fraction, so the small diameter difference (EC>SC, IC) indicates that new capillaries have formed. (From Black, J.E., Sirevaag, A.M., & Greenough, W.T. [1987]. Complex experience promotes capillary formation in young rat visual cortex. *Neuroscience Letters, 83,* 351–355; reprinted by permission from Elsevier Science.)

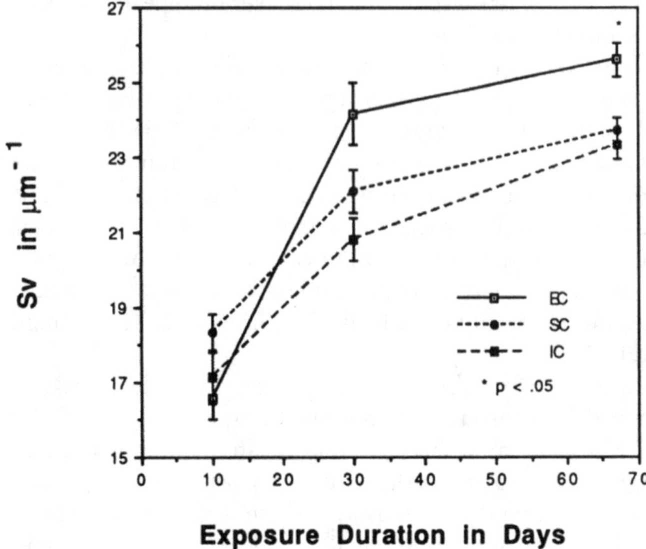

Figure 11.11. Sv, the ratio of astrocyte surface to total tissue volume, indicates the "working capacity" of astrocytes. In this experiment, astrocyte Sv was measured after 10, 30, and 60 days in EC, SC, or IC housing. There were no statistical differences after 10 days, although after 30 days EC rats had greater astrocyte surface. (From Sirevaag, A.M., & Greenough, W.T. [1991]. Plasticity of GFAP-immunoreactive astrocyte size and number in visual cortex of rats reared in complex environments. *Brain Research, 540,* 273–278; reprinted by permission from Elsevier Science.)

Mechanisms of experience-dependent change allow us to learn from our experience. Thus, scientists can use measures of how brain cells change with experience to see how learning affects the brain. A question one might ask is whether learning has a different effect on the brain than does mere physical activity.

We began to answer this question by comparing brains of animals that learned a lot, but were otherwise relatively inactive, with the brains of animals that were highly active but learned relatively little (Black, Isaacs, Anderson, Alcantara, & Greenough, 1990). In this experiment, one group of adult rats was actively engaged in learning motor tasks. They learned to negotiate obstacles. One might think of these animals as in training for a rodent gymnastics meet, although their relative energy output was more at the level of billiards or golf and not at the level of aerobic exercise. Two separate groups of animals spent time on treadmills (e.g., involuntary activity) or activity wheels (e.g., voluntary activity), where they were physically active but learned very little. A fourth group of rats, the "cage potatoes," that neither learned nor were active, served as a control group. How did these three groups of animals differ in the density of blood vessels and the number of synapses per neuron?

The animals that exercised either voluntarily (activity wheel) or involuntarily (treadmill) had a higher density of capillaries in their brain (in this case cerebellar cortex paramedian lobule) than did either the learning or the inactive animals (see Figure 11.12). The learning and inactive animals did not differ in the density of capillaries. Based on this experiment, activity but not learning causes vascular changes in the brain. In contrast, however, the animals that learned the acrobatic tasks showed a significant increase in the number of synapses per neuron, whereas the active animals were indistinguishable from the inactive animals in the number of synapses per neuron (see Figure 11.12). Thus, learning, but not mere activity, causes synapses to form.

So, although both changes in vasculature and synapses per neuron are responsive throughout the life span to the demands that the organism places on the brain, they are responsive to different things. If we need to learn and to acquire skills, we develop synapses. If we need stamina, we grow blood vessels.

One might wonder what the long-term effects of learning might be on the brain. Specifically, one might ask: What happens in the brains of ani-

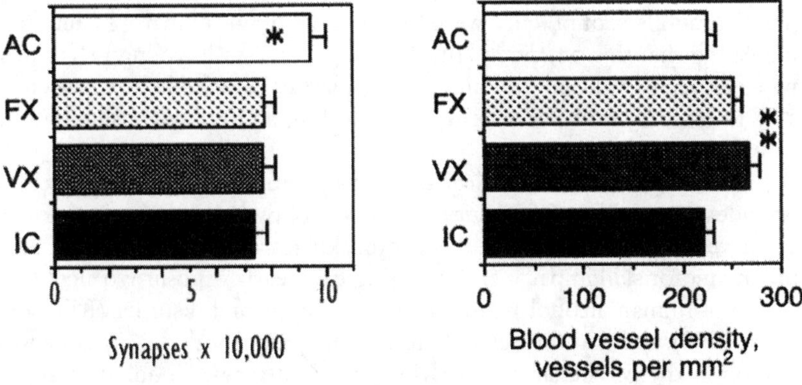

Figure 11.12. Blood vessel density results for groups described in Figure 11.12. Acrobats did not differ from inactive rats. Both exercise groups showed increased vascularization (right panel). Synapse per neuron results for groups described in Figure 11.12. In contrast to blood vessels, synapse number was selectively elevated in the animals that had learned motor skills (left panel). (Modified from Black, J.E., Isaacs, K.R., Anderson, B.J., Alcantara, A.A., & Greenough, W.T. [1990]. Learning causes synaptogenesis, whereas motor activity causes angiogenesis, in cerebellar cortex of adult rats. *Proceedings of the National Academy of Sciences [USA], 87,* 5568–5572; reprinted by permission. From Isaacs, K.R., Anderson, B.J., Alcantara, A.A., Black, J.E., & Greenough, W.T. [1992]. Exercise and the brain: Angiogenesis in the adult rat cerebellum after vigorous physical activity and motor skill learning. *Journal of Cerebral Blood Flow and Metabolism, 12,* 110–119; reprinted by permission.)

mals that learn skills but do not practice them? Do the synapses formed during learning continue to exist if the skills are not used or do they disappear? In other words, if animals do not *use* the newly formed synapses, do they *lose* them?

An experiment that compared brain changes in three groups of rats provides an interesting answer to this question (Kleim, Vij, Ballard, & Greenough, 1997). One group of rats learned motor skills for 10 days, after which they were sacrificed and their brains examined. A second group of rats learned motor skills and practiced them for 38 days before they were sacrificed and their brains examined. A third group of animals learned and practiced motor skills for 10 days and then were put into retirement for 4 weeks. At the end of their retirement (38 days from when the learning began) these animals were retested on the skills they had learned, then sacrificed and their brains examined.

Lack of practice did have an effect on the animals' brains. Absence of sustained practice or performance of the learned skills caused the amount of astrocyte, a supportive glial cell, per neuron to decrease. Astrocytes fell back to prelearning levels (not shown). However, the new synapses that resulted from learning did not fall back to original levels with lack of practice. As Figure 11.13 shows, the synaptic changes persisted in the face of nonpractice of the skills. These patterns of change following learning, practice, and lack of practice were found in the brains of mature adult rats, indicating that this synaptic plasticity is not just seen in young rats. Thus, we again see that the adult brain remains plastic, modifiable by experience, able to learn from experience throughout life, and relatively stable in its response to learning.

Finally, the motor skill learning manipulation noted previously also provides a model for *therapeutic intervention* following early brain damage. We have found that exposure to the motor skill learning procedure can rehabilitate motor skill impairments resulting from early exposure to alcohol, a model of human alcohol-related neurodevelopmental disorder (Klintsova et al., 1998), and that this rehabilitation is associated with new synapse formation in the cerebellar cortex (Klintsova, Matthews, Goodlett, Napper, & Greenough, 1997). These rehabilitative results, as with the original effects of motor skill training, occurred in the brains of adult rats well after the alcohol-induced damage had occurred.

These results, together with what scientists have learned about the importance of synapse elimination for normal development, should cause us to question simplistic appeals to the oft-cited maxim about synapses of "use them or lose them." With experience-expectant brain change (associated with critical or sensitive periods) losing synapses is an expected and crucial part of normal brain development. With experience-dependent brain

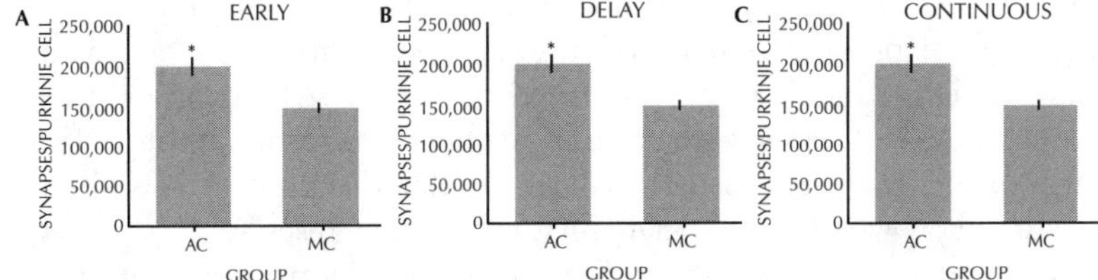

Figure 11.13. Effect of 10 days' brief EARLY training, brief early training followed by a 28-day DELAY and CONTINUOUS training for the entire 38 days of the experiment on synapse number per neuron in acrobat (AC) rats versus a motor control (MC) that ran in an alley. Synaptic effects of AC (i.e., more synapses per neuron than MC) were at the same level after 10 and 38 days of training. Moreover, synapse number did not decline more than 28 days of nonpractice in the delay group. These results indicate that the experience-dependent synaptic effects of learning are stable for reasonably long periods of time. (From Kleim, J.A., Vij, K., Ballard, D.H., & Greenough, W.T. [1997]. Learning dependent synaptic modifications in the cerebellar cortex of the adult rat persist for at least four weeks. *Journal of Neuroscience, 17,* 717–721; reprinted by permission from the Society for Neuroscience.)

change, synapses formed during learning persist over the long term, even if the learned skills are not practiced, that is, even if the synapses are not used to perform what was learned.

CONCLUSION

From this basic neuroscience, there are a number of bottom-line conclusions we can take away to help us think critically about critical periods and about the effects of experience on early brain development. These conclusions run counter to many of the statements that we read in popular articles, policy recommendations, and some early childhood literature.

First, experience-expectant development relies on eliminating synapses. Early in life, developmental synaptogenesis often results in excess synapses that subsequent experience eliminates. The amount of overproduction and loss is probably greater than is estimated by counting absolute number of synapses at periodic points, because synapses may be simultaneously generated and lost, as seen in the whisker barrel system.

Synaptic loss is a normal and necessary part of brain development. Moreover, as we see from the research on fragile X, more synapses do not necessarily equate to higher intelligence. And the notion that one benefits from preserving, through early stimulation, synapses that would normally be lost has no basis in neuroscience research.

Experience-dependent development involves the addition of synapses. However, this kind of brain modification is a lifelong process or at least one that does not end early in life. The brain is a dynamic organ that constantly adjusts to the demands that activity and learning place on it. Activity affects the brain's vasculature and glial support structures. Learning increases the number of synapses per neuron and these synaptic changes are long lasting, even when learned skills are not practiced or used. "Use them or lose them" claims should be treated with caution in the short term, although long-term nonpractice of skills usually will lead to deterioration of the skills and this quite likely would be associated with loss of synapses.

What might the positive implications be of scientists' current understanding of how experience affects brain development? Critical or sensitive periods do occur in the development of sensory and motor systems, among them aspects of vision and first language acquisition (see Chapters 3, 4, and 9). The good news is that the stimulation children need—the experience that their brains expect—for normal development of these systems is ubiquitous in any reasonably typical human environment. It is not something that parents and caregivers must make a special effort to provide. Developmental problems in these areas are almost always the result of problems with the child's sensory systems (see Chapters 3 and 4). They are seldom the result of deficiencies in the child's environment. The positive implication of this research is to make sure children's sensory receptors—their eyes and ears—are functioning properly and to remedy deficiencies as early as possible. Children cannot use the ubiquitously available experience to tune their sensory and motor systems if they cannot sense it properly.

Experience-dependent change occurs throughout our lifetime. We can expect that humans—adults and children—can benefit from exposure to complex learning environments throughout their lives. What people learn is a function of the living and learning environments they inhabit. Our emerging understanding of lifelong brain plasticity raises the question of what kind of environments we might provide to people of any age to maximize their learning and development. Research in the behavioral sciences can already inform how we might optimize learning environments. It is conceivable that in the not too distant future brain science might also contribute to this design project.

If indeed what people learn is a function of the environments they inhabit, the larger policy challenge is to decide which living and learning environments to foster and which to discourage. This is a complex political and moral challenge that brain science, no matter how far it advances, will never be able to meet alone.

REFERENCES

Black, J.E., Isaacs, K.R., Anderson, B.J., Alcantara, A.A., & Greenough, W.T. (1990). Learning causes synaptogenesis, whereas motor activity causes angiogenesis, in cerebellar cortex of adult rats. *Proceedings of the National Academy of Sciences (USA), 87*, 5568–5572.

Black, J.E., Polinsky, M., & Greenough, W.T. (1989). Progressive failure of cerebral angiogenesis supporting neural plasticity in aging rats. *Neurobiology of Aging, 10*, 353–358.

Black, J.E., Sirevaag, A.M., & Greenough, W.T. (1987). Complex experience promotes capillary formation in young rat visual cortex. *Neuroscience Letters, 83*, 351–355.

Boothe, R.G., Greenough, W.T., Lund, J.S., & Wrege, K.S. (1979). A quantitative investigation of spine and dendrite development of neurons in the visual cortex (area 17) of *Macaca nemestrina* monkeys. *Journal of Comparative Neurology, 186*, 473–490.

Comery, T.A., Harris, J.B., Willems, P.J., Oostra, B.A., Irwin, S.A., Weiler, I.J., & Greenough, W.T. (1997). Abnormal dendritic spines in fragile X knockout mice: Maturation and pruning deficits. *Proceedings of the National Academy of Sciences, 94*, 5401–5404.

Consortium, D.B.F.X. (1994). Fmr1 knockout mice: A model to study fragile X mental retardation. *Cell, 78*, 23-33.

Cragg, B.G. (1975). The development of synapses in the visual system of the cat. *Journal of Comparative Neurology, 160*, 147–166.

Green, E.J., Greenough, W.T., & Schlumpf, B.E. (1983). Effects of complex or isolated environments on cortical dendrites of middle-aged rats. *Brain Research, 264*, 233–240.

Greenough, W.T., Black, J.E., & Wallace, C.S. (1987). Experience and brain development. *Child Development, 58*(3), 539–559.

Greenough, W.T., & Chang, F.L.F. (1988). Dendritic pattern formation involves both oriented regression and oriented growth in the barrels of mouse somatosensory cortex. *Developmental Brain Research, 43*, 148–152.

Hart, B., & Risley, T.R. (1995). *Meaningful differences in the everyday experience of young American children.* Baltimore: Paul H. Brookes Publishing Co.

Horn, G., Bradley, P., & McCabe, B.J. (1985). Changes in the structure of synapses associated with learning. *Journal of Neuroscience, 5*, 3161–3168.

Horton, J.C., & Hocking, D.R. (1996). An adult-like pattern of ocular dominance columns in striate cortex of newborn monkeys prior to visual experience. *Journal of Neuroscience, 15*(5), 1791–1807.

Huttenlocher, P.R. (1979). Synaptic density in human frontal cortex—developmental changes of aging. *Brain Research, 163*, 195–205.

Huttenlocher, P.R. (1990). Morphometric study of human cerebral cortex development. *Neuropsychologia, 28*(6), 517–527.

Huttenlocher, P.R., & Dabholkar, A.S. (1997). Regional differences in synaptogenesis in human cerebral cortex. *Journal of Comparative Neurology, 387*, 167–178.

Huttenlocher, P.R., de Courten, C., Garey, L.J., & van der Loos, H. (1982). Synaptogenesis in human visual cortex—evidence for synapse elimination during normal development. *Neuroscience Letters, 33*, 247–252.

Huttenlocher, P.R., & de Courten, C. (1987). The development of synapses in striate cortex of man. *Human Neurobiology, 6*, 1–9.

Juraska, J.M., Greenough, W.T., Elliott, C., Mack, K.J., & Berkowitz, R. (1980). Plasticity in adult rat visual cortex: An examination of several cell populations after differential rearing. *Behavioral and Neural Biology, 29*, 157–167.

Kleim, J.A., Vij, K., Ballard, D.H., & Greenough, W.T. (1997). Learning dependent synaptic modifications in the cerebellar cortex of the adult rat persist for at least four weeks. *Journal of Neuroscience, 17*, 717–721.

Klintsova, A.Y., Cowell, R.M., Swain, R.A., Napper, R.M.A., Goodlett, C.R., & Greenough, W.T. (1998). Therapeutic effect of complex motor skill learning on neonatal alcohol-induced motor performance deficits: I. Behavioral results. *Brain Research*, *800*, 48–61.

Klintsova, A.Y., Matthews, J.T., Goodlett, C.R., Napper, R.M.A., & Greenough, W.T. (1997). Therapeutic motor training increases parallel fiber synapse number per Purkinje neuron in cerebellar cortex of rats given postnatal binge alcohol exposure: Preliminary report. *Alcoholism: Clinical and Experimental Research*, *21*, 1257–1263.

Kolb, B., Gorny, G., & Gibb, R. (1994). Tactile stimulation enhances recovery and dendritic growth in rats with neonatal frontal lesions. *Society for Neuroscience Abstracts*, *20*, 1430.

LeVay, S., Wiesel, T.N., & Hubel, D.H. (1980). The development of ocular dominance columns in normal and visually deprived monkeys. *Journal of Comparative Neurology*, *191*, 1–51.

Sirevaag, A.M., & Greenough, W.T. (1991). Plasticity of GFAP—immunoreactive astrocyte size and number in visual cortex of rats reared in complex environments. *Brain Research*, *540*, 273–278.

Stryker, M.P., & Harris, W.A. (1986). Binocular impulse blockade prevents the formation of ocular dominance columns in cat visual cortex. *Journal of Neuroscience*, *6*, 2117–2133.

Turner, A.M., & Greenough, W.T. (1985). Differential rearing effects on rat visual cortex synapses. I. Synaptic and neuronal density and synapses per neuron. *Brain Research*, *329*, 195–203.

Volkmar, F.R., & Greenough, W.T. (1972). Rearing complexity affects branching of dendrites in the visual cortex of the rat. *Science*, *176*, 1445–1447.

12

Critical Periods and Early Intervention

Dale C. Farran

Much of the increased interest in the development of young children has been predicated on the assumption that there may be new neuroscientific evidence supporting the notion of critical periods in the development of brain and behavior. The first 3 years of life have been portrayed as a critical period for human development. The attempt to specify critical periods is not new but has been a recurring area of interest in developmental psychology. The notion of critical periods in human cognitive development, however, is new and is resonating with those advocating early intervention, especially for children of low socioeconomic status. This chapter addresses 1) the neuroscience underpinnings for the possibility of critical periods in early childhood development, 2) several alternative models for how a critical period hypothesis might work, and 3) powerful environmental influences with demonstrable positive or negative influences on development. These findings are related to the research from the past 30 years in early intervention for young children of low socioeconomic status.

BRAIN ORGANIZATION CHARACTERISTICS IMPORTANT FOR INTERVENTION

The development of the cerebral cortex in humans can be divided into two major phases, according to Huttenlocher (1994). The first phase involves

---

With profound gratitude to Ford Ebner for his willingness to discuss complex neuroscience issues with me and to read drafts of this chapter. Any misunderstandings I still have, though, are not his fault.

the birth and migration of cortical neurons (nerve cells), which take place early in pregnancy and occur only once (Elman et al., 1997). The timing of cell birth and migration is sensitive to conditions in the embryonic environment, suggesting benefits from interventions to prevent conditions that slow down or prevent the timing of proper developmental processes (e.g., poor prenatal care, malnutrition, exposure to alcohol). This chapter focuses on the second phase Huttenlocher outlines for cerebral cortex development—the refinement of cortical connections, or active synaptogenesis.

Period of Active Synaptogenesis

Among primates, the process of synaptogenesis has been thoroughly documented in Macaque monkeys (Huttenlocher, 1994; see Chapter 2). The process has been summarized by Goldman-Rakic, Bourgeois, and Rakic (1997) and in a review by Nelson (2000). Shortly before and immediately after birth there is an explosion of synapse formation that leads to a level of synapses, far above that of an adult, in cortex at 1–2 years after birth. Most of the overproduction takes place in the asymmetric synapses, those associated with excitatory signals, while the smaller number of inhibitory symmetric synapses are not so wildly overproduced. In Macaque monkeys, the density of synapses plateaus about 2 months after birth and then remains the same, with higher levels of density than are in an adult, until puberty (Goldman-Rakic et al., 1997). Huttenlocher (1994) asserted that initially the connections among axons and dendrites may have a high proportion of local randomness. Axons can make more contacts with a target cell than they end up maintaining. There are trillions of synapses in cortex but only 50,000–100,000 genes; therefore, more creative mechanisms must be brought to bear to specify the final arrangements of synapses. Individual synapses cannot be genetically programmed for exact locations, which is actually beneficial to the brain as it prepares for the next step in synaptogenesis.

Loss of Synapses

"The major changes that occur [in the human CNS] between the ages of 2 and 12 years are in the interconnection of neurons, largely through a decrease in the number of synapses, as well as an increase in the complexity of their dendritic arborizations" (Kolb & Fantie, 1997, p. 26). This selective pruning takes place as a result of sensory experience when some connections are stabilized while others are eliminated or suppressed (Neville, 1991). Characterizing the process at birth, Byrnes and Fox (1998) noted that sets of neurons are genetically programmed to communicate with each other, waiting for the stimulation to enable them to adjust their connections. The multiplicity of synaptic connections becomes reorganized through the elimination of many of them, "provided the system is subjected to incoming signals that have repeating patterns" (Huttenlocher, 1994, p. 139).

Two different types of postnatal brain plasticity exist for the storage of information originating in the environment. Greenough and his colleagues use the terms *experience-expectant* and *experience-dependent* to define the two types of responses to postnatal stimulation (Greenough, Black, & Wallace, 1987). Experience-expectant environmental information storage is a response to the types of stimulation expected to be universally available to the species. Another term, *species-typical environment*, is used by Johnson (1993). A typical environment for a human includes stimulation such as patterned light, gravity, and exposure to spoken language.

Johnson (1993) argued that most of what is known about the environment's effect on cortical structure has involved gross disturbances of the species-typical environments for other animals—for example, rearing kittens in a dark room. Experience-expectant information storage by the brain in response to standard environmental input begins to determine which of the surplus neuronal connections will survive after birth. Vision and hearing have been the focus of intense research on the effects of sensory deprivation on experience-expectant information storage. Work with congenitally deaf kittens who were given cochlear implants has shown that auditory cortex can be recaptured for auditory input months after birth despite early auditory deprivation (Klinke, Kral, Heid, Tillein, & Hartmann, 1999). This plasticity does not maintain for adult animals, however.

Experience-dependent information storage, however, relates to interactions with the environment that are unique to individuals (or in Johnson's terms, individual-specific environments). This capability allows mammals to take advantage of information in their own environment (to attend to English in English-speaking homes). Greenough et al. (1987) believed that individual survival depends in large part on this aspect of the nervous system. Experience-dependent plasticity allows the organism to strengthen old and to develop new synaptic connections in response to environmental events (e.g., learning). In rats, Greenough (1993) demonstrated that while the adult brain retains the ability to generate new synapses, it may lose the flexibility to support those synapses through increased blood flow (capillary formation that helps the transfer of nutrients from the blood to the brain).

To summarize this important process of experience-dependent synaptogenesis: In response to various types of environmental stimulation, the absolute number of synapses in human and other primate brains begins to decrease, gradually approaching adult levels. It is important to note that dendrites are growing and producing new synaptic sites with spines ready to be innervated (stimulated). Thus, in addition to pruning some of the random connections present at birth, there also is enormous restructuring and reorganization of synapses. It is fallacious to claim, as some policy makers have, that the goal in early childhood should be to hold on to as many synapses as possible. According to Huttenlocher (1994), synapse elimination as a developmental process seems to escalate with increasing complexity of the neural system. The smaller number of connections that remain, however, are organized into functional circuits in coherent ways.

Higher Cortical Functions

In Macaques, synaptogenesis and subsequent pruning appear to take place in all areas of the brain simultaneously, and Goldman-Rakic et al. (1997) argue that the process in monkeys may be preprogrammed and relatively impervious to minor differences in the environment. In other words, development in monkeys may be a product of experience-expectant information storage and not from experience-dependent storage. After years of research with monkeys and great apes, the Premacks assert that individualized teaching among monkeys and apes, either from parent to offspring or among members of a troop, does not occur, except rarely when apes are in captivity (Premack & Premack, 1996). Learning from individualized instruction involves experience-dependent information storage, a process important in humans.

Even though not enough evidence has been collected to determine the synaptogenesis pattern in human development, it appears that different areas of the human cortex undergo synaptogenesis and sculpting by experience at different times and with different postnatal trajectories. In humans, synapse elimination in the visual cortex begins around 1 year of age and continues until about age 10. Huttenlocher (1994) speculated that the time frame for the frontal cortex (involved in organizing behavioral responses) is slower. He proposed that synapse elimination for frontal cortex does not begin until age 7 and then continues through adolescence. This difference between humans and other primates highlights the importance of species-specific studies. It is likely that the human brain has longer developmental periods of increased sensitivity to environmental influence, especially with regard to higher cortical functions.

ACTIVELY SEARCHING FOR REGULARITIES

"The brain does something different from any other organ: It processes information" (Kosslyn & Koenig, 1992, p. 17). How the brain actively processes and encodes information has been a subject of interest to cognitive and developmental psychologists as well as those involved with artificial intelligence. In the late 1990s, a new form of computer simulation was created that involved something called connectionist-computation, which more closely resembled the workings of the human brain than previous computer simulations. Old computer simulations differed from human brains in that they could only do one thing at a time, they operated as explicitly instructed, they could not discover new strategies, and they made a clear distinction between material they stored and the operations they used with that material (Kosslyn & Koenig, 1992).

The new system, based on nonlinear dynamics, allows the program to be able to respond both to materials it has seen before and to novel stimuli as well. These computers have begun to model actual learning from sensory experience. The final learning product is determined by the initial structure of the system, the rate of learning, and the data to which it was exposed. The data do not have to be completely clear and whole; the program searches for regularity in bits and pieces of the data presented to it (Bates & Elman, 1993).

Real neural networks are more complex than any current models, and the environment to which the human infant is exposed is more complex than data yet presented to the new simulations. "In human beings, the first years of learning and development take place in a nervous system that is noisy and unstable" (Elman et al., 1997, p. 316). Therefore, human beings must be active processors of environmental information even as infants. Experiments with infants' understanding of word boundaries indicate that by 11 months of age infants were sensitive to word boundaries in fluent speech (Myers et al., 1996), while other infants of 13 and 18 months of age remembered new names for objects 24 hours after being exposed to the label only nine times in 5 minutes. By 6 months of age, infants have formed a perceptual map of their native language and are sensitive to the same phonetic contrasts as adult speakers of the language (Kuhl, 1998).

Dynamic perception is a primary characteristic of early life in which behavior is selected from an array of possibilities, rather than being imposed (Thelen & Smith, 1995) and may be related to the higher proportion of excitatory synapses present in the young child. Both Karmiloff-Smith (1992) and Kuhl (1998) have argued that the brain is not prestructured with ready-made representations about the world (as in a language acquisition device) but progressively develops representation through the interactions of the information coming from the external environment, the capabilities of the child's internal environment, and the child's own motor activity.

This filling-in-the-blanks aspect of human cognition has been demonstrated in cognitive research. Payne, Neuschatz, Lampinen, and Lynn (1997) presented adults with lists of thematically related words. The subjects remembered other words meaningfully associated with the experimental group of words even though they had not been presented. Similarly, when subjects were presented a story that centered on an unnamed theme, they named a theme and remembered nonpresented actions, even though they were not part of the original story. Searching for regularities and filling in missing data is an efficient strategy for human brains and one they retain throughout life. Filling in missing data also is a characteristic of cortical activity in other animals. The deaf kittens with cochlear implants described before (Klinke et al., 1999) received a degraded auditory stimulus, not an electrical code, equivalent to normal hearing, but the kittens' brains were "clever enough to figure out the rest" (Rauschecker, 1999, p. 1687).

Attention and Emotional Regulation

A new area of research focuses on the factors that affect children's attention to environmental input, which may contribute to how well children dynamically map new representations. Fox and Bell (1993) proposed a possible similarity between frontal lobe regulation of emotional involvement and its regulation of aspects of attention. Arguing from the adult neuropsychological data, Harman and Fox (1997) asserted that specific regions of the left and right frontal lobes are responsible for different emotions. They characterized the left frontal region as controlling the emotions that are approach behaviors while the right frontal region is associated with behaviors that could be termed withdrawal behavior.

Irritability and response to calming stimuli are related to attention according to the model proposed by Harman and Fox (1997). In order to be soothed, infants must develop flexible attention strategies; they must learn to look away from distressing stimuli and turn to calming stimuli. In the second year of life, infants engage in joint attention with adults, both initiating joint attention episodes and responding to initiations from others, a phenomenon thought to be an important context for language acquisition as well as other learning (Mundy, Card, & Fox, 1999). In a short-term longitudinal study, Mundy et al. found that higher left frontal activation at 14 months was associated with more initiations of joint attention at 18 months. The field does not have ways to measure brain activity in young children precisely, and there are few methods for relating observed activity to behavior. Further exploration of the paradigm suggested by Fox and his group could provide important information.

Other evidence indicates that asymmetries in frontal lobe activation may be a function of early experiences in the home. Dawson, Hessl, and Frey (1994) found that when mothers with clinical depression failed to provide sufficient levels of stimulation their infants were at risk for not developing adequate means for regulating their own arousal and emotion. This is an area of investigation that could have important implications for children's early learning and one that should be explored further. It is consistent with the earlier Sameroff, Seifer, and Zax (1982) finding that a predictor of later learning difficulties and behavior problems for children was living with a mother who was clinically depressed in early childhood.

This brief review of major nervous system processes operating in the first years of life suggests several important areas for future investigation:

1. Critical periods are a feature of development for input from species-typical environments—experience-expectant information storage. These sensitive periods appear early in the organism's development, within a short time after birth. They relate to areas of development such as vision and hearing (and, for humans, language) for which an external stimulus is required within a narrow window of time to trigger the next steps of central nervous system development (Klinke et al., 1999).
2. No neuroscience researcher has suggested that critical periods exist for experience-dependent information storage or that the first 3 years are the most important for this process. Both the behavior of the brain and its reorganization in response to specific individual environments appear to be more complex.
3. The best evidence suggests that children are active organizers of the information coming to them from their environments, searching for regularities among a large mass of "messy" data.
4. Depending on the complexity of the stimuli (e.g., language, memory), synapse elimination and reorganization may take place over a long period of time, with the frontal cortex continuing to be involved in the process at least through early adolescence. Little is known, however, about how flexible and responsive the evolving patterns remain in humans.
5. Evidence is emerging to suggest that infants may show early individual differences in attention and soothability—perhaps in response to emotional aspects of their environment—and these characteristics may be linked to learning complex skills.

ALTERNATIVES FOR CRITICAL PERIODS AND INTERVENTION

The notion of critical periods in early development supports the idea of early intervention for children at risk because of their low socioeconomic status. If it could be established that the early years are critical for development and that, once those years pass, impairments cannot be overcome, public policy could be influenced to provide funding for enriched learning experiences for children of low socioeconomic status and, perhaps, intervention efforts for those with disabilities. Furthermore, the critical periods hypothesis has been invoked for media campaigns (e.g., I Am Your Child) to convince parents to engage in early stimulation—reading to their children, playing classical music, and so forth. Even if one assumed the importance of early experience, there are alternate perspectives on how experiences exert effects, and not all of them invoke neuroscience for support. They range from a strict critical periods perspective to a looser idea of early foundations for later learning. The alternative possibilities for the importance of intervening early are explored in this section.

CLASSIC DEFINITION: CLOSING WINDOWS OF OPPORTUNITY

"A critical period for any behavior is defined as a specific phase of the life cycle of an organism in which there is enhanced sensitivity to experience, or to the absence of a particular experience" (Doupe & Kuhl, 1999, p. 609). The term *critical period* for human development has been replaced by the term *sensitive period.* Sensitive periods are times during development when the organism is "especially sensitive to particular types of experience" (Elman et al., 1997, p. 283), and there is reduced responsivity before and after the experience.

The argument that there are specifically defined periods when certain types of learning can develop, and, moreover, if they do not occur, they are followed by detrimental consequences, is linked to a modular view of brain development. In 1983, Fodor published *The Modularity of the Mind,* in which he argued that certain parts of the brain process specific and separate types of stimulation. Thus, a module would process certain types of information and ignore others. Moreover, these modules were described as innately specified, as Karmiloff-Smith says, like "special purpose computers with proprietary data bases" (1992, p. 3). Each module might have its own critical period, like windows opening and closing at different times.

Neville's work with individuals who have congenital deafness has come close to making a sensory-modality specific modular argument for certain aspects of language. She argued that the acquisition of syntax appears to be more vulnerable to environmental input at specified ages than is the acquisition of semantics (Neville, 1991). Similarly, in their classic study of second-language learning, Johnson and Newport (1989) asserted that early in life human beings have a superior capacity to acquire language, a capacity that declines or disappears with maturation. This research has led to the notion that second language learning should occur before puberty and that if it occurs after puberty, because of the closing window for plasticity related to syntax, the second language cannot be mastered as well. And, the argument goes, if there is an established critical or sensitive period for second language acquisition, it makes sense that there would be similar periods of optimal development for other areas of development. The evidence for a critical end point for second language learning is, however, not as clear as the earlier studies presented.

In a study of second language speakers, Perani et al. (1998) demonstrated that, rather than age of acquisition, proficiency in the second language was the critical factor. Individuals who were equally proficient in their second language showed the same pattern of brain activation during positron emission tomography scans for the second language as they did for their first, no matter what the age of acquisition. Those individuals with poorer second language acquisition showed different patterns of brain activation. It appeared that the subjects with low proficiency recruited multiple and variable brain regions to handle aspects of the second language that were different from the first. As proficiency increased, so did anatomical overlap in the brain areas used to process the two languages. Few studies before this had directly controlled for proficiency in the second language. The authors hastened to add that their measure of language proficiency was related to language comprehension and that language production might be a different phenomenon. Even if comprehension and production follow different pathways, this study makes the argument for a single critical period for second language acquisition less tenable.

The Perani et al. research has implications for other areas of study in which brain activation has appeared to be different for those more proficient in a skill (e.g., reading). Groups who differ in proficiency are certain to have different areas of brain activation as they engage in the skill, differences that could disappear if the less proficient were to practice the skill. Conclusions drawn from these studies—that brain organization actually leads to or causes differences in proficiency—are unwarranted at this point in the developing knowledge base concerning brain–behavior connections.

CRITICAL PERIODS AS DECREASING PLASTICITY

A milder version of sensitive periods has been offered by Doupe and Kuhl (1999), one supported by the new connectionist model of neural functioning of Elman et al. (1997). Doupe and Kuhl cited evidence for decreasing capability in learning language through early childhood. Sufficient plasticity exists in the brain at very early ages for it to recover from traumas such as lesions and tumors in brain areas thought to be responsible for language. The upper limit to that plasticity appears to be 3–6 years for major damage and 8 years to puberty for less severe injuries. Moreover, Doupe and Kuhl cited studies of second language learning indicating that the speed of learning the second language declines when the language is learned later (a fact that may influence the ultimate proficiency acquired). Similarly, Klinke et al. (1999) cited research demonstrating a lack of responsivity in congenitally deaf human adults to cochlear implants (in stark contrast to the responsivity of children).

A less stringent sensitive period argument asserts that learning itself may be a determining (and terminating) factor in how easily new skills in an area can be acquired. "At some point, the old learning is entrenched to the point in which certain kinds of new learning can no longer take place, i.e., a 'point of no return'" (Elman et al., 1997, p. 283). For example, the speech maps of infants are incomplete at birth, but as infants respond to the language heard around them, they gradually develop a neural commitment to that language, making future learning more difficult, especially if the second language is very different from the first (Doupe & Kuhl, 1999). Doupe and Kuhl, however, never discussed a point of no return; rather, they argued that the end of the sensitive period is characterized by an increased need for intense and arousing stimulation if new learning is to occur. Biologically, this transition would be expected if the cellular inhibition in the cortical areas involved matured to adult levels, thus raising the bar for synaptic plasticity without eliminating plasticity. This difference is a crucial one for thinking about early intervention.

CRITICAL TIMING OF EVENTS: SOCIETALLY IMPOSED COMPETENCY REQUIREMENTS

The timing of learning provides another view of early experience that emphasizes the importance of early skill development through intervention without asserting a critical period in brain development. The timing argument is that children need to learn certain skills early because of the societally imposed requirement of school entry. School performance, it can be argued, depends on the acquisition of prerequisite, foundational skills on which formal instruction builds (e.g., expressive and receptive language skills, knowledge of the alphabet and number system, how to respond to behavioral demands of classrooms). Children who enter school without those readiness skills will be behind their peers, and, the timing notion asserts, the gap between them will only widen as the school years progress. The longitudinal study of Alexander and Entwisle (1988) lends support to this view. They found that the first grade was a critical year for school achievement; if children were behind in achievement at the end of the first grade, it was difficult for them to alter their learning trajectory.

Although this position is appealing, there is little evidence that later differences in achievement between children rest solely on differences in the ability they have when they enter school. In a natural experiment, for example, Morrison, Griffith, and Alberts (1997) showed that the youngest children in a first-grade classroom progressed typically over the school year, just slightly behind the achievement levels of the oldest children in the classroom. Most interestingly, the youngest first graders made more progress in achievement than the oldest kindergartners, those who missed the age cutoff for first grade by a few days. Morrison et al. concluded that entrance age is not a major factor in school achievement. In a follow-up study, Morrison's colleagues demonstrated that achievement differences that existed at the end of first grade between oldest and youngest children were gone by the end of third grade and did not reemerge through the eighth grade (Bachman & Kienstra Friese, 2000).

A further difficulty with the timing perspective is defining prerequisite skills. As is apparent later in this chapter, there does not appear to be an advantage for children of low socioeconomic status from intervention programs entering public schools with higher scores on standard IQ or readiness tests. Those scores tend to plateau by the second or third year of formal schooling, which does not give the impression that the skills assessed on those instruments served as a foundation for later learning. An alternate view of readiness has been developed by Watson (1996), who asserted that young children are naive theorists about various domains of knowledge. They encounter formal theories of systematized knowledge in school that require them to revise and examine their earlier understandings. Watson argued that to engage in learning in schools children must be ready for formal instruction, a sentiment echoed by kindergarten teachers when they are interviewed about what skills they want children to possess when they enter kindergarten (Cooper & Farran, 1988). The skills listed by the teachers were related to knowing how to participate in a formal environment than to possessing discreet pieces of information. Helping children to participate in learning through formal instruction would seem to be a simple and obtainable goal—one that could be addressed in kindergarten itself—better than remediating presumed deficits in readiness, unalterable once school begins.

SIMILAR OUTCOMES AT DIFFERENT AGES REQUIRE DIFFERENT LEARNING PATHWAYS

A much less explored hypothesis related to critical periods is the idea that learning at one point in time may rely on one pathway, but mastering the same learning at a later point may require different neural pathways. Thus, the illusion of an earlier critical period would be maintained if the later learner were exposed only to the same stimulation and instruction provided to the younger learner. This explanation would support the large number of studies showing that when children are retained in the early grades in school they experience more negative outcomes than children with the same achievement profile who were promoted (Meisels & Liaw, 1993). Typically, children who are retained are exposed to the same classroom learning environment that had not been successful the first time.

Thelen and Smith (1995) demonstrated how unpredictable and chaotic behavioral pathways appear the closer one gets to the individual learner, asserting that in normal development multiple pathways lead to the same behavioral outcomes. Clay's Reading Recovery program is based on the assumption that different learning pathways are used by individual children. Children who have not learned to read with standard instruction are given alternate instruction in an intensive fashion to allow them to quickly become full members of the classroom (Clay, 1996). Moreover, this instruction is different and individualized for each low achiever. Clay asserted that most of the children having difficulties can master reading if the process of instruction is based on the unique characteristics of each child (thus, different pathways to the same outcome). In her various research studies, only about 1% of the children need more specialized instruction than Reading Recovery provides.

In sum, there are alternate hypotheses about the way critical periods might operate for human behavior, none has the unequivocal support of empirical research. The old notion of a critical developmental period was derived from work with animals and humans who were deprived of essential elements of species typical environments; the results were clear and consistent. When organisms were deprived of information the nervous system expected to receive, those neural areas were taken over by other functions, leaving the original area different and unresponsive even if the information was finally presented.

For experience-dependent information storage, such clear-cut effects have not been achieved. The process appears to be more complex, especially for humans and for higher order cognitive functions like language and learning. It does appear that the process of learning reduces the responsivity of the brain to contrary stimulation, but reducing responsivity is not the same as eliminating it. An area that needs to be explored is whether intense learning experiences, perhaps via different pathways, could produce new learning past the sensitive and normal window.

MAJOR INTERVENTIONS LINKED TO OUTCOMES

The fact that early experiences are important for development is indisputable. Over many years, natural variations in developmental environments among humans and experimental variations imposed on animals have been associated with different developmental outcomes in offspring. The interventions tend to be total immersion experiences that rearrange the organism's entire environment, they tend to be continuous over a long period of time, and they tend to be associated with natural consequences that sustain the changes in behavior by the organism.

Positive Environmental Effects

Early Adoption Major studies of adoption have shown that adopted children's IQ scores 8–10 years after adoption were higher than would have been expected (Scarr & Weinberg, 1976, 1983; Schiff & Lewontin, 1986; Weinberg, Scarr, & Waldman, 1992). Adoption studies are used to investigate environmental versus genetic contributions to intelligence, usually through a series of correlations of IQ test scores obtained from the adoptees and various others: biological parents (often just their educational level), adoptive parents, adoptive siblings, and so forth. The correlations between the scores of the adoptive children and their adoptive parents are lower than between the adoptees and whatever score is available from their biological parent. These analyses are irrelevant, however, to the issue of how malleable development is in a different environment. In these same studies, the mean level of the IQ scores increased for the group of adoptees, clearly demonstrating response to a positive developmental environment.

The effects of such a massive, positive early intervention were reviewed by Locurto (1991b) as a contrast to the effects achieved by preschool early intervention projects such as the Perry Preschool. (The preschool programs operated for a few hours a day for 1–2 years before school entry, following which children entered the same public schools they would have attended.) Locurto summarized results from the major adoption studies as showing that 1) the IQ changes achieved appeared to be relatively permanent; 2) these changes were accompanied by gains on standardized achievement tests, school grades, and other measures of competence that also appeared to be permanent; and 3) the predictive relationship between achievement and IQ test scores and real-world outcomes was the same for the group of adopted children as obtained in nonadopted populations. Locurto argues that adoptive parents are successful because they are sensitive to their individual child's developmental needs. Relating these conclusions to the earlier discussion of brain organization, it is possible to think of adoptive parents as creating individually specific environments that are responsive to the presenting characteristics of their new children but intense enough to provoke the establishment of new neural patterns. When this combination is present in experience, intervention appears to work and is linked to long-lasting change.

Early Mothering Levine (1957) and Denenberg (Zarrow, Campbell, & Denneberg, 1972) demonstrated that rats who had been handled by humans in the first few weeks of life showed reduced responses to stress later in their lives into adulthood. These experimental studies are taken as animal models supporting the importance of early stimulation (see Chapter 6). In a follow-up to those studies, Meaney and his colleagues have shown that the effects of early handling on rats were mediated through the effects on the mother–pup interactions (Liu et al., 1997). Rat pups who were handled by humans received more licking, grooming, and arched-back nursing from their mothers when they were returned to their cages. Meaney et al. searched for naturally occurring variations in those mothering patterns and compared their offspring to those of mothers who were naturally low in those mothering behaviors. They found that the greater the frequency of maternal licking and grooming in infancy, the lower the response to stress in adulthood, without handling as a contributing variable.

The Meany et al. research generates ideas for possible applications to humans. It may be that patterns of early parenting in humans are associated with later behaviors of their children. If it is possible to generalize from the animal studies to humans, the Liu et al. study suggests that an avenue to explore might be emotional functioning, not necessarily school performance and achievement. A second application is to think of the parenting behaviors of the mother rats as a buffer, protecting the handled pups from the consequences of their stressful experiences. The maternal behaviors compensated for the early experience and had a salutary effect. If that is a possibility, it would be useful to examine the protective actions of human parents when their children have stressful experiences to search for analogous positive effects. In other words, the response of the parents to dangerous or threatening situations for their children may be a critical factor for long-term successful outcomes (see, for example, Shahinfar & Fox, 1997).

Maternal Education Positive developmental outcomes in all domains (e.g., health, schooling, adult success) are achieved by children around the world when their mothers have more education (Stein, 1997). This holds true regardless of the mean level of maternal education in the country; in countries where the average maternal education is third grade, child outcomes are better for mothers who have a fifth-grade education. Thus, the relationship between good child outcome and maternal education is not a function of the specific knowledge possessed by the mothers per se. Rather, it seems to be a function of how competently the mother is functioning relative to others in her country.

Within specific subgroups in the United States, maternal education has proven to be a predictor of how well their children succeed. For example, in searching for family factors that might predict which former Head Start children were high academic achievers, Robinson, Weinberg, Redden, Ramey, and Ramey (1998) identified maternal education as one of the primary factors. Babies with low birth weights born to mothers of higher education had better long-term outcomes than those born to less educated mothers in the Infant Health Program and Development Study, irrespective of whether they received intervention (Duncan, Brooks-Gunn, & Klebanov, 1994). In Werner's seminal longitudinal study of an entire birth cohort in Kauai, Hawaii, maternal education was identified as a protective factor especially for males well into their thirties (Werner & Smith, 1992). In general, Werner and Smith found that better educated parents had children who had better problem-solving and reading skills at age 10, and who were healthier with fewer school absences or repeated serious illnesses. Higher education in parents also has been linked to how quickly and easily children recover from trauma (Shahinfar & Fox, 1997).

The phenomenon appears to be genuine, but scant attention has been paid by researchers to the process by which higher maternal education exerts its influence. Most early intervention programs, for example, have focused on changing the children's readiness for school, with little attention to such parental characteristics as education. Even Start is one exception. It is a national program emphasizing increasing levels of parental education, as well as early childhood education and parenting skills. Unfortunately, the one published national evaluation of the program showed few effects on levels of parental education and also few long-term effects on child achievement (St. Pierre & Swartz, 1996).

Life-Course Alterations in Adulthood In Werner and Smith's prospective study of an entire birth cohort, one third of the children were designated as high risk because they were born into poverty, experienced moderate to severe perinatal stress, or lived in a family environment troubled by multiple risk factors. Of these children, two thirds were exposed to four or more risk factors by age 2 and went on to develop learning disabilities or behavior problems by age 10 or had delinquency records, mental health problems, or pregnancies by age 18. (The potent effect of experiencing four or more major risk factors early in life is well recognized. See, for example, Sameroff, Seifer, Barocas, Zax, & Greenspan, 1987.)

The value of longitudinal work is shown by the life-course changes experienced by the majority of these high risk children when they became adults. In their twenties and thirties, individuals achieved dramatic and permanent changes in their life situations. These changes were achieved by total immersion experiences such as the military or fundamentalist religious conversion. "Among the most potent forces for positive change for high risk youths on Kauai in adulthood were: education at community colleges, educational and vocational skills, acquired during service in the armed forces, and active involvement in a church or religious community" (Werner & Smith, 1992, p. 206). Clearly, malleability and recovery from early childhood experiences can occur well into adulthood, though those avenues for intervention rarely have been tapped. One of the unfortunate consequences of emphasizing the importance of the first years of life might be to decrease funding for these avenues associated with later adult malleability.

Positive evidence of the power of the environment in changing individual developmental outcomes for the better exists. A common characteristic of positive environments is that they involve the immersion of the organism in a changed environment. Adoption is an example of a complete change in the environment, but maternal education could signify a substantially different environment from that provided by less educated mothers. The children of Kauai joined the military or became involved in fundamentalist religious groups, experiences that would remove them from one environment and place them in a restructured one (or in the case of religion, provide powerful support for a changed perspective in the individual). Each of these empirically established, effective, positive interventions has the characteristics identified by Doupe and Kuhl (1999) as necessary for later changes in previously learned patterns of behavior—they are powerful and intense learning situations inculcating an alternative pattern of behavior. Those experiences that occurred early in children's lives, such as adoption, might support a notion of an early critical period, but it is hard to merge a critical period hypothesis with the changes Werner and Smith identified in the life-course trajectories of adults despite multiple early risk factors.

Negative Environmental Effects

Institutional Rearing A negative total immersion experience comparable to adoption involves institutionalized rearing for individuals with disabilities. Over the years, various facets of the institutionalized experience, from maternal deprivation to stimulus deprivation, have been proposed as the operative factors producing negative results. Regardless of which factors carry the predictive weight, the effects are irrefutable. For example, until the 1970s children with Down syndrome routinely were placed in institutions at birth. In 1929, the life expectancy for individuals with Down syndrome was 9 years; by 1947 it was 12 years (Carr, 1995). Today, individuals with Down syndrome are reared in homes with families, may live into their sixties, and function at higher developmental levels. One could hardly find a more compelling example of the potency of the environment. This potency has been reflected in other studies of the negative effects of orphanage rearing (Skuse, 1988), as well as studies of the effects of institutionalization on Romanian orphans (see Chapter 7).

Feral Rearing Another negative rearing condition is feral rearing or rearing in extreme social isolation. Each of the cases of feral rearing is unique, yet in each case the children had similar characteristics (Skuse, 1988). The children were socially withdrawn, inappropriate in their social interactions, and had poor language skills. Perceptuomotor skills were relatively unaffected by the deprivation. Progress, however, was rapid once the children were brought into a social environment. Gains in language appeared to be linked to the development of an attachment relationship with the new caregivers. Skuse concluded that the amount of intervention effort did not seem to be the important factor in bringing about recovery; rather, it was the intensity of the social relationship formed—or the qualitative aspect of the intervention—that was critical to developing new language and cognitive skills. None of these children has been able to function completely normally despite intervention.

Maternal Depression Maternal depression, especially in the first few years of the child's life, has been linked to a variety of problematic outcomes for children. Sameroff et al. (1982) found that maternal depression was linked to more negative child outcomes than maternal schizophrenia. Negative outcomes include academic difficulties (Coghill, Caplan, Alexandra, Robson, & Kumar, 1986) and behavior problems (Ghodesian, Zajicek, & Wolkind, 1984). The possible mechanisms underlying the relationship between depression and negative outcomes have been outlined by Dawson and her colleagues (Dawson, Hessl, et al., 1994; Dawson, Frey, Panagiotides, Osterling, & Hessl, 1997). They have shown that depressed mothers have less positive and more negative affect when interacting with their children. Dawson speculated that infants may have difficulty learning to regulate their own emotional arousal and they may imitate the mother's affective state.

In two different samples, Dawson, Frey, et al. (1997) and Dawson, Hessl, et al. (1994) have demonstrated that infants of depressed mothers showed reduced left frontal EEG alpha activity, a finding most pronounced in infants whose mothers were currently depressed, but still present to a lesser degree in those infants whose mothers' depression was in remission. EEG activity patterns were more discriminative of children whose mothers were or were not depressed than direct observations of the infants' emotional states or behaviors. Further research is needed to determine if the condition remediates with continued and sustained improvement in the mother's emotional state. These findings support the idea of a link between emotional arousal and attention and could help account for the long-term effects of maternal depression on both child learning and behavior that have been found by others.

Abuse and Trauma Conditions that are the opposite of depression and nonresponsiveness are children's experiences of abuse and stress, experiences marked by violent, unpredictable adult behavior and threat. LeDoux (1998) proposed that stress causes malfunctions in the hippocampus, a major part of the brain involved in learning and memory. In a stressful situation, another part of the brain, the amygdala, instructs the hypothalamus to tell the pituitary and adrenal glands to secrete stress hormones. This action by the amygdala involves an emotional response to stimulation independent of the higher processing systems of the brain. The hippocampus is responsible for a cognitive appraisal of the stress situation ("Is this adult jumping out at me about to yell 'happy birthday' or about to hit me?"). If the appraisal is benign, the hippocampus sends messages to counter the instructions of the amygdala. However, LeDoux argued that, if the stress persists too long, the hippocampus has difficulty maintaining its ability to control the release of the stress hormones. Severe but temporary stress results in the shriveling of some dendrites in the hippocampus, while prolonged stress causes irreversible changes such that cells in the hippocampus begin to degenerate, leading to permanent memory loss. LeDoux cited evidence of shrunken hippocampuses (found in autopsies) in children who have experienced repeated abuse and in Vietnam veterans who suffered from posttraumatic stress syndrome.

The pathway LeDoux outlined is the Hypothalamic-Pituitary-Adrenal (HPA) axis, and disturbances in this pathway are associated with depression in adults, according to Kaufman et al. (1997). Assessing children, Kaufman et al. found that evidence of disturbance in the HPA axis was obtained only in children who were depressed and experiencing ongoing chronic adversity (e.g., abuse, marital discord). As more children have early experiences with violence, either directly or through exposure to various media sources, it is important to determine whether there are both short- and long-term biological effects on hippocampal activity. These effects could be linked to behaviors in children from stressful environments, such as inattention, poor memory, and inadequate learning strategies. Once again, little is known about the remediability of these effects if the negative conditions are removed (Nelson & Carver, 1998).

Recent investigations of the effects of stress on primate mothers during different periods of their pregnancies suggest that infants also may be responsive in utero to stressful experiences. Schneider, Roughton, Koehler, and Lubach (1999) subjected pregnant rhesus monkeys to stress early in pregnancy or during the middle to late stages of pregnancy. While there were few effects on the mothers' health, measured by weight gain, length of pregnancy, and number of still births, the two stress groups of infants showed different, flatter learning curves after birth compared to controls born to nonstressed mothers. Both the early- and later-stressed groups of monkeys displayed altered attention and motor immaturity, but the early-stressed group also showed lower birth weight and more pervasive disorders than the later-stressed group. The authors believed that sensitivity to stress peaks during early pregnancy, as the nerve cells are being produced and migrating but decreases during later pregnancy. They speculated that the time of neuronal migration may be a sensitive period in fetal growth. Long-term follow-up of these monkeys will be important to help determine if the effects of such early stress maintain or dissipate. Humans have shown far greater plasticity in their recovery from early trauma than monkeys have, and thus it is difficult to know how applicable these findings are for human infants. Nonetheless, prudence would suggest caution in terms of the amount of stress pregnant mothers are exposed to, particularly early in their pregnancies.

Poverty Another pernicious environment for young children has been living in poverty in America in the latter half of the 20th century. Persistent poverty is linked to more detrimental outcomes than transitory poverty and is evidenced in a 9.1 decrease in IQ scores and higher scores on both internalizing and externalizing disorders (Duncan et al., 1994). There is disagreement on whether when poverty is experienced makes a difference to the outcomes. Duncan et al. did not find any differences in outcome for experiencing poverty early in a child's life or later; the differences were due to how long the poverty lasted and were worse if the family's neighborhood also was poor. Dubow and Ippolito (1994), however, found that early poverty was more associated with lower math and reading scores than later poverty, though they also found that the most negative factor for the development of children was the number of years the family had lived below the poverty line.

The detrimental effects of poverty for young children on both cognitive and health outcomes are well established (Smith, Brooks-Gunn, & Klebanov, 1997), but Starfield (1992) argued that the studies to date have been primarily descriptive and not analytical. She argued that the mechanisms by which poverty affects outcomes are not understood. For example, she cited evidence that women who were once poor are likely to bear low birth weight babies, even if they are currently not living in poverty. She cited other British data that indicate an independent effect of poverty on shorter adult stature even after adjustments are made for, among other things, the effects of parental height and the child's birth weight. Her assertion was that science does not know how these effects are obtained, so intervention efforts are likely to be ineffective.

Macro-Societal Influence: Racism in America A pervasive and pernicious environmental state that also is understudied and misunderstood is membership in a minority group (e.g., African Americans) in the United States. Disproportionally more minority families are poorer than majority families, which leads to the assumption that poverty is the primary factor in low birth weights, poor school achievement, and high rates of delinquency for minority children. It is true that African American families are both more likely to be poor and poor for a longer time than Caucasian families (Duncan et al., 1994), but poverty alone is not a sufficient explanation for the effects, as the following examples for two different outcomes demonstrate.

In 1971, Scarr-Salapatek published an analysis in *Science* of the heritability estimates for Philadelphia school children who were twins using available achievement data from the school system. Comparing the correlations of test scores between dizygotic (i.e., fraternal) twins to the scores achieved by monozygotic (i.e., identical) twins is a strategy for behavioral geneticists interested in calculating heritability estimates. The Philadelphia children were heterogeneous with respect to social class (as estimated from census tract information where the children lived) and were classified in school records as either Caucasian or African American.

The findings were complex, but Scarr-Salapatek's primary finding was that she could not estimate the genetic component of the variance in achievement scores of the disadvantaged groups for either racial group, but the least similar to each other were the African American twins. She concluded that minority status acted as a suppressor variable for the achievement of African American children. Minority status reduced the variability among the test scores for African Americans at all socioeconomic levels so that the children appeared to be similar to each other. This suppressor effect reduced the average level of achievement for the group as well as individual differences within the group. Furthermore, she concluded that "no study of human family correlations to date has looked at all of these effects of suppressive environments" (Scarr-Salapatek, 1971, p. 1293).

Through a series of studies concerning hypertension, Anderson and Scott (1999) also demonstrated the negative effects of racism in America. African Americans have higher rates of hypertension than any other group in the world according to Anderson and Scott. The prevalence of hypertension in African Americans is twice that of Caucasians even when social class is controlled. The high rates of hypertension lead to higher rates of morbidity and mortality among African Americans from heart disease, strokes, and renal disease. They argued that African Americans may have genetic predispositions for retaining sodium and for blood pressure reactivity. However, these only lead to phenotypic differences in blood pressure "in the presence of sufficient psychosocial or behavior stressors. The model predicts that ethnic group differences in biological functioning are due principally to differences in social and environmental factors, especially greater exposure to psychosocial stressors (e.g., residential stressors, racial discrimination) and lower SES [socioeconomic status] in Blacks" (Anderson & Scott, 1999, p. 8). They cited experimental work that shows that reactions to racism, such as rage suppression, augment the effects of racism on stressful reactions while other behaviors, such as increased exercise and social support, may reduce the effects.

The Anderson and Scott model has received empirical support from the Multi-City Study of Urban Inequality (O'Connor, 2000). This seven-volume study is the result of surveys of 9,000 households and 3,500 employers in four cities between 1992 and 1994. This work reveals that racial stereotypes and attitudes remain crucial factors in the labor market, with African Americans suffering the worst. The study concluded that racial stereotyping is deeply entrenched in America with a pervasive influence on everything from housing to schooling to employment.

To summarize, the negative environmental factors described here have similar characteristics to the positive environments described before in that they are pervasive and involve the total immersion of the organism. Given the dearth of neuroscience research with children, it would be speculative to try to link the experiences of individuals within negative environments to the neurological processes occurring during synaptogenesis and the storage of environmental information through the experience-dependent process. Clearly, these environments represent individual situations. One might assume that such environments present repetitive patterns of stimulation that are different from typical and salutatory environments, or conversely that, in the case of abusive conditions, environmental stimulation is presented in a too disorganized a fashion to allow the child to determine the regularities.

All of the negative environments may exert their influences through another, separate factor they have in common; they all may involve the HPA axis. All are stressful but unavoidable. The environments with the most significant long-lasting effects were present early in the child's life and lasted a long time. They occurred at a time when the child might be learning from stressful experiences but not in a conscious way (LeDoux, 1998). These early experiences could predispose the child behaviorally to react in certain ways in the future, for example, with greater reactivity, impulsivity, and lessened attention. The distinction between this interpretation and the one in the preceding paragraph is important. The first explanation argues that the way the child's brain has been organized has been permanently affected by negative environmental input. The second explanation proposes that the involvement of the child's emotional system has given the child behavioral responses that influence his or her actions and interpretations of later situations.

Clearly, these negative environments are powerful enough to have effects on biological as well as cognitive reactions—height, life span, and blood pressure. There is no way to know from the current research how the environment exerts its effects, and therefore no way to know how to intervene to prevent those effects. The next section will show that these factors have seldom been included as targets in early intervention programs mounted for children who live in environments marked with the negative characteristics described previously.

EARLY INTERVENTION PROGRAMS FOR CHILDREN IN POVERTY: A 30-YEAR OVERVIEW

History

Early intervention programs for children living in poverty were begun in the 1960s in response to a new view about the malleability of intelligence and a newly developed commitment to education as the route out of poverty. Hunt's (1961) book entitled *Intelligence and Experience* convinced scientists and advocates that intelligence was affected by the postnatal environment and was not strictly genetically determined. At the same time, Benjamin Bloom was arguing from correlational data (erroneously, as Scott-Jones, 1992, points out) that the first 4 years of a child's life were the most crucial for development, a critical period, in fact, for environmental variation (Bloom, 1964).

In the early 1960s, the political and social climate of the country encouraged psychologists and social workers to establish preschool programs for children from low socioeconomic backgrounds (detailed in The Consortium for Longitudinal Studies, 1983). Many of these programs were mounted as research programs and were developed and run by psychologists or educators in university settings. As Gray, Ramsey, and Klaus (1982) noted, the early studies were begun with a great deal of hope and a profound belief in the educability of children from disadvantaged backgrounds. The field of psychology traditionally has been individualistic, searching for laws that govern the behavior of individuals and for causes of behavior inside the individual (Berscheid, 1999). It is understandable that the focus of these early programs was on fixing the child (often the child's deficits) and not on changing broader, ongoing environmental contributions to developmental functioning levels. The assumption of these programs was that the child's natural environment was not facilitative, and the solution was to remove children from the environment for at least part of the day to supplement and enrich their experiences to make them better prepared for school. Those assumptions continue to dominate the field of early intervention even in the so-called two generation intervention programs (Smith & Sigel, 1995).

The field also has been marked by a rush to implement national programs before effectiveness has been demonstrated or replicated at a local level. Head Start was begun in 1965 after Sargent Shriver visited Susan Gray's Darcee Program in Nashville, Tennessee, and suggested that it be tried on a national level (Shriver, personal communication, October 1996). Even Start was begun in 1988 (St. Pierre, Swartz, Murray, & Deck, 1996) during the Ronald Reagan administration because members of his administration were fond of a program developed in Kentucky to work in counties with both high unemployment and high numbers of adults who had not graduated from high school. It was implemented in cities across the country which might have had neither of those characteristics. The Comprehensive Child Development Program also was developed in 1988 to improve the functioning of children of low socioeconomic status by intervening with the family. The assumptions behind the program were detailed by St. Pierre, Layzer, Goodson, and Bernstein (1997) in their report on the national impact of the program. There were strong beliefs—but little empirical validation—that the best way to help families in poverty would be to coordinate existing social services at the community level. Moreover, the focus should be on families with young children because of the critical nature of early experiences.

CONCLUSIONS FROM 30 YEARS OF INTERVENTION WITH CHILDREN IN POVERTY

I have reviewed the research evidence on the effectiveness of early intervention programs for children reared in poverty—one from 1977 to 1987 (Farran, 1990) and one from 1987 to 1997 (Farran, 2000)—and came to similar conclusions in both reviews.

1. The tested developmental performance of the children involved in individual programs, especially those created in university settings, was raised immediately and was high at age 3 where early intervention seems to produce an inflated, but unsustainable, test score. The tested performance of children in the intervention programs did not continue to show effects after the first 1–3 years of public school experience.
2. Children in the control groups tested behind the experimental children beginning in the middle of the second year of life for programs that began in infancy (e.g., the Abecedarian Project [Campbell & Ramey, 1995; Ramey & Campbell, 1984] and the Infant Health Program and Development Study [Brooks-Gunn, Liaw, & Klebanov, 1992]) and immediately for those that began in preschool (e.g., the Darcee Project [Gray et al., 1982] and the Perry Preschool [Schweinhart, Barnes, & Weikart, 1993]).
3. The test scores of children in the control group gradually caught up to experimental subjects so that by the second, third, or fourth grades the differences between them were neither statistically nor educationally significant.
4. Projects that included home visiting as an additional component did not achieve any stronger effects, and the provision of home visiting as the only intervention (exemplified in only one study with a small sample) was associated with negative outcomes for the children (Ramey, Bryant, Sparling, & Wasik, 1985).
5. Early intervention that began in infancy did not have significant or longer lasting effects than intervention efforts that began in the preschool years.
6. There may be a few longer lasting effects on other outcomes, such as avoiding grade retention and special education placement in school, but these have been questioned by other researchers (Locurto, 1991a).
7. Almost all of the intervention programs were effective when initially developed, especially if they were conceived during a heightened period

of belief that a new solution to a developmental problem had been found.

8. Generalization to policy has not proven effective. The achievement levels of the children in Head Start, Even Start, and the Comprehensive Child Development Program never matched those levels obtained by children in the specialized, individual programs.
9. The strongest claims for the effectiveness of early intervention have come from the researchers who initially developed the programs and from which they continue to benefit (e.g., the High Scope Educational Research Foundation). For example, the Infant Health Program and Development Study modeled its intervention on the Abecedarian Project and used the same curriculum, but the effects were modest and disappeared earlier than those of the original program (Brooks-Gunn et al., 1994).

None of the early intervention programs have undergone a serious assessment by independent investigators. It may be that the field is ready for a new consortium, a group that could organize the projects developed since the 1960s; collect standard, comparable data from each of them; report the full results (not in line graphs or tables of percentages); and make them available for scrutiny.

One exception to the pattern of developers conducting research on their own programs was rediscovered: the sustained set of studies by Miller and her colleagues of four preschool programs in which the children were followed into tenth grade in the St. Louis school system (Miller & Bizzell, 1983, 1984; Miller & Dyer, 1975). Miller had not developed any of these intervention models (she assessed Darcee, Bereiter-Englemann, Montessori, and what she termed traditional appears similar to the Bank Street College program). The majority of the children were African American and half of the families were recipients of Aid to Families with Dependent Children (AFDC). From the outset, the male children in the sample who had been in the Montessori preschool scored better on the outcome measures than males in the other three programs. Those program differences became significant, favoring Montessori for males, at the end of second grade and were maintained through the tenth grade (the opposite of plateauing found in other programs). The Darcee program was associated with the strongest positive effects for females.

Miller and Bizzell (1984) speculated that because girls tend to mature faster than boys during the preschool years, girls may have been ready to process information from the types of verbal instruction provided by Darcee, while the boys needed more "kinesthetic methods of instruction" (p. 1586) and hands-on manipulation of the learning materials provided by the Montessori approach. These findings have had little effect on policy—

they were not accompanied by press conferences, specialized training programs for teachers, or other self-promoting activities and have not had the attention they deserve.

POSSIBLE EXPLANATIONS FOR LACK OF SUSTAINED EFFECTS FOR CHILDREN IN POVERTY

There are several reasons why most of these programs have not been successful. The first relates to the differences between intervention programs and environments with demonstrable positive or negative effects described earlier in this chapter. All of the preschool intervention programs lacked a contextual focus. Even when parents were enlisted as a part of the intervention, the objective was to fix their parenting as well as the child's development (for example, the Parent-Child Development Centers, Johnson & Walker, 1991). There appears to be a lack of recognition of the intimate relationship between parenting and context; parenting grows out of the contexts in which parents are functioning. None of the programs reviewed here made any difference to the income, housing conditions, or employment of the parents involved, despite the fact that the families often were chosen because they had low incomes. A substantial proportion of the mothers involved in those intervention programs that measured depression tested clinically depressed, a finding confirmed in a survey of parents of Head Start graduates (Robinson et al., 1998). Depression scores also were unaffected by the intervention. Thus, the larger environments in which the children functioned were unchanged by the intervention. Those environments contained factors for which there is empirically established evidence of long-term negative effects.

Second, the content of the interventions themselves may have been a problem. Most provided activities and a curriculum that were generically maturational in focus. Goals chosen were general and based on the skills children are naturally developing at specific ages. As Scott-Jones (1992) noted, the aspects of development that were presumed to be affected by the intervention also were globally described (e.g., language and cognitive competencies). Thus, it is difficult to connect the intervention with specific targeted outcomes in the children. Even if one were to adopt the weaker sensitive-period hypothesis that asserts early skills are important because they are foundational for later learning, there is little evidence that these programs based their curricular focus on essential foundational skills. Instead most programs taught children concrete skills and pieces of information that enabled them to perform better on readiness tests when they entered school but may not have given them a knowledge base with enough depth to sustain continued performance in a school setting.

Byrnes and Fox (1998) asserted that most school-like tasks like reading and math are complex Functions (with a capital F) composed of multiple lower-order functions (lowercase f). Some of these lower-order functions are redundant and allow children to accomplish the complex tasks in a variety of individually specific ways. Byrnes and Fox asserted that

> The task for educational psychologists is to discover all the lower-order functions that operate within a higher-order Function for school-based skills [such as competent language performance or reading] . . . as well as specify how all of the lower-order functions work together to produce competent performance. (1998, p. 316)

That kind of experimentation was not done by the researchers who mounted the early intervention programs described here. If early preschool experiences are to be provided for children, it is incumbent upon the scientific and educational community to create and assess alternative ideas about which foundational skills and experiences are required to be successful in school when the school curriculum profoundly changes at third and fourth grade (Chall, Jacobs, & Baldwin, 1990; Snow, Barnes, Chandler, Goodman, & Hemphill, 1991). The goal of a child is not merely to become 5 years of age and "ready" for school—an entirely different set of skills may be required in order to be successful later in school when an understanding of the content of more difficult materials is required.

The most troubling explanation for the lack of effects relates to the last negative environmental effect described earlier—the macro-social environment experienced from being a member of a minority group in this culture. Scott-Jones (1992) cited work by Laosa and Washington demonstrating that the percentage of children who were African American and Hispanic in Head Start was twice the percentage of African American and Hispanic children living in poverty. Right from the beginning these intervention programs were aimed not just at children of low socioeconomic status but at *minority* children of low socioeconomic status. Furthermore,

> The subordinate status of poor minority families and children is illustrated in the pejorative language that characterized 1960s descriptions of poor minority families. Some of these terms, for example, *disadvantaged, deprived, deficient* are being resurrected in current discussions. These terms assume some underlying stable trait beyond poverty and minority status. These are not terms that poor minority communities would use in describing themselves. (Scott-Jones, 1992, p. 91)

The absolute number of Caucasian children living in poverty is greater than the number of Hispanic or African American children in poverty. Programs for children of low socioeconomic status should be serving majority and minority children in the same proportions they exist below the poverty level. Confounding poverty and minority status in the minds of teachers and policy makers could have unfortunate effects on the types of programs developed and delivered. Given the unrecognized extent of racism in America and the effects early experiences of racism may have on the HPA axis, one wonders why these kinds of interventions have been primarily targeted at minority children and families and what perceptions are being conveyed—unwittingly—to those involved.

CONCLUSION

The sooner more facilitative environments are provided for young children the better. However, despite 30 years of mounting various programs with only modest success, early intervention has not been approached from a scientific perspective. As Vernon-Feagans (1997) pointed out in her description of the history of the Abecedarian Project, the hypothesis about what caused the poor school performance of children of low socioeconomic status was inaccurate and based on a deficit model. More sophisticated understanding of children's learning strategies could be employed to develop new intervention efforts (Bransford, Brown, & Cocking, 1999).

Unfortunately, the new emphasis on the importance of the first 3 years of life as a critical period for brain growth and development may serve to distract the field even further. If neuroscience is used to justify expanding the availability of existing intervention models to families of low socioeconomic status, past data would suggest the effects will be minimal. If neuroscience has anything to tell the field of intervention, it would seem to be that children are active learners from their total environments. Impoverished environments contain negative elements associated with developmental risk. Income transfer programs that change the economic and living conditions of families are likely to be associated with more beneficial and wholesale changes in children's development than preschool intervention programs.

Moreover, neuroscience also suggests that the cerebral cortex associated with more complex cognitive skills develops for a longer period in humans than in other primates. Emphasizing preschool programs and ignoring early school instruction is not warranted. There have been sustained efforts to develop intervention programs that operate in the early years of school, several of which appear to be successful. The Kamehameha Early Education Program developed a culturally compatible approach for instruction in the early grades of part-Hawaiian children that proved successful and exportable to public schools (with training support) (Au, 1997; Tharpe & Gallimore, 1988). James Comer's efforts with high poverty schools in New Haven, Connecticut, were effective in improving the achievement levels of the children who attended (Comer, 1999; Comer, Haynes, Joyner, & Ben-Avie, 1996). Reading Recovery (Clay, 1996) and the Success for All programs have been subjected to extensive investigation and comparison (Ross, Smith, Casey, & Slavin, 1995) and both have proven to be effective with children of low socioeconomic status in early school grades. These programs demonstrate that public education can work for children of low socioeconomic status—it has to be tried (Berliner & Biddle, 1995).

Educational outcomes may be poorer for children of low socioeconomic status not because of deficits resulting from deprivation during the first 3 years of their lives, but because of the condition of their school environments when they are 6, 7, and 8 years old. The General Accounting Office concluded in 1995 that 14 million students attended one third of American schools that required extensive repair or replacement of one or more buildings (Natriello, 1996). Schools in inner cities and those with a minority enrollment of 50% or greater were more likely to be in physically poor condition. Neither children nor teachers can learn or teach in such crumbling, dangerous, and demoralizing physical structures. Environment is important, not only for what it communicates about respect for and belief in those who must occupy it during the day but also because children learn best in organized settings that communicate clear expectations.

Experience-dependent information storage involves learning from the particular environments organisms inhabit. Such learning begins early, at least in infancy, if not in utero, but it also continues for a long time, well into adulthood. The longer the organism remains in a similar environment the more committed the neural system is to certain patterns of learning and responding to stimulation. In order to make changes at later ages, environmental stimulation has to be more intense. There is little evidence that a few hours a day of general preschool instruction for a year or two is sufficiently intense to make much impact initially or to be sustained long term. In order to change the trajectories of the lives of children from impoverished environments, stronger, more intense, immersion-type alterations in their environments may be required. The critical period for development may not be the first 3 years of life, but there are important consequences of some early childhood experiences. Subjecting children to poor instruction, terrible physical settings, and situations that produce fear is likely to produce negative outcomes for children, and the longer the situations last, the more negative the outcomes are likely to be.

REFERENCES

Alexander, K., & Entwisle, D. (1988). Achievement in the first 2 years of school: Patterns and processes. *Monographs of the Society for Research in Child Development, 53*(2, Serial No. 218).

Anderson, N., & Scott, P. (1999). Making the case for psychophysiology during the era of molecular biology. *Psychophysiology, 36*, 1–13.

Au, K. (1997). A sociocultural model of reading instruction: The Kamehameha Elementary Education Program. In S. Stahl & D. Hayes (Eds.), *Instructional models in reading* (pp. 181–202). Mahwah, NJ: Lawrence Erlbaum Associates.

Bachman, H., & Kienstra Friese, M. (2000, April). *The long term effects of entrance age on academic achievement: Interactions with IQ and social skills*. Paper presented at the Biennial Conference on Human Development, Memphis, TN.

Bates, E., & Elman, J. (1993). Connectionism and the study of change. In M. Johnson (Ed.), *Brain development and cognition*. Oxford, England: Blackwell.

Berliner, D., & Biddle, B. (1995). *The manufactured crisis: Myths, fraud, and the attack on America's public schools*. Reading, MA: Addison Wesley Longman.

Berscheid, E. (1999). The greening of relationship science. *American Psychologist, 54*, 260–266.

Bloom, B. (1964). *Stability and change in human characteristics*. New York: John Wiley & Sons.

Bransford, J.D., Brown, A.L., & Cocking, R.R. (1999). *How people learn: Brain, mind, experience, and school*. Washington, DC: National Academy Press.

Brooks-Gunn, J., Liaw, F., & Klebanov, P. (1992). Effects of early intervention on cognitive function of low birth weight preterm infants. *The Journal of Pediatrics, 120*, 350–359.

Brooks-Gunn, J., McCarton, C., Casey, P., McCormick, M., Bauer, C., Bernbaum, J., Tyson, J., Swanson, M., Bennett, F.C., Scott, D., Tonascia, J., & Meinert, C. (1994). Early intervention in low birth-weight premature infants. *Journal of the American Medical Association, 272*, 1257–1262.

Byrnes, J., & Fox, N. (1998). The educational relevance of research in cognitive neuroscience. *Educational Psychology Review, 10*, 297–342.

Campbell, F., & Ramey, C. (1995). Cognitive and school outcomes for high risk African-American students at middle adolescence: Positive effects of early intervention. *American Educational Research Journal, 32*, 743–772.

Carr, J. (1995). *Down's syndrome children growing up*. Cambridge, England: Cambridge University Press.

Chall, J., Jacobs, V., & Baldwin, L. (1990). *The reading crisis: Why poor children fall behind*. Cambridge, MA: Harvard University Press.

Clay, M. (1996). Accommodating diversity in early literacy learning. In D. Olson & N. Torrance (Eds.), *Education and human development: New models of learning, teaching and schooling* (pp. 202–224). Cambridge, MA: Blackwell Publishers.

Coghill, S., Caplan, H., Alexandra, H., Robson, K., & Kumar, R. (1986). Impact of maternal postnatal depression on cognitive development of young children. *British Medical Journal, 292*, 1165–1167.

Comer, J. (1999). *Child by child: The Comer process for change in education*. New York: Teachers College Press.

Comer, J., Haynes, N., Joyner, E., & Ben-Avie, M. (1996). *Rallying the whole village: The Comer process for reforming education*. New York: Teachers College Press.

The Consortium for Longitudinal Studies. (1983). *As the twig is bent: Lasting effects of preschool programs*. Mahwah, NJ: Lawrence Erlbaum Associates.

Cooper, D., & Farran, D.C. (1988). Behavioral risk in kindergarten. *Early Childhood Research Quarterly, 3*, 1–20.

Dawson, G., Frey, K., Panagiotides, H., Osterling, J., & Hessl, D. (1997). Infants of depressed mothers exhibit atypical frontal brain activity: A replication and extension of previous findings. *Journal of Child Psychology and Psychiatry, 38*, 179–186.

Dawson, G., Hessl, D., & Frey, K. (1994). Social influences on early developing biological and behavioral symptoms related to risk for affective disorder. *Development and Psychopathology, 6,* 759–779.

Doupe, A., & Kuhl, P. (1999). Birdsong and human speech: Common themes and mechanisms. *Annual Review of Neuroscience, 22,* 567–631.

Dubow, E., & Ippolito, M. (1994). Effects of poverty and quality of the home environment on changes in the academic and behavioral adjustment of elementary school-age children. *Journal of Clinical Child Psychology, 23,* 401–412.

Duncan, G., Brooks-Gunn, J., & Klebanov, P. (1994). Economic deprivation and early childhood development. *Child Development, 65,* 296–318.

Elman, J., Bates, E., Johnson, M., Karmiloff-Smith, A., Parisi, D., & Plunkett, K. (1997). *Rethinking innateness*. Cambridge, MA: The MIT Press.

Farran, D.C. (1990). Effects of intervention with disadvantaged and disabled children: A decade review. In S. Meisels & J. Shonkoff (Eds.), *Handbook of early intervention*. Cambridge, England: Cambridge University Press.

Farran, D.C. (2000). Another decade of intervention for disadvantaged and disabled children: What do we know now? In J.P. Shonkoff & S.J. Meisels (Eds.), *Handbook of early childhood intervention* (2nd ed., pp. 510–548.). New York: Cambridge University Press.

Fodor, J.A. (1983). *The modularity of the mind: An essay on faculty psychology*. Cambridge, MA: The MIT Press.

Fox, N., & Bell, M. (1993). Frontal function in cognitive and emotional behaviors during infancy: Effects of maturation and experience. In B. de Boysson-Bardies, S. de Schonen, P. Jusczyk, P. McNeilage, & J. Morton (Eds.), *Developmental neurocognition: Speech and face processing in the first year of life* (pp. 199–210). Dordrecht, Netherlands: Kluwer Academic/Plenum Publishers.

Ghodesian, M., Zajicek, E., & Wolkind, S. (1984). A longitudinal study of maternal depression and child behavior problems. *Journal of Child Psychology and Psychiatry, 25,* 91–109.

Goldman-Rakic, P.S., Bourgeois, J.P., & Rakic, P. (1997). Synaptic substrate of cognitive development: Life-span analysis of synaptogenesis in the prefrontal cortex of the nonhuman primate. In N.A. Krasnegor, G.R. Lyon, & P.S. Goldman-Rakic (Eds.), *Development of the prefrontal cortex: Evolution, neurobiology, and behavior* (pp. 27–47). Baltimore: Paul H. Brookes Publishing Co.

Gray, C.W., Ramsey, B., & Klaus, R. (1982). *From 3 to 20: The Early Training Project*. Baltimore: University Park Press.

Greenough, W. (1993). Brain adaptation to experience: An update. In M. Johnson (Ed.), *Brain development and cognition: A reader* (pp. 319–322). Oxford, England: Blackwell.

Greenough, W., Black, J., & Wallace, C. (1987). Experience and brain development. *Child Development, 58,* 539–559.

Harman, C., & Fox, N.A. (1997). Frontal and attentional mechanisms regulating distress experience and expression during infancy. In N.A. Krasnegor, G.R. Lyon, & P.S. Goldman-Rakic (Eds.), *Development of the prefrontal cortex: Evolution, neurobiology, and behavior* (pp. 191–208). Baltimore: Paul H. Brookes Publishing Co.

Hunt, J.M. (1961). *Intelligence and experience*. New York: Ronald Press.

Huttenlocher, P. (1994). Synaptogenesis in human cerebral cortex. In G. Dawson & K. Fischer (Eds.), *Human behavior and the developing brain*. New York: The Guilford Press.

Johnson, D., & Walker, T. (1991). A follow-up evaluation of the Houston Parent-Child Development Center: School performance. *Journal of Early Intervention, 15*, 226–236.

Johnson, J., & Newport, E. (1989). Critical period effects in second language learning: The influence of maturational state on the acquisition of English as a second language. *Cognitive Psychology, 21*, 60–99.

Johnson, M. (1993). Constraints on cortical plasticity. In M. Johnson (Ed.), *Brain development and cognition*. Oxford, England: Blackwell.

Kagan, J. (1998). *Three seductive ideas*. Cambridge, MA: Harvard University Press.

Karmiloff-Smith, A. (1992). *Beyond modularity*. Cambridge, MA: The MIT Press.

Kaufman, J., Birmaher, B., Perel, J., Dahl, R., Moreci, P., Nelson, B., Wells, W., & Ryan, N. (1997). *Biological Psychiatry, 42*, 660–679.

Klinke, R., Kral, A., Heid, S., Tillein, J., & Hartmann, R. (1999). Recruitment of the auditory cortex in congenitally deaf cats by long-term cochlear electrostimulation. *Science, 285*, 1729–1733.

Kolb, B., & Fantie, B. (1997). Development of the child's brain and behavior. In C. Reynolds & E. Fletcher-Janzen (Eds.), *Handbook of clinical child neuropsychology*. New York: Kluwer Academic/Plenum Publishers.

Kosslyn, S., & Koenig, O. (1992). *Wet mind: The new cognitive neuroscience*. New York: The Free Press.

Kuhl, P. (1998). Language, culture and intersubjectivity: The creation of shared perception. In S. Braten (Ed.), *Intersubjective communication and emotion in early ontogeny* (pp. 297–315). Cambridge, England: Cambridge University Press.

LeDoux, J. (1998). *The emotional brain*. New York: Touchstone.

Levine, S. (1957). Infantile experience and resistance to physiological stress. *Science, 126*, 405–406.

Liu, D., Diorio, J., Tannenbaum, B., Caldji, C., Francis, D., Freedman, A., Sharma, S., Pearson, D., Plotsky, P., & Meaney, M. (1997). Maternal care, hippocampal, glucocorticoid receptors, and hypothalamic-pituitary-adrenal responses to stress. *Science, 277*, 1659–1662.

Locurto, C. (1991a). Beyond IQ in preschool programs. *Intelligence, 15*, 295–312.

Locurto, C. (1991b). Hands on the elephant: IQ, preschool programs, and the rhetoric of inoculation: A reply to commentaries. *Intelligence, 15*, 335–349.

Meisels, S., & Liaw, F. (1993). Failure in grade: Do retained students catch up? *Journal of Educational Research, 87*, 69–77.

Miller, L., & Bizzell, R. (1983). Long-term effects of four preschool programs: Sixth, seventh, and eighth grades. *Child Development, 54*, 727–741.

Miller, L., & Bizzell, R. (1984). Long term effects of four preschool programs: Ninth and tenth grade results. *Child Development, 55*, 1570–1587.

Miller, L., & Dyer, J. (1975). Four preschool programs: Their dimensions and effects. *Monographs of the Society for Research in Child Development, 40*(5–6, Serial No. 162).

Morrison, F., Griffith, E., & Alberts, D. (1997). Nature-nurture in the classroom: Entrance age, school readiness and learning in children. *Developmental Psychology, 33*, 254–262.

Mundy, P., Card, J., & Fox, N. (1999). *The development of joint attention and cortical activity in the second year*. Unpublished paper, University of Miami at Coral Gables.

Myers, J., Jusczyk, P., Kemler-Nelson, D., Charles-Luce, J., Woodward, A., & Hirsch-Pasek, K. (1996). *Journal of Child Language, 23*, 1–30.

Natriello, G. (1996). Diverting attention from conditions in American schools. *Educational Researcher, 25*(8), 7–9.
Nelson, C. (2000). The neurobiological bases of early intervention. In J. Shonkoff & S.J. Meisels (Eds.), *Handbook of early childhood intervention* (2nd ed., pp. 204–227). Cambridge, England: Cambridge University Press.
Nelson, C., & Carver, L. (1998). The effects of stress and trauma on brain and memory: A view from developmental cognitive neuroscience. *Development and Psychopathology, 10,* 793–809.
Neville, H. (1991). Neurobiology of cognitive and language processing: Effects of early experience. In K.R. Gibson & A.C. Peterson (Eds.), *Brain maturations and cognitive development.* Hawthorne, NY: Walter de Gruyter.
O'Connor, A. (2000). *The multi-city study of urban inequality.* New York: Russell Sage Foundation. (Available on www.russellsage.org)
Payne, D., Neuschatz, J., Lampinen, J., & Lynn, S. (1997). Compelling memory illusions: The qualitative characteristics of false memories. *Current Directions in Psychological Science, 6,* 56–60.
Payne, K., & Biddle, B. (1999). Poor school funding, child poverty, and mathematics achievement. *Educational Researcher, 28,* 4–13.
Perani, D., Paulesu, E., Galles, N., Dupoux, E., Dehaene, S., Bettinardi, V., Cappa, S., Fazio, F., & Mehler, J. (1998). The bilingual brain: Proficiency and age of acquisition of the second language. *Brain, 121,* 1841–1852.
Premack, S., & Premack, A. (1996). Why animals lack pedagogy and some cultures have more of it than others. In D. Olson & N. Torrance (Eds.), *Education and human development: New models of learning, teaching and schooling* (pp. 302–323). Cambridge, MA: Blackwell Publishers.
Ramey, C., Bryant, D., Sparling, J., & Wasik, B. (1985). Project CARE: A comparison of two early intervention strategies to prevent retarded development. *Topics in Early Childhood Special Education, 5,* 12–25.
Ramey, C., & Campbell, F. (1984). Preventive education for high-risk children: Cognitive consequences of the Carolina Abecedarian Project. *American Journal of Mental Deficiency, 88,* 515–523.
Rauschecker, J. (1999). Making brain circuits listen. *Science, 285,* 1686–1687.
Robinson, N., Weinberg, R., Redden, D., Ramey, S., & Ramey, C. (1998). Family factors associated with high academic achievement among former Head Start children. *Gifted Child Quarterly, 42,* 148–156.
Ross, S., Smith, L., Casey, J., & Slavin, R. (1995). Increasing the academic success of disadvantaged children: An examination of alternative early intervention programs. *American Educational Research Journal, 32,* 773–800.
Sameroff, A., Seifer, R., Barocas, R., Zax, M., & Greenspan, S. (1987). IQ scores of 4-year-old children: Social-environmental risk factors. *Pediatrics, 79,* 343–350.
Sameroff, A., Seifer, R., & Zax, M. (1982). Early development of children at risk for emotional disorder. With commentary by Norman Garmezy. *Society for Research in Child Development Monographs, 47* (7, Serial No. 199).
Scarr, S., & Weinberg, R. (1976). IQ test performance of black children adopted by white families. *American Psychologist, 31,* 726–739.
Scarr, S., & Weinberg, R. (1983). The Minnesota adoption studies: Genetic differences and malleability. *Child Development, 54,* 260–267.
Scarr-Salapatek, S. (1971). Race, social class, and IQ. *Science, 174,* 1285–1295.
Schiff, M., & Lewontin, R. (1986). *Education and class: The irrevelance of IQ genetic studies.* Oxford, England: Clarendon.

Schneider, M., Roughton, E., Koehler, A., & Lubach, G. (1999). Growth and development following prenatal stress exposure in primates: An examination of ontogenetic vulnerability. *Child Development, 70,* 263–274.

Schweinhart, L., Barnes, H., & Weikart, D. (1993). Significant benefits: The High/Scope Perry Preschool study through age 27. *Monographs of the High/Scope Educational Research Foundation, 10.* Ypsilanti, MI: The High/Scope Press.

Scott-Jones, D. (1992). Family and community interventions affecting the development of cognitive skills in children. In T. Sticht, M. Beeler, & B. McDonald (Eds.), *The intergenerational transfer of cognitive skills: Vol. I. Programs, policy and research issues.* Norwood, NJ: Ablex Publishing Co.

Shahinfar, A., & Fox, N. (1997). The effects of trauma on children: Conceptual and methodological issues. In D. Chicchetti & S. Toth (Eds.), *Developmental perspectives on trauma: Theory, research and intervention.* Rochester, NY: The University of Rochester Press.

Skuse, D.H. (1988). Extreme deprivation in early childhood. In D. Bishop & K. Mogford (Eds.), *Language development in exceptional circumstances.* Edinburgh, Scotland: Churchill Livingstone.

Smith, J., Brooks-Gunn, J., & Klebanov, P. (1997). Consequences of living in poverty for young children's cognitive and verbal ability and early school achievement. In G. Duncan & J. Brooks-Gunn (Eds.), *Consequences of growing up poor* (pp. 132–189). New York: Russell Sage Foundation.

Smith, S., & Sigel, I. (1995). *Two generation programs for families in poverty: A new intervention strategy* (pp. 251–270). Norwood, NJ: Ablex Publishing Company.

Snow, C., Barnes, W., Chandler, J., Goodman, I., & Hemphill, L. (1991). *Unfulfilled expectations: Home and school influences on literacy.* Cambridge, MA: Harvard University Press.

St. Pierre, R.G., Layzer, J., Goodson, B., & Bernstein, L. (1997). *National impact evaluation of the Comprehensive Child Development Program: Final Report.* Cambridge, MA: Abt Associates, Inc.

St. Pierre, R.G., & Swartz, J. (1996). *The Even Start family literacy program: Early implementation.* Cambridge, MA: Abt Associates, Inc.

St. Pierre, R.G., Swartz, J., Murray, S., & Deck, D. (1996). *Improving family literacy: Findings from the national Even Start evaluation.* Cambridge, MA: Abt Associates, Inc.

Starfield, B. (1992). Effects of poverty on health status. *Bulletin of the New York Academy of Medicine, 68,* 17–24.

Stein, J. (1997). *Empowerment and women's health: Theory, methods and practice.* London: Zed Books.

Tharpe, R., & Gallimore, R. (1988). *Rousing minds to life.* Cambridge, England: Cambridge University Press.

Thelen, E., & Smith, L. (1995). *The dynamic systems approach to the development of cognition and action.* Cambridge, MA: The MIT Press.

Vernon-Feagans, L. (1997). *Children's talk in communities and classrooms.* Cambridge, MA: Blackwell Publishers.

Watson, R. (1996). Rethinking readiness for learning. In D. Olson & N. Torrance (Eds.), *Education and human development: New models of learning, teaching and schooling* (pp. 148–172). Cambridge, MA: Blackwell Publishers.

Weinberg, R., Scarr, S., & Waldman, I. (1992). The Minnesota transracial adoption study: A follow-up of IQ test performance and achievement. *Intelligence, 16,* 117–135.

Werner, E., & Smith, S. (1992). *Overcoming the odds: High risk children from birth to adulthood*. Ithaca, NY: Cornell University Press.

Zarrow, M., Campbell, P., & Denneberg, V. (1972). Handling in infancy: Increased levels of the hypothalamic corticotropin releasing factor (CRF) following exposure to a novel situation. *Procedures of the Society for Experimental Biological Medicine, 356*, 141–143.

13

The Concept of Critical Periods and Their Implications for Early Childhood Services

Robert B. McCall

Bradford W. Plemons

A national media campaign in the spring of 1997 announced that new research on the development of the human brain reveals that stimulation of infants and young children contributes to the development of adult characteristics that help to define success and fulfillment of individuals in American society. Some scientists and journalists have claimed that brain development occurs through a sequence of critical periods in which each period offers a window of opportunity for environmental stimulation to support and enhance development, and without such stimulation important potential capabilities for learning, thinking, feeling, and loving may be lost forever. But some of these claims and conclusions seem contradictory. For example, after admonishing parents to stimulate their infants and children before these windows of opportunity close, parents are told not to feel guilty if they have not provided enough stimulation to their infants because

The preparation of this chapter was supported in part by an Urban Community Services Program Grant No. P252A50226 awarded by the federal Department of Education to the University of Pittsburgh Office of Child Development.

The authors are indebted to Ross A. Thompson, whose unpublished paper entitled *Early Brain Development and Early Intervention* provided much of the empirical basis for this chapter. The authors also appreciate the contributions and insight of Mark S. Strauss.

it is never too late to encourage the development of one's children. If early experience is crucial for later skills, why does early stimulation often not have permanent benefits?

This chapter attempts to formulate general principles concerning critical periods of development; reconcile the apparent contradictions regarding the necessity of early stimulation and the permanence of such experiences; and consider the implications these principles have for practitioners, policy makers, and parents, especially with respect to stimulation of and programming for young children. The hope is to provide justification and guidance to programming, but it is recognized that in the process important limitations, exceptions, and qualifications in the technical literature will be ignored.

THE BASICS OF BRAIN DEVELOPMENT

Two Fundamental Principles

Two fundamental principles of brain development must be acknowledged. First, except for minor reflexes, essentially all human behavior—looking, listening, speaking, thinking, loving, worshiping, imagining, and socializing—is governed by the brain. Therefore, it should not be surprising that any experience that changes the behavior of an infant, child, or adult also produces a change in the brain of that individual.

Consequently, it should *be expected* that 1) providing rats with toys to play with instead of barren cages produces bigger and better brains (Greenough & Black, 1992; Hebb, 1949, Rosenzweig, Krech, Bennett, & Diamond, 1962), 2) the brains of neglected children are smaller than those of advantaged children (Chase, Canosa, Dabiere, Welch, & O'Brien, 1974; Winick & Rosso, 1969), 3) the more experiences and stimulation given to an animal or child will increase the number of brain cell connections (Greenough & Black, 1992), and 4) the brain areas associated with the control of finger movements are larger in experienced string instrument musicians than in other individuals (Elbert, Pantev, Wienbruch, Rockstroh, & Taub, 1995).

The latest brain research shows that experience that produces changes in behavior produces changes in the brain (Johnson, 1990). The availability of new technologies allows researchers to locate those changes in specific areas and nerve cells in the brain. The fact that the brain reflects these experiences, however, is not news, is not remarkable, and does not validate the importance of certain experiences. Most of the current brain research *illustrates* what child development psychologists, child care professionals, and parents already knew, and it *confirms* the nature of good parenting and child care, rather than redirecting researchers to do something different.

The second fundamental principle is that a lot of brain research shows the consequences of poor and atypical stimulation and environments on the brain development of animals and humans. No research, however, shows that extreme amounts of stimulation or rich environments produce a superior brain and human being. Specifically, the new brain research confirms that abusive and neglectful treatment of infants and young children produces serious and sometimes permanent deficits in the brains and behavior of these victims. But it does not show that bombarding infants and young children with sights, sounds, language, social interaction, music, games, and other experiences will produce a super child. Indeed, too much stimulation and experiences that are not developmentally appropriate may hinder infant development, turn a child off to learning, and impede other opportunities for growth. More, or even earlier, stimulation may not always be better. How much stimulation is enough, whether earlier is always better, and when more stimulation is beneficial are the focus of what follows.

THE DEVELOPMENTAL TASK

Even if many of the principles of development are not new, the neurological process of brain development is one of the most incredible phenomena in the universe. For example, the brain of every human being contains approximately 100 billion neurons, each of which is formed between the sixth week and the fifth month of prenatal life (Rakic, 1988, 1996). This means that approximately a quarter to half a million nerves are created every minute during this period of time (Cowan, 1979), and no additional nerve cells are generated after this point in development. It is almost inconceivable to know how these nerves become wired to permit learning, imagination, and loving. New brain research is beginning to reveal how this takes place.

Neural Proliferation

Brain development occurs in a sequence of overlapping stages. The first stage is neural proliferation, in which 100 billion nerve cells, called neurons, are created by the end of the fifth prenatal month (Rakic, 1988, 1996). Barring unfavorable conditions, these neurons are produced in every infant according to biological instructions (Nelson & Bloom, 1997). Basically, this phase produces the neurological wires and hardware of the brain.

Neural Migration

Shortly after neural proliferation begins, the second phase, called neural migration, begins. This phase is completed during prenatal life (Rakic, 1971, 1972, 1988, 1996). Neural migration, in the language of telephone networks, is the "reach out and touch someone" phase. By a process not yet understood, nerves grow and send long arms through the brain to different areas and make contact with one another. This migration establishes trunk lines, which, for example, allow a call to be made between Pittsburgh and Seattle, but do not connect a specific telephone in Seattle.

Synaptogenesis and Differentiation

When neural migration is nearly complete, the third phase—neural synaptogenesis and differentiation—starts. *Synaptogenesis* means that different nerve cells connect (at places called *synapses*) to form a network of linkages that provide the opportunity to dial specific telephone numbers in Seattle. As a result of these connections, different neurons, which start out the same, become differentiated to perform one function instead of another—for example, hearing, rather than seeing (Nowakowski, 1987).

This neural synaptogenesis and differentiation does not occur at the same time in every area of the brain, and consequently different functions develop at different times (Huttenlocher, 1990, 1994a). For example, the peak activity of development occurs in the region associated with hearing during the first postnatal months, in the region associated with vision during the third and fourth months of postnatal life, and in areas responsible for cognition and intelligence (prefrontal cortex and association areas) at 1 year through adolescence (Huttenlocher, 1994b). This sequencing of development is part of the neurological basis for providing stimulation and pertinent experiences specifically for different skills and functions at different times in a child's life, in short for developmentally appropriate practices.

Neural Overproduction

In the process of making all of these connections, the brain overproduces connections. That is, it makes more connections than it needs (Kandel, Schwartz, & Jessell, 1991). For example, a human infant in the first few months of life is capable of distinguishing between every pair of sounds that occurs in any language in the world (Werker & Lalonde, 1988; Werker & Polka, 1993; Werker & Tees, 1984). Moreover, infants are sensitive to speech sounds as opposed to other kinds of sounds (Eimas, Siqueland, Jusczyk, & Vigorito, 1971).

Selective Elimination and Degeneration

Most brain growth is governed by biology, but sometimes experience and stimulation are needed. Such experience and stimulation produce connections between neurons and selective elimination and degeneration of connections, in what is called a "use it or lose it" developmental process (Kolb, 1989). For an infant living in the United States and hearing English, the connections in the brain that help the infant distinguish the sounds (phonemes) of English are used when the infant hears those sounds; but sounds that are unique to Japanese or to Russian are not heard, and those neural connections literally wither and die. So, while all infants are born with the ability to distinguish "r" and "l" sounds within the first 6 months of life, infants in Japan can no longer distinguish between these two sounds because they do not exist in Japanese, whereas infants reared in English-language homes are able to distinguish these sounds (see Werker & Lalonde, 1988; Werker & Polka, 1993; Werker & Tees, 1984). This is the neurological basis for the advice to parents to talk to their infants, even if their infants cannot understand their words. Also, this allows infants to recognize their parents' voices more quickly.

Selective elimination, or use it or lose it, is a strategy of nature. It may be one of the first, if not most crucial, components of the ability of human beings to adapt to their environments. The fact that nerve connections die if not used is often invoked as the basis for the claim that certain capabilities not nurtured at particular times in early development (e.g., critical periods or windows of opportunity) are lost and cannot be developed later. This is only partly true.

Some abilities are lost unless they are nurtured with specific stimulation at specific times during development. For example, unless an infant sees light during the first 6 months of life, the nerves leading from the eye to the visual cortex of the brain that will process those signals will degenerate and die (Wiesel & Hubel, 1963). As a consequence, an infant born with total cataracts that are not removed for several months will be blind for the rest of his or her life, because the nerves from the eye to the brain will die from disuse. In contrast, an adult who develops cataracts later in life and has them removed will not be blind because the nerves of the visual system developed at an appropriate time and remain intact.

However, not every set of connections and every capability is permanently lost if not stimulated early. Actually, few human functions are lost forever from lack of stimulation. For some abilities, connections that once degenerated can be recreated when the environment changes (Diamond, 1991; Greenough & Black, 1992; Kandel et al., 1991). In adults, when a part of the brain normally responsible for a certain function is injured, some other part of the brain, normally responsible for another function, sometimes comes to the rescue and compensates for the lost ability (Neville, 1988, 1990, 1991).

Myelination

The last stage of brain development is called myelination. *Myelination* is the process by which nerve cells become coated with a layer of fatty cells (myelin) that insulates the cells and speeds neural conduction. Whereas synaptogenesis produces the functional capability of the brain and synaptogenic proliferation and elimination fine-tunes and differentiates those capacities, myelination contributes speed and efficiency to the functioning of the brain. Myelination occurs at varying rates, with primitive and survival-related cognitive processing structures becoming myelinated first (e.g., early postnatal development) and nonprimitive and executive functioning structures becoming myelinated later (e.g., as late as adolescence and early adulthood) (Gibson, 1991). Although myelination occurs from infancy to early adulthood, maternal malnutrition during the last trimester of pregnancy can have adverse effects on the maturation and myelination of neurons (Morgan & Gibson, 1991).

THE ROLE OF EXPERIENCE

Parents, child care professionals, and policy makers can do little about biology, so their primary concern is the role of experience in the developing brain. How much stimulation is necessary? When is it necessary? Is earlier better? When, if ever, is it too late? Is more stimulation better? What are the right activities to promote the development of children? What kind of programming should be offered to children and at what ages? The answers depend on the particular functions and capabilities researchers want to promote.

Basic Functions

One of the principles of brain development is that it occurs in a sequence of stages, and such stages are arranged in a hierarchical order. Specifically, functions that are necessary for survival, which essentially every human being acquires in basic form, tend to develop first. These functions require some experience at particular times to develop normally. But the necessary experience is minimum and is common in the typical environments of human infants and children. Therefore, almost every human infant and child receives the minimum amount of experience necessary, and more experience usually does not improve the development of these capabilities (Diamond, 1991; Greenough & Black, 1992).

For example, it was said previously in the chapter that the visual system needs light to develop normally. Experience with light must occur during the time that the nerves from the eye to the brain are developing most rapidly, typically in the first 4 months of life (Held, 1985, 1990). This is a fairly short window of opportunity, and if light is not available to the infant, these nerves will die and the infant will be permanently blind. However, essentially every infant is exposed to light at the proper time during development. A minimum amount of light is needed and more than the minimum does not improve vision (see Chapters 3 and 4).

But what about more complex visual behavior than being able to see light? Experience with visual patterns—lines, angles, forms, and contrasts—also is necessary for an infant to visually distinguish shapes, geometric forms, and recognize a parent's face from that of another person (Held, 1990; Johnson, 1993; Turkewitz & Kenny, 1982, 1985). In contrast to light, which must be experienced early, experience with patterns can occur over a longer window of time. Monkeys, for example, that are permitted only light but no pattern vision during the first 6 months of life and then are given normal visual experience behave at 6 months exactly like normal newborn monkeys with respect to their ability to distinguish between visual objects, reach for an object, and so forth (Riesen, 1958). But, thereafter, they develop at the same rate, just 6 months delayed, as do monkeys given normal experience from birth. So, for this slightly higher visual function, the window of opportunity is longer and more forgiving.

Humans are social beings; and having a warm, caring, stable relationship with another human being, usually a parent, is a crucial component of early experience, without which the ability to care, love, socialize, empathize, and so forth may not develop normally (Carlson et al., 1995, Carlson & Earls, 1997; see Chapter 7). Attachment between infant and parent starts early and should be nurtured from the beginning (Ainsworth & Marvin, 1995). But the window is long—children probably must have such a relationship before reaching 4 to 6 years of age, otherwise severe long-lasting problems will likely occur because of timing alone (Rutter, 1979).

In contrast to lower animals, humans are more flexible in the nature and timing of necessary stimulation. For example, a chick inside its egg must rest its head on its chest at a certain point in development before hatching so that the beating of the heart pushes the chick's head up and down with each beat. Without this prenatal experience, the chick will not accurately peck at seeds on the ground to obtain food (Kuo, 1932). In this case, a highly specific event must occur at a particular time for normal eating behavior to develop. Even so, nature sees to it that almost every chick is exposed to this crucial prenatal experience. Very little in human development requires that such highly specific stimuli are needed at particular times.

Higher Functions

In contrast to the previously described functions that essentially every human acquires, higher functions are those that some people become better at than others. They include social, emotional, and mental skills, such as language fluency, intelligence, social relations, and loving. Higher functions require certain stimulation and experience to occur, but the necessary experiences are likely to be unique to the individual and not shared with all other people. In addition, the window of opportunity is longer, and the necessary experiences may not be tied to the particular period in which the brain that governs that function is developing most rapidly.

For example, language development is actually a combination of basic and higher processes. Human beings, who are biologically disposed to developing language, need to experience a responsive language environment before they will develop basic language (Bloom, 1998). Consequently, children tragically reared in closets for the first 6 years of life, for example, do not walk out of closets speaking a language (Davis, 1947). Also, children confined to a room with a television set do not develop language unless they have the opportunity to talk with other people who respond to their language initiatives (Dale, 1972). Except for these unusual catastrophes, every child experiences *a responsive language environment* and develops basic language.

When does a child need to experience a responsive language environment before it's too late? It is a good idea for parents to talk to their infants because they can come to recognize their parents' voices (DeCasper & Spence, 1986) and, by selective degeneration, infants will focus on the sounds of the particular language spoken to them. Yet, infants do not fail to develop normal language or the ability to sing or appreciate music even when special efforts are not made to talk and sing to them in the first months or year of life. Experience with a responsive language environment probably needs to occur during the first 8–10 years of life (Johnson & Newport, 1989; Newport, 1991) or perhaps by puberty (see Chapter 9), which is a very long window of opportunity before permanent dysfunction in developing a language is likely to occur. The child mentioned previously who had been locked in a closet until age 6 had three guttural words when discovered; but after 18 months of tutoring, the child developed a vocabulary, language fluency, and an IQ score within the normal range (Davis, 1947; Mason, 1942). The child was permanently affected and earlier stimulation would have produced improved functioning, but nature has provided flexibility when stimulation needs to occur for basic language to develop.

Children differ in their ability to use language, think and conceptualize abstractly, solve problems, and so forth. Such higher skills—which are important for success in school and in the development of intelligence—also require experience, but not every child receives the same type and amount of the relevant experience, so children differ in these abilities. Furthermore, such experience does not have to occur at specific periods of time in development. Even rats that were given special toys as infants and grew to have larger brains did not necessarily have to experience those toys as infants; rats deprived of such experience until adulthood and then given toys to play with developed the same larger brains (Diamond, 1991; Greenough & Black, 1992).

Consequently, higher skills, which include capabilities that human beings value most about life and that contribute to success in modern society, do not require highly specific experiences at particular ages for their development. They do require a great variety of developmentally appropriate stimulation that is delivered both early and over a prolonged period of time. Therefore, one should not worry about how early stimulation is given or how much of it is provided lest the brain die and the function be lost forever. One should worry about providing a variety of developmentally appropriate experiences both early and throughout childhood, adolescence, and adulthood.

SOME FUNDAMENTAL QUESTIONS

Given the distinction between basic and higher functions noted in this chapter, several of the major questions concerning the role of experience in early childhood need to be discussed.

Is Earlier Better?

Earlier stimulation is essential for basic functions; it is better but not essential for higher functions. That is, the windows of opportunity are shorter for basic functions and longer for higher functions.

Essential early experiences include exposure to light (Wiesel & Hubel, 1963) and establishing a stable relationship with another human in the first 4–6 years of life (Rutter, 1979). Experiences that can occur later in life include pattern vision (Riesen, 1958) and exposure to a responsive language environment in the first 8–12 years of life (Johnson & Newport, 1989; Newport, 1991). But exposure to more complicated language, thought processes, problem-solving strategies, and abstract reasoning can occur over a long window of opportunity, perhaps decades in length.

Even if the windows of opportunity are long, there is something compelling about the idea that earlier is better. In fact, earlier can be better, even for higher functions. Developmentally appropriate stimulation should begin when a window opens, even if it may be years before that window closes.

Nature has given us at least 4–6 years to experience a stable human relationship (see Chapter 7), but that does not mean to wait until then to experience such a relationship. It is best to start at the beginning of that window—at birth (if not sooner). Nature gives us 8–12 years to experience a responsive language, but that does not mean avoiding talking to infants—even fetuses.

Early stimulation has been shown to produce better social relationships, language, and intelligence later. Children adopted by Western parents from orphanages providing minimal social relationships experience long-term socioemotional impairments the longer they have stayed in the orphanage beyond 6–18 months (see Chapter 7). Children who learn a second language earlier in their lives do better at that language than those who wait until adolescence or adulthood to learn it (see Chapter 10). But adolescents and adults can learn a second language, albeit with greater difficulty, and if they are thoroughly immersed in the new language environment, they can learn it well, even if they don't start until adulthood. So, it is better and efficient to start earlier, but it is not too late to start for many characteristics.

Furthermore, early educational programs for low-income children have produced some lasting benefits even when the special stimulation stopped by age 6 (Ramey & Ramey, 1992). In some programs these children were less likely to fail a grade, need special education services, become pregnant or delinquent as teenagers, and need public assistance as young adults.

Is More Stimulation Better?

Sometimes more stimulation is better. For basic functions, a modest amount of stimulation is all that is required and more is not better. For progressively higher functions, however, varied stimulation over a prolonged period of time is likely to produce corresponding results—that is, more is better.

More stimulation than the minimum necessary to maintain and promote basic functions is not always beneficial and can be harmful (e.g., when such stimulation is forced on children and it becomes aversive). In terms of raw stimulation necessary to keep the eyes and ears operating, children of low socioeconomic status get more to look at and hear because they tend to live in closer quarters with many people than infants of high socioeconomic status who tend to have their own bedrooms and fewer people in the house. But the sensory skills of infants of low socioeconomic status are no better than those of infants of high socioeconomic status. Indeed, nature has built the human infant to shut out excessive stimulation by closing the eyes; turning the head away; arching the back; and crying when someone talks too much, too loudly, and without pauses. The appropriate auditory stimulation of an infant is one that is distinctive (e.g., sounds that stand out from a quiet background), delivered up close and personal to the baby, and followed by a long pause, which allows the infant to absorb the stimulation and respond to it.

But, for higher functions, more developmentally appropriate stimulation is better. Fluid language, abstract thinking, higher mathematics, exceptional social skills, and so forth need a great deal of nurturing with progressively more complex, developmentally appropriate stimulation over a long period of time. This is why quality educational services are important and why schooling takes so many years.

How Much Is Enough?

How much stimulation is enough again depends on the specific function. For basic functions, little stimulation at the right time in development is enough to produce permanent benefits. But for higher functions, more stimulation over longer periods of time is required to develop and maintain the ability.

So, a little light early in life will keep the visual neurons functioning for the rest of one's life, even if light is not available later (e.g., perhaps because of cataracts at age 60). But for fluid language and intelligence, more is needed over a longer period of time and early stimulation may produce only modest long-term benefits without continuing stimulation to maintain the ability.

The latter principle is important for public policy because it says that for many higher functions, including school and life success, the inoculation model of early experience is not true. That is, one cannot expect to vaccinate children at age 4, for example, with language and mental stimulation (e.g., Head Start) and expect that to immunize those children for the rest of their lives against the subsequent effects of poor environments (Entwistle, 1995). To support Head Start while ignoring the quality of the schools that Head Start children later attend is futile. Earlier has certain advantages, but continuous environmental support of higher functions also is needed.

What Should Be Done?

Given the distinction between basic and higher functions and the role of experience in early childhood development described in this chapter, what should practitioners, policy makers, and parents do? The practical implications are not revolutionary; instead, they validate contemporary beliefs and principles of parenting and intervention programs.

GENERAL ACTION PRINCIPLES

Five general principles for action follow.

1. Basic and higher functions and capabilities will develop normally if a child is reared in a typical environment. Being neglected or having a dysfunctional parent because of alcohol, drug abuse, or psychopathology is not a typical environment. Such families need help to provide their children with a typical environment, and some of these children may need out-of-home experiences or care to develop typically. This is what many contemporary intervention programs attempt to accomplish.

2. Love and responsive communication provide stimulation to an infant. Having a good time with an infant by talking, responding, and listening is one of the most important things a parent can do. A parent should follow his or her instincts and be sensitive to the way his or her infant communicates. Intervention may be necessary when parents do not provide a typical environment for their child.
3. There are some advantages to beginning earlier for higher functions, but earlier is only better if it is matched in a developmentally appropriate manner to an infant's or child's capabilities and interests at the moment. Consequently, it is necessary to provide quality experiences that match the brain's stage of development at every age throughout life, which is the neurological basis behind the educational practice of developmentally appropriate practices. To match experience to an infant's or young child's abilities and motivations, parents and caregivers should respond to rather than stimulate their children. One of the best ways to respond appropriately is to imitate the child's action, perhaps with slight variations. Then the adult is doing something the child understands. The simple advice is that if the child is relaxed, attentive, and responsive, and parent and child are having a good time together, chances are those activities are developmentally appropriate.
4. Many of the important skills and human characteristics need long-term and varied nurturing from parents, caregivers, teachers, and friends. As a nation, investment is disproportionate in education beginning at approximately age 6. There should be a commitment to invest more in early childhood education and family programs because parents need them, and crucial child functions (e.g., attachment, human relationships) have early windows and other functions (e.g., language, intelligence) begin and can be nurtured easily and efficiently. Given the premises that some benefit is associated with developmentally appropriate stimulation early in the window of opportunity of a given function and that as a society there is less programmatic effort during the early years when the windows for many mental and socioemotional skills are first open and the brain is developing rapidly, more investment should be made in the early years.
5. Society should not try to inoculate children with a shot of early quality education before age 6 and then send children of low socioeconomic status to inferior schools for the remainder of their educational careers and expect them to perform at the national average. The most crucial human characteristics benefit from early and continuing nurturing that is paced and tailored to the changing developmental and motivational needs of children and adolescents. Indeed, Entwistle (1995) argued that the effects of early childhood programs are temporary because children of low socioeconomic status are placed in inferior schools and into low

achievement tracks from which it is difficult to escape. Consequently, there should be an effort to improve the schools in communities of low socioeconomic status. The new brain research highlights the development of the human mind, and although that mind needs certain environmental food early on, it also requires nutrition throughout its existence to produce the intellectual, social, and emotional benefits children need.

Principles of Action for Early Childhood and Family Programming

These five general principles suggest that the nation should increase its investment in early childhood intervention and educational programming for young children, not only to compensate for inferior environments but also to improve the educational and socioemotional potential of children, especially children of low socioeconomic status. The data on critical periods suggest that interventions have the potential for accomplishing these goals, even though continued nurturing beyond the early childhood period may be necessary to sustain those early benefits. Although public programs, such as Head Start, have shown documented success, they have not been as successful in producing benefits in children as professionals had hoped. What does the literature say with respect to early childhood programming? This literature has been reviewed numerous times (Behrman, 1995; Farran, 1990; Guralnick, 1997; Ramey & Ramey, 1992; Shonkoff & Hauser-Cram, 1987; see Chapter 12), so the focus here will be on general conclusions without details of empirical documentation, which can be obtained from these literature reviews.

Early childhood programs can accomplish many of their short-term and some of their long-term goals. It is helpful to distinguish between the *potential* of early childhood programs and what they *actually* accomplish. What they can accomplish is demonstrated by flagship research demonstration projects (Weiss, 1988), whose purpose is to create the best and most intensive interventions possible and document their developmental benefits to children. What early intervention programs do accomplish is represented by the results of fleet (Weiss, 1988) programs that are often publicly supported and provided as public services for all eligible children (often on the basis of income alone).

The data from the flagship programs clearly show that such interventions can produce the following benefits.

1. *There can be an increase in IQ scores, language fluency, and other early mental and academic skills.* Many of these gains, relative to children who do not receive the intervention, diminish within 3 years of the early childhood program because the children receiving the intervention decline

in average performance and those children not receiving the early intervention catch up in mental performance, as a result of attending school (see Chapter 12). The latter fact suggests that some of the benefits of early childhood programming can be achieved at age 6, which casts doubt on the strong version of the principle that earlier is better in this context.

2. *High-quality early childhood education programs can minimize academic problems in grade and high school, including the reduction of class failure, dropout rates, rates of grade retention, and use of remedial and special education services.* These intervention programs do produce some long-term educational benefits.
3. *Relative to home-reared comparisons, children 3–5 years of age who have attended early childhood programs are more socially mature and independent.* Such benefits depend on whether the program makes a deliberate attempt to improve social development and teaches appropriate peer behavior. There is a tendency to get what you pay for—you get mental performance improvements when the program focuses on cognitive development and you get social improvements when the program concentrates on social behavior. Such benefits also diminish across the group in the years after the intervention program because treatment children decline and comparison children improve when they experience school.
4. *A few long-term follow-up studies show program children who engage in less noncompliant and delinquent behavior, have fewer teen pregnancies, graduate at higher rates, and are employed and less dependent on welfare after high school.* Again, long-term benefits are observed, but in both cases they consist of the prevention of disasters in some children, not average benefits for all children. The cost of such disasters, especially criminality, can be so great that preventing them can make the early intervention programs cost-effective.

Fleet programs are less effective than flagship programs. Despite the potential demonstrated by the flagship programs, fleet programs—those publicly available early childhood services—produce similar benefits but to a lesser extent. Head Start, for example, produces benefits that are qualitatively similar to those of the flagship early childhood education programs, but the size of the benefits, persistence over developmental time, and the consistency with which they are found from study to study is often smaller. In short, public service programs *can*, but they typically *don't*, produce the same level of outcome benefits as the demonstration programs upon which they are based and that are used to justify public investment. The question is why? The answer requires an examination of the characteristics of successful programs, especially the flagship programs.

Reduced to a single concept, successful early childhood programming provides a higher dosage of treatment, both quantitatively and qualitatively.

1. *Successful programs deliver a greater quantity of intervention treatment.* The more time children spend in the intervention program, the better the results, and in some cases the longer lasting the benefits. Indeed, for a fleet program in Chicago funded by Title I, Reynolds (1994) showed that at least 4 years in a preschool-through-third-grade educational support program were necessary to produce noticeable benefits on education measures at program termination and 2 years following termination, with improvements increasing with 5 and 6 years in the program. Also, it is not clear that the earlier the intervention the better the outcome. This is because the amount of services is often greater for programs that start earlier (Barnett, 1995; Bryant & Maxwell, 1997; Frede, 1995). Also, Reynolds (1994) demonstrated that years spent in the program were more strongly related to educational outcomes than whether the program was initiated when the children were 3, 4, or 5 years of age.
2. *Successful programs deliver better quality experiences to children.* Specifically, better outcomes for children are associated with
   - Smaller groups of children, lower ratios of children-to-staff, and developmentally appropriate practices
   - Well-trained personnel who are closely monitored and supervised
   - More involvement of parents in the program

More is better in terms of the quantity and quality of services in an early childhood program. Barnett (1995) made one of the more profound yet obvious observations in this domain—*unless the treatment program represents an improvement over the home environment in ways related to the desired outcome, it represents no intervention or treatment at all.* If early childhood intervention programming is simply custodial care, it is unlikely to produce the benefits described above. Finally, quantity and quality of the program complement each other, so improvements in either respect have the potential of improving outcomes for children.

Fleet programs are less successful than flagship programs because they usually do not provide the same dosage of treatment (Chubrick & Kelley, 1994; Frede, 1995; Haskins, 1989; Woodhead, 1988). Head Start, for example, is typically a half-day program for 9 months of the year for 1 or 2 years. In general, fleet programs have lower staff-to-child ratios, less parental involvement, and less well-trained personnel, largely because they have lower budgets. A classic example of low dosage, even in a flagship demonstration program, is the Comprehensive Child Development Program, which managed to provide substantial amounts of services to parents but only 2 extra hours per day of early childhood services for children, and most of those services were of the custodial rather than the educational variety. It is not surprising that major child benefits were not found for the Comprehensive Child Development Program (McCall, Ryan, & Plemons, in press; St. Pierre, Layzer, Goodson, & Bernstein, 1997).

POLICY ISSUES

Because economics tend to drive child and family policies and programming, it is important to determine whether quality matters in early childhood programming. The economic realities of welfare reform, in particular, require public support for early childhood services for the children of women of low socioeconomic status who are forced into employment. The government provides services at a minimum cost, which means custodial services are offered rather than higher quality educational programs.

That the government should invest a relatively small increment of funds to upgrade custodial programs to be more educationally and developmentally enriching rests on the proposition that quantitative and qualitative dosage are important ingredients in producing beneficial outcomes for children. Early returns from the National Institute of Child Health and Human Development (NICHD) Early Child Care Research Project show that family and parental factors account for more variance in child outcomes than quality of care environments (Child Care Network, 1999). It is easy to conclude from these data that an investment in quality would produce minimum return.

But this result appears to contradict the majority of the early childhood programming literature. Why? For one thing, outcomes at this point have only been reported through age 3, and even the correlations between family socioeconomic status and child mental performance at age 3 are modest (e.g., approximately .35; McCall, 1979), suggesting that it is not likely that enrichment programs will have a major effect that is measurable at this age. Second, it is not clear how many of the early childhood experiences the NICHD sample of children received were actually better than what they experienced at home. The early childhood educational literature is based almost solely on deliberate attempts to improve upon the home environment, whereas the NICHD sample represents early childhood services that exist naturally in the community that parents select. Third, the NICHD study has the advantage that the sample represents nearly the entire range (minus the lowest income strata) of the American population, but only a small portion of that sample consists of families of low socioeconomic status that are eligible for publicly supported intervention programs. These families are likely to benefit from quality early childhood programs, which are likely to provide environments that are better than the home environments of their children. It is possible, then, that the NICHD study will not show substantial effects for quality, because most of its sample provides an adequate home environment and does not benefit additionally from quality early childhood services.

It has been concluded that it is best to start appropriate stimulation when a window of opportunity opens rather than waiting until later in that window. Yet, successful programs are not confined to those beginning in the first 3 years of life. Early programming may have its benefits, perhaps in promoting parent–child relationships by engaging parents in child-rearing practices that contribute to their children's life chances after the program ends. But there is little evidence that a critical period for higher functions has lapsed by age 3, 4, or 5 years, especially if the children's early experience before the intervention is not poor. Early Head Start, for example, was begun partly under the premise that earlier is better and that regular Head Start may actually be too late. For children from the most depressed environments, intervention should begin earlier than age 3, and perhaps parental engagement during the first 3 years of their children's lives will have short- and long-term benefits. But it is unlikely that Early Head Start will produce substantial benefits that are observable in the children at age 3. They may be visible later, but benefits can fade unless high quality programming is continued. Intervention programs that begin early and are sustained over time are more beneficial than programs that do not begin early and are not sustained over time (Campbell & Ramey, 1994; Gomby, Larner, Stevenson, Lewit, & Behrman, 1995; Lee, Brooks-Gunn, Schnur, & Liaw, 1990; Ramey et al., 1992). Services must be increased in public programs if benefits are to be observed for children of low socioeconomic status. This can be done qualitatively by increasing the opportunities, as well as the requirements, for training of child care providers. This is not only true for staff of Head Start but for home care providers who, if even registered, may be required to have little more than training in first aid and CPR. Quantitatively, dosage can be increased by linking early childhood programs with public schools to provide seamless programming for children from the earliest years through the primary grades. Title I could serve as the administrative and financial vehicle for doing so, perhaps being linked with Head Start and Early Head Start as well as other public and private programs that serve children who are at risk. The Chicago Parent-Child Program reported by Reynolds (1994) and funded largely with Title I money represents a successful model fleet program that linked services and is conducted at affordable costs.

CONCLUSION

In early childhood programming researchers are much less a victim of critical periods than of dosage. Researchers have provided too little for too short a duration, rather than starting the intervention too late, to promote the development of children. From a policy standpoint, more dosage—which comes at a higher cost—is needed.

REFERENCES

Ainsworth, M., & Marvin, R. (1995). On the shaping of attachment theory and research: An interview with Mary D.S. Ainsworth. In E. Waters et al. (Eds.), *Caregiving, cultural, and cognitive perspectives on secure base behavior and working models: New growing points in attachment theory. Society for Research in Child Development (SRCD) Monograph, 60* (2-3, Serial No. 244).

Barnett, W.S. (1995). Long-term effects of early childhood programs on cognitive and school outcomes. In R.E. Behrman (Ed.), *The future of children: Long-term outcomes of early childhood programs, 5*, 25–50. Los Angeles: The David and Lucile Packard Foundation.

Behrman, R.E. (Ed.). (1995). *The future of children: Long-term outcomes of early childhood programs, 5*. Los Angeles: The David and Lucile Packard Foundation.

Bloom, L. (1998). Language acquisition in the context of development. In W. Damon (Series Ed.) & D. Kuhn & R. Siegler (Vol. Eds.), *Handbook of child psychology: Cognition, perception, and language, 5*, 309–370. New York: John Wiley & Sons.

Bryant, D., & Maxwell, K. (1997). The effectiveness of early intervention for disadvantaged children. In M.J. Guralnick (Ed.), *The effectiveness of early intervention* (pp. 23–46). Baltimore: Paul H. Brookes Publishing Co.

Campbell, F.A., & Ramey, C.T. (1994). Effects of early intervention on intellectual and academic achievement: A follow-up study of children from low-income families. *Child Development, 65*, 684–698.

Carlson, M., Dragomir, C., Earls, F., Farrell, M., Macovei, O., Nystrom, P., & Sparling, J. (1995). Effects of social deprivation on cortisol regulation in institutionalized Romanian infants. *Society of Neuroscience Abstracts, 218*, 12.

Carlson, M., & Earls, F. (1997). Psychological and neuroendocrinological sequelae of early social deprivation in institutionalized children in Romania. In C.S. Carter & I.I. Lederhendler (Eds.), *The integrative neurobiology of affiliation. Annals of The New York Academy of Sciences, 807*, 419–428. New York: New York Academy of Sciences.

Chase, H.P., Canosa, C.A., Dabiere, C.S., Welch, N.N., & O'Brien, D. (1974). Postnatal undernutrition and human brain development. *Journal of Mental Deficiency Research, 18*, 355–366.

Chubrick, R.E., & Kelley, M.F. (1994). Head Start expansion in the 1990's: A critique. *Focus on Early Childhood, 6*, 1–3.

Cowan, W.M. (1979). The development of the brain. *Scientific American, 241*, 112–133.

Dale, P.S. (1972). *Language development: Structure and function*. Hinsdale, IL: Dryden Press.

Davis, K. (1947). Final note on a case of extreme isolation. *American Journal of Sociology, 45*, 554–565.

DeCasper, A.J., & Spence, M.J. (1986). Prenatal maternal speech influences newborns' perception of speech sounds. *Infant Behavior and Development, 9*, 133–150.

Diamond, M.C. (1991). Environmental influences on the young brain. In K.R. Gibson & A.C. Petersen (Eds.), *Brain maturation and cognitive development* (pp. 107–124). Hawthorne, NY: Walter de Gruyter.

Eimas, P.D., Siqueland, E.R., Jusczyk, P., & Vigorito, J. (1971). Speech perception in infants. *Science, 171*, 303–306.

Elbert, T., Pantev, C., Wienbruch, C., Rockstroh, B., & Taub, E. (1995). Increased cortical representation of the fingers of the left hand in string players. *Science, 270,* 305–307.

Entwistle, D.R. (1995). The role of schools in sustaining early childhood benefits. In R.E. Behrman (Ed.), *The future of children: Long-term outcomes of early childhood programs, 5,* 133–144. Los Angeles: The David and Lucile Packard Foundation.

Farran, D.C. (1990). Effects of interventions with disadvantaged and disabled children: A decade review. In S.J. Meisels & J.P. Shonkoff (Eds.), *Handbook of early childhood intervention* (pp. 501–539). Cambridge, England: Cambridge University Press.

Frede, E.C. (1995). The role of program quality in producing early childhood program benefits. In R.E. Behrman (Ed.), *The future of children: Long-term outcomes of early childhood programs, 5,* 115–132. Los Angeles: The David and Lucile Packard Foundation.

Gibson, K.R. (1991). Myelinization and behavioral development: A comparative perspective on questions of neoteny, altriciality, and intelligence. In K.R. Gibson & A.C. Petersen (Eds.), *Brain maturation and cognitive development* (pp. 29–63). Hawthorne, NY: Walter de Gruyter.

Gomby, D.S., Larner, M.B., Stevenson, C.S., Lewit, E.M., & Behrman, R.E. (1995). Long-term outcomes of early childhood programs: Analysis and recommendations. In R.E. Behrman (Ed.), *The future of children: Long-term outcomes of early childhood programs, 5,* 6–24. Los Angeles: The David and Lucile Packard Foundation.

Greenough, W.T., & Black, J.R. (1992). Induction of brain structure by experience: Substrates for cognitive development. In M.R. Gunnar & C.A. Nelson (Eds.), *The Minnesota Symposia on Child Psychology: Vol. 24. Developmental behavioral neuroscience* (pp. 155–200). Mahwah, NJ: Lawrence Erlbaum Associates.

Guralnick, M.J. (Ed.). (1997). *The effectiveness of early intervention.* Baltimore: Paul H. Brookes Publishing Co.

Haskins, R. (1989). Beyond metaphor: The efficacy of early childhood education. *American Psychologist, 44*(2), 127–132.

Hebb, D.O. (1949). *The organization of behavior.* New York: John Wiley & Sons.

Held, R. (1985). Binocular vision: Behavioral and neuronal development. In J. Mehler & R. Fox (Eds.), *Neonate cognition: Beyond the booming, buzzing confusion* (pp. 37–44). Mahwah, NJ: Lawrence Erlbaum Associates.

Held, R. (1990). Development of binocular vision revisited. In M.H. Johnson (Ed.), *Brain development and cognition* (pp. 159–166). Oxford, England: Blackwell.

Huttenlocher, P.R. (1990). Morphometric study of human cerebral cortex development. *Neuropsychologia, 28,* 517–527.

Huttenlocher, P.R. (1994a). Synaptogenesis in human cerebral cortex. In G. Dawson & K.W. Fischer (Eds.), *Human behavior and the developing brain* (pp. 137–152). New York: The Guilford Press.

Huttenlocher, P.R. (1994b). Synaptogenesis, synapse elimination, and neural plasticity in human cerebral cortex. In C.A. Nelson (Ed.), *The Minnesota Symposia on Child Psychology: Vol. 27. Threats to optimal development: Integrating biological, psychological, and social risk factors* (pp. 35–54). Mahwah, NJ: Lawrence Erlbaum Associates.

Johnson, J.S., & Newport, E.L. (1989). Critical period effects in second language learning: The influence of maturational state on the acquisition of English as a second language. *Cognitive Psychology, 21,* 60–99.

Johnson, M.H. (1990). Cortical maturation and the development of visual attention in early infancy. *Journal of Cognitive Neuroscience, 2,* 81–95.

Johnson, M.H. (1993). Constraints on cortical plasticity. In M.H. Johnson (Ed.), *Brain development and cognition* (pp. 703–721). Oxford, England: Blackwell.

Kandel, E.R., Schwartz, J.H., & Jessell, T.M. (1991). *Principles of neural science, Third Edition.* New York: Elsevier.

Kolb, B. (1989). Brain development, plasticity, and behavior. *American Psychologist, 44,* 1203–1212.

Kuo, Z.Y. (1932). Ontogency of embryonic behavior in aves: II. The mechanical factors in various stages leading to hatching. *Journal of Experimental Zoology, 62,* 453–487.

Lee, V.E., Brooks-Gunn, J., Schnur, E., & Liaw, F.R. (1990). Are Head Start effects sustained? A longitudinal follow-up comparison of disadvantaged children attending Head Start, no preschool, and other preschool programs. *Child Development, 61,* 495–507.

Mason, M.K. (1942). Learning to speak after six and a half years of silence. *Journal of Speech Disorders,* 7, 295–304.

McCall, R.B. (1979). The development of intellectual functioning in infancy and the prediction of later IQ. In J.D. Osofsky (Ed.), *Handbook of infant development* (pp. 707–741). New York: John Wiley & Sons.

McCall, R.B., Ryan, C.S., & Plemons, B.W. (in press). Some lessons learned on evaluating community-based two-generation service programs: The case of the Comprehensive Child Development Program (CCDP). *Journal of Applied Development Psychology.*

Morgan, B., & Gibson, K.R. (1991). Nutritional and environmental interactions in brain development. In K.R. Gibson & A.C. Petersen (Eds.), *Brain maturation and cognitive development* (pp. 91–106). Hawthorne, NY: Walter de Gruyter.

Nelson, C.A., & Bloom, F.E. (1997). Child development and neuroscience. *Child Development, 68*(5), 970–987.

Neville, H.J. (1988). Cerebral organization for spatial attention. In J. Stiles-David, M. Kritchevsky, & U. Bellugi (Eds.), *Spatial cognition* (pp. 327–341). Mahwah, NJ: Lawrence Erlbaum Associates.

Neville, H.J. (1990). Intermodal competition and compensation in development: Evidence from studies of the visual system in congenitally deaf adults. In A. Diamond (Ed.), *The development and neural bases of higher cognitive function* (pp. 71–91). New York: New York Academy of Sciences.

Neville, H.J. (1991). Neurobiology of cognitive and language processing: Effects of early experience. In K.R. Gibson & A.C. Petersen (Eds.), *Brain maturation and cognitive development* (pp. 355–380). Hawthorne, NY: Walter de Gruyter.

Newport, E.L. (1991). Contrasting conceptions of the critical period for language. In S. Carey & R. Gelman (Eds.), *The epigenesis of mind: Essays on biology and cognition* (pp. 111–130). Mahwah, NJ: Lawrence Erlbaum Associates.

NICHD Child Care Network. (1999, April). *Effect sizes from the NICHD study of early child care.* Paper presented at the meeting of the Society for Research in Child Development, Albuquerque, NM.

Nowakowski, R.S. (1987). Basic concepts of CNS development. *Child Development, 58,* 568–595.

Rakic, P. (1971). Guidance of neurons migrating to the fetal monkey neocortex. *Brain Research, 33,* 471–476.

Rakic, P. (1972). Mode of cell migration to the superficial layers of fetal monkey neocortex. *Journal of Comparative Neurology, 145,* 61–84.

Rakic, P. (1988). Specification of cerebral cortical areas. *Science, 241,* 170–176.

Rakic, P. (1996). Development of the cerebral cortex in human and non-human primates. In M. Lewis (Ed.), *Child and adolescent psychiatry* (2nd ed., pp. 9–30). Baltimore: Lippincott, Williams & Wilkins.

Ramey, C.T., Bryant, D.M., Wasik, B.H., Sparling, J.J., Fendt, K.H., & LaVange, L.M. (1992). Infant Health and Development Program for low birth weight, premature infants: Program elements, family participation, and child intelligence. *Pediatrics, 3,* 454–465.

Ramey, S.L., & Ramey, C.T. (1992). Early educational intervention with disadvantaged children: To what effect? *Applied and Preventive Psychology, 1,* 131–140.

Reynolds, A.J. (1994). Effects of a preschool plus follow-up intervention for children at risk. *Developmental Psychology, 30,* 787–804.

Riesen, A.H. (1958). Plasticity of behavior: Psychological aspects. In H.F. Harlow & C.N. Woolsey (Eds.), *Biological and biochemical bases of behavior* (pp. 425–450). Madison: University of Wisconsin Press.

Rosenzweig, M., Krech, D., Bennett, E.L., & Diamond, M. (1962). Effects of environmental complexity and training on brain chemistry and anatomy: A replication and extension. *Journal of Comparative and Physiological Psychology, 55,* 429–437.

Rutter, M. (1979). Maternal deprivation, 1972-1978: New findings, new concepts, new approaches. *Child Development, 50,* 283–305.

Shonkoff, J.P., & Hauser-Cram, P. (1987). Early intervention for disabled infants and their families: A quantitative analysis. *Pediatrics, 80,* 650–658.

St. Pierre, R.G., Layzer, J.I., Goodson, B.D., & Bernstein, L.S. (1997, June). *National impact evaluation of the Comprehensive Child Development Program: Final report.* Cambridge, MA: Abt Associates.

Turkewitz, G., & Kenny, P.A. (1982). Limitations on input as a basis for neural organization and perceptual development: A preliminary theoretical statement. *Developmental Psychology, 15,* 357–368.

Turkewitz, G., & Kenny, P.A. (1985). The role of developmental limitations of sensory input on sensory/perceptual organization. *Developmental and Behavioral Pediatrics, 6,* 302–306.

Weiss, H.B. (1988). Family support and education programs: Working through ecological theories of human development. In H.B. Weiss & F.H. Jacobs (Eds.), *Evaluating family programs.* Hawthorne, NY: Walter de Gruyter.

Werker, J.F., & Lalonde, C.E. (1988). Cross-language speech perception: Initial capabilities and developmental change. *Developmental Psychology, 24,* 672–683.

Werker, J.F., & Polka, L. (1993). The ontogeny and developmental significance of language-specific phonetic perception. In B. de Boysson-Bardies, S. de Schonen, P. Jusczyk, P. McNeilage, & J. Morton (Eds.), *Developmental neurocognition: Speech and face processing in the first year of life* (pp. 275–288). Dordrecht, Netherlands: Kluwer Academic Publishers.

Werker, J.F., & Tees, R.C. (1984). Cross-language speech perception: Evidence for perceptual reorganization during the first year of life. *Infant Behavior and Development,* 7, 49–63.

Wiesel, T.N., & Hubel, D.H. (1963). Single-cell responses in striate cortex of kittens deprived of vision in one eye. *Journal of Neurophysiology, 26,* 1003–1017.

Winick, M., & Rosso, P. (1969). Head circumference and cellular growth of the brain in normal and marasmic children. *Journal of Pediatrics, 74,* 774–778.

Woodhead, M. (1988). When psychology informs public policy: The cases of early childhood interventions. *American Psychologist, 43,* 443–454.

14

Critical Periods

Reflections and Future Directions

Donald B. Bailey, Jr.
Frank J. Symons

In preparing this book, we asked each author to present his or her own perspective on critical periods in a defined area of expertise or development. We did not set out necessarily to draw a single conclusion or reach consensus. Rather, we wanted the full range of perspectives as substantiated by existing data. Thus, we have assembled an array of chapters, each of which addresses the concept of critical periods from a different point of view. What have we learned from this?

The first message that will likely be taken from this book is that the concept of *critical periods* in its purest sense—a defined period of time during which it is essential for normal development that certain experiences occur—probably is not the most appropriate term to describe early human development or to justify policy decisions regarding practices with children. And this is not just a lesson in semantics—reflecting disagreements over whether one term (e.g., critical period, sensitive period, window of opportunity) is most appropriate. We have too much evidence about the remarkable ability of humans to change and learn from experience at virtually every age to conclude that the early childhood years are necessarily more important than other years. Thus, caution is clearly warranted in the use of this term and the arguments we make to support efforts to improve quality of early care and education for children.

Having said that, however, there is unanimous agreement that human learning begins at least at birth, if not before. From the moment a child enters this world, he or she forms perceptions about the nature of life and relationships with others. Even if we cannot justifiably apply the term *critical period* to the earliest years, experience is the unquestioned basis by which these perceptions are formed. To use the analogies suggested by several authors in this book, the windows of opportunity begin to open at birth. It logically follows that when a window of opportunity opens, we should take advantage of it, even if we don't have evidence that doing so now is necessarily better than later. We certainly do not have any evidence whatsoever that once a window opens, later is better.

Several future directions for research and practice are clear. First, different windows open at different times. Thus, teachers and parents need to know general developmental milestones so that we know when it is and is not appropriate to focus on specific skills. Although we know a great deal about development already, research is needed to clarify when windows of opportunity generally open for certain specific skills, and this information needs to be made available to parents and teachers in a much more accessible format.

Second, each child follows a unique developmental course. Thus, knowing general developmental milestones does not ensure that we know when to begin to provide certain kinds of experiences for an individual child. Effective parents and teachers are aware of each child's level of development and provide experiences that are challenging enough to promote development but not so challenging that they result in constant failure or frustration. Research is needed on how best to identify individual opportunities for learning, and tools are needed that parents and teachers can use with individual children.

Third, there is no point in trying to teach something if the window is not yet open. For example, a 12-month-old child is not ready to learn letters of the alphabet. Thus, providing these experiences earlier would make little sense and, in fact, could easily be harmful. We need research that helps us understand the potential negative consequences of too much stimulation of the wrong type, and this information needs to be made more accessible for families and teachers.

Finally, it is clear that inequity exists in our society in the extent to which children have opportunities for access to various experiences after certain windows open. For example, when the language window opens (probably at birth), almost all children have access to sufficient sounds and social interactions to develop language. But, some children have access to more complicated language and more supportive language than others. The inequity magnifies when the windows of opportunity for learning to read begin to open. Some children have dramatically more opportunities to be read to and to experience books and printed materials than other children. Research is needed on effective programs that help eliminate such societal inequities, and policies need to be enacted that make such programs a reality.

This book continues to affirm the importance of appropriate experiences during the early childhood years. Indeed, as the first period during which humans have extensive interactions with and feedback from the environment, the early childhood years constitute our first opportunity as parents and as a society to influence development. Although opportunities for influence continue throughout the life span, they begin during early childhood; and, thus, early childhood constitutes a period during which we should pay close attention to what children experience and how these experiences shape later development. The real issue is the vast differences in opportunities for children today to develop needed skills, even though the window of opportunity for this development is quite long. Children living in impoverished and other high-risk environments often miss out on important learning opportunities provided for more advantaged children in today's society, putting them at risk for substantial delay in development and setting a pattern of educational failure that is difficult to overcome. Thus, while we contend that there is no magical critical period, early intervention for children at risk of school failure remains an important national goal.

The ultimate purpose for thinking critically about critical periods is to improve our understanding of the mechanisms regulating early development. By understanding what we know and do not know about early development from both a brain and behavior perspective, informed and rational interventions designed to alter development can be tested. The goal from an applied practice and policy perspective is to improve the health and welfare of children whose development is at risk for any number of reasons. Among the chapters in this book, none was definitive regarding practice or policy initiatives. We hope that this fact alone will help us all to realize the strength of multiple perspectives working together and aimed at the common goal of understanding the early development of young children and the factors that *can* interfere with optimal development. It is important to note the italicized "can," because much of what we know from the biological perspective is based on controlled experimental studies with different species, with findings that are suggestive but not necessarily absolute when the human condition is considered. Moreover, studies from the behavioral and social sciences share problems common to sampling limitations, quasi-experimental designs, and correlational data. The point is that the methods used by different domains of inquiry have strengths and weaknesses. Thinking critically about how our knowledge is generated can help us learn more about what we already know, what we do not know, and what we need to know. As research continues and new possibilities for early intervention evolve, the intersections between basic brain science and the behavioral and social sciences will become busy places full of promises and pitfalls. Intervention work will continue to be one of the most visible contexts for exploring the difficult questions raised by basic researchers and seized on by policy makers.

We hope that this book has helped clarify for the field the nature of the arguments surrounding critical periods and has provided a basis for the next generation of research. This research should not focus so much on trying to prove that critical periods do or do not exist, because this will be virtually impossible to determine, but rather on what is the nature of developmental risk in today's society that potentially could be addressed through programs of prevention and education.

Index

Page references followed by *f* indicate figures; those followed by *n* indicate notes; and those followed by *t* indicate tables.